The Agony of Heroes

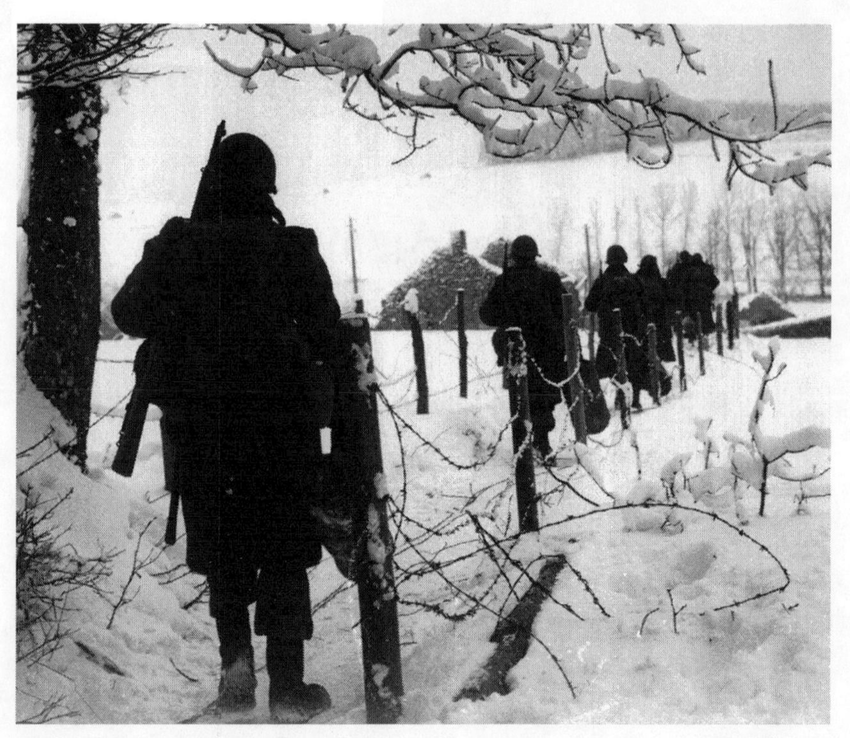

Thomas S. Helling

The Agony of Heroes

Medical Care for America's
Besieged Legions from
Bataan to Khe Sanh

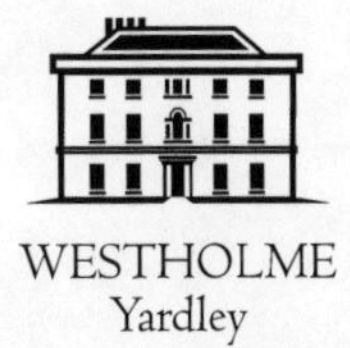

WESTHOLME
Yardley

Facing title page: 3rd Infantry Division soldiers moving toward a Belgian village in January 1945 following the relief of Bastogne. (*National Archives*)

First Westholme Trade Paperback 2024

Westholme Publishing, LLC
904 Edgewood Road
Yardley, Pennsylvania 19067
Visit our Web site at www.westholmepublishing.com

ISBN: 978-1-59416-418-7
Also available as an eBook

Printed in the United States of America.

For Walt

And for the men and women who endured. . . .

Talk not thou to me of flight, for I deem thou wilt not persuade me. Not in my blood is it to fight a skulking fight or to cower down; still is my strength steadfast.

Homer, Iliad V, 249-253

Contents

List of Maps

Preface

HISTORY IS WRITTEN NOT MERELY TO DESCRIBE BUT TO UNDERSTAND. And at its most granular, history portrays the range of human emotions that produced actions—good or bad—that shaped destiny. In that sense it is a study of behavior—individual and collective—motivated by deep-seated beliefs, desires, and social conscience in response to stresses internal and external. Most palpably, history defines a nobleness or wretchedness that brings forth the finest and vilest of mortal character. Endurance, perseverance, and survival are qualities repeatedly summoned for those caught up in whirlwinds of time, particularly in times of great conflict. Some embrace, others reject. They are stories of moments—indefinable stretches—that assembled in total call forth again and again the immortal words of Charles Dickens: "the best of times . . . the worst of times."

And at the extreme are the life-and-death struggles of armed human conflict. Warfare propels individuals into these most uncertain periods. We who examine from the safety of history will never fully appreciate men and women trapped in the dread of doom. But the finite spans of hours, days, or weeks that they bore register far into their moral fiber as if the rest of a lifetime was merely preparation and recovery. It is this we seek to milk from the pages of history, noble or ignoble passages and not just uninspiring recitations of chronology.

This book seeks to remember these heroes—and understand. They are stories with beginnings and ends, but, more importantly, they are stories of images and feelings and commemorations. Graphic impressions seared into minds know not time and space; dates and hours and minutes soon melt away—only instances remain. Huddled under jungle canopies or bullet-ridden tents or in icy shacks, men and women, devoted to caring only for others, found themselves beyond the boundaries of human tolerance, sometimes staring helplessly to watch unrequited suffering. Many, long dead, will never see these pages. But their memories inspire and reassure that we humans are all connected. That extensions of ourselves have existed before. That we would hope our actions could match heroics of those who came before. That this world continues to be a better place because of them.

It is the specific focus of this work to examine an ordinariness about the human condition that becomes extraordinary—not just the idea of combat itself, although enough of a traumatic event in its own right, but the immediate peril of annihilation, whether from sudden explosion, a sniper's bullet, or capture and subjugation. These are circumstances of entrapment and siege, settings where hope and mercy have evaporated, and all face the inevitability of destruction. War has produced sieges for centuries as an effective form of brutal capitulation. One can imagine the tribulations of men at arms: surrounded, hungry, desperate. But what of the noncombatants? What of the mercy workers whose intent is to save and not destroy? Let us exam them in their valor and equal desperation. Of all the tragedies history might furnish, let us focus on five: Bataan, Anzio, Bastogne, Chosin, and Khe Sanh. Each presented different challenges: climate, geography, tactics, and resources that assailed the resiliency of its defenders. The Bataan Peninsula, a singularly unattractive locale for defense, was hot, humid, and disease ridden. The deprivations of all vital material were soon lacking. Besiegement was complete. Capitulation virtually assured. Anzio was a military blunder salvaged only by superhuman efforts at resistance and resilience, and by a uniquely robust supply chain seaward that kept the beachhead lifelines open. At Bastogne, encirclement by a rabid, fanatical enemy spelled disaster, aggravated by extremes of cold and demoralizing absence of casualty care. The Chosin retreat, fought in frigid temperatures, might have ended in complete annihilation—and basically did so for many of the combatants—were it not for the sturdy leadership and dogged tenacity of Marine infantry. French capitulation at Dien Bien Phu a dozen years earlier loomed large for the Khe Sanh garrison, as Vietnamese regulars crept dangerously close to their perimeter, and their tenuous lifeline was a hazardous airborne journey into bullet-filled airspace. In those horrid places, American boys and girls bled real blood, endured endless bombardments, fought ravaging disease, followed familiar frigid footpaths, and vied for dwindling rations. In those tents and trenches and dugouts—be they doughboy or jarhead, medic or corpsman, doctor or nurse—they would wonder like the besieged from the times of Troy what minute what hour what day would be their last. What manner of brutality would usher in their demise? What ghastly miscalculation brought them this destiny? Could we rise to superhuman intensities as they had? Could we still exude compassion and caring and patience for those *in extremis* as they did? Immersed in their personal agony, could we be as noble as they?

FROM THE SECOND WORLD WAR ON, American combat casualty care involved early surgical intervention for those with life-threatening injuries—as close to the battlefield as prudent. "Nontransportables" they were called—men so unstable that any attempt to evacuate would likely prove fatal. Drs. Edward Churchill and Michael DeBakey, army surgery consultants, devised teams with seasoned surgeons to link with field hospitals as mobile units following troops. By the Korean conflict they were called mobile Army surgical hospitals. A minority of wounded needed their services. Most wounds were mercifully not life threatening, even though urgent care was desirable. For those, delays could be tolerated—to an extent. But inability to extract any wounded—particularly seriously wounded—affected all casualties sooner or later. Failure to stop hemorrhage, improper or negligent cleansing (debridement), and source control of sepsis took a toll, often leading to crippling complications and even mortality. This was the conundrum of siege: the dual needs for early surgical intervention and prompt evacuation. Logistics held the key. Supply and extraction ultimately meant the difference between life and death, between resistance and capitulation.

Heavy combat consumed medical material: blood, bandages, plasma, morphine. Resupply became a practical and psychological issue. Doctors and nurses needed fresh stocks, and the battle wounded needed hope. That wounds could be inspected, cleaned, and dressed in a timely fashion was paramount to surgeons and nurses, but also to patients. The illusion that doctors could resurrect the dying was key to maintaining a fighting spirit, key to necessary risk taking. Without it, when comrades were seen to suffer needlessly, when soldiers were surrounded by the dead, resolve weakened. For medical staff under fire, the focus on the wounded was therapeutic, a welcome distraction from danger about which most could do little. Yet siege imposed limitations. "Meatball" surgery—carving away of devitalized tissue—might be sufficient for the majority of cases and might be possible under even the most austere of conditions, but complex repairs could be impossible. For these patients, the slow spiral to death was uniquely unsettling—a direct consequence of circumstances, not science or ability. And all became painfully aware of it.

Nooses that tightened around Bataan, Anzio, Bastogne, Chosin, and Khe Sanh generated tales of individual resilience and valor. Medics, nurses, and doctors reached beyond their own welfare and safety to uncover a courage few were aware they possessed. Stamina, ingenuity, and devotion kept medical care in motion, even if treatments degenerated to their most rudimentary forms. What is even more remarkable, these men and women were not normally endowed with superhuman qualities. Many were simple people, committed to the medical professions but distinctly ordinary in their ambitions and expectations. An awareness of country and duty—some would call this patriotism—led to a military leaning. And war caught them up, with its unbridled violence and injustice. And now, in an arena distinctly different than their civilian practices, skill sets were needed that had to be honed as much from intuition as from empiricism, as much from humanism as from science. Were they unwitting heroes? No doubt it would be an abhorrent label they would discard. Heroes, it would be said, were combatants who fell victim, who had risked their lives in incomprehensible circumstances of high jeopardy.

But indeed they were heroes. And it was their agony, too. Not just providers but consumers, some were felled by the same savagery. They suffered as all suffered, in the loneliness and misery of abandonment. Ordinary folk in extraordinary settings. With fortitude and resilience no different than their combatant counterparts. Fear, loathing, dread? Of course, these emotions coursed throughout their veins as in any human being, mortality a palpable terror. Did some cower, sulk, despair? Of course, but sooner or later, there surfaced a sharper focus on compassion and benevolence. Few ran—as if there were anywhere to run—almost all knelt beside their patients and tended as from the times of Aesculapius.

Part 1

Bataan

"I have not the slightest intention in the world of surrendering. . . ."—General Douglas MacArthur, 1942

1

America's Colony, Las Islas Felipinas

In 1909, a diminutive, thirty-year-old hunchback named Homer Lea, twice rejected by the US military because of his frailty, published a prophetic diatribe on American foreign policy, *The Valor of Ignorance.* In it he brilliantly outlined Japan's quest for domination in Asia, its desire for supremacy over mainland China and procurement of sea corridors along East Asia. Vital to its success, he claimed, was the conquest of the Philippine Islands. "The Philippines command the Asian coast from the Formosan Strait to Cape Cameo," he wrote. "Sovereignty over the Philippines is not only imperative to Japan in her overlordship of Asia and the Pacific, but is essential to the very preservation of her national existence." And the United States, meekly equipped with a Pacific navy and far, far from Asian battlefields, would be powerless to defend its new possession, the first child of a colonial empire. "The conquest of these islands [the Philippines] by Japan will be less of a military undertaking than was the seizure of Cuba by the United States. . . . Manila will be forced to surrender in less than three weeks." The lack of a standing army in the Philippines, the inability to reinforce that garrison, and a paucity of warships that could rush to aid beleaguered troops would ensure a swift victory, Lea foretold. He even outlined the invasion route: "As the conquest of Cuba was accomplished by landing forces distant from any fortified port so will the Philippines fall. Lingayen Gulf on the north coast of Luzon, or Polilo Bight on the east coast, will form the Guantanamo Bays of the Japanese." The American army "would be in a position wherein their capitulation could alone prevent their complete destruction." Sadly, Lea's prophesies were decried by critics and panned by pacifists. While few copies of his book were sold in America, over eighty-four thousand were distributed in Japan, its tacticians fascinated by his strategy. Only a rather obscure but rising star, Brigadier General Douglas MacArthur, superintendent of West Point, recognized Lea's brilliance and felt his book should be required reading for cadets.[1] MacArthur, already a veteran of Philippine insurrections, was fully aware of the strategic position of these islands.

Years later, the tall, regal-appearing figure opened the doors to his balcony, stepped out, and stared across the placid waters of Manila Bay at the distant shores of Bataan's wilderness, a view worthy of Kodachrome picture postcards. General Douglas MacArthur, commander of the newly formed United States Army Forces Far East, housed himself in lodgings fit for an emperor, the six-room penthouse suite of the Manila Hotel, situated on broad Dewey Boulevard with a sweeping view of the Bay and the old Spanish walled city of Intramuros. MacArthur had settled in among mahogany and marble and leather and portraits of Foch and Pershing, and dined on *lapu-lapu* wrapped in banana leaves brought to him by a host of deferential Filipino servants.[2] He ruled over a small force of Americans sent by President Franklin Roosevelt to hold sway over a dwindling colonial empire wrestled by the United States from Spain at the close of the nineteenth century. He was enamored with the islands, his father and now he wedded to the Filipino people, their history, and the fledgling government of President Manuel Quezon. MacArthur had been appointed field marshal by Quezon in 1936 and then commanding general (USAFFE), by Chief of Staff General George Marshall in 1941. It was now early December of that year. There was every concern the Japanese would strike the Philippines soon. His army was all that stood between a looming Nippon empire and its conquest of the Southwest Pacific. It was the "key that unlocks the door to the Pacific,"[3] he had said. And now, on the eve of a great national crisis it is this man, Douglas MacArthur, who will bear the burden of his genius and his folly in that nightmarish jungle across the bay and, like all tragic figures, suffer the intense conviction of his miscalculations.[4]

His father, Brigadier General Arthur MacArthur, had participated in the American expedition to Luzon in 1898, forcing, more or less, a prearranged capitulation of Spanish forces. The Spanish, besieged in their walled city by angry Filipino insurrectionists, preferred a more civilized resolution and chose American occupation over Philippine nationalists.

The elder MacArthur was then appointed provost marshal general of Manila and lived in the royal palace at Malacanan. He then chased Filipino insurgents out of Manila in their confrontation with American forces for Philippine independence. The insurgents, under Emilio Aguinaldo and his lieutenant, nineteen-year-old Manuel Quezon, dispersed throughout Luzon, Quezon to the wilds of the Bataan Peninsula, where malaria and malnutrition almost killed him. Aguinaldo was captured in northern Luzon, and Quezon was coaxed out of the jungle to surrender to MacArthur in 1901. In 1935, Quezon became the first president of the Philippines Commonwealth.

Douglas MacArthur had fallen in love with the Philippine Islands, perhaps because of his father's involvement, perhaps his own experiences, or perhaps he seemed to be enraptured by this tropical paradise:

> The Philippines charmed me. The delightful hospitality, the respect and affection expressed for my father, the amazingly attractive result of a mixture of Spanish culture and American industry, the languorous laze that seemed to glamorize even the most routine chores of life . . . fastened me with a grip that has never relaxed.[5]

He had served with an engineering unit as a young lieutenant just out of West Point in 1903, while his father was still military governor, again in the 1920s to command an infantry brigade, and again in 1935 as military adviser to Quezon. That flattering appointment by Roosevelt at the behest of Quezon may have blinded him to the reality of possibilities the Filipino government had to defend the islands. It would be he, Douglas MacArthur, who would shore up Quezon's young island nation.

MacArthur vowed to make the Philippines impregnable. The Philippine National Defense Act of 1935 allowed conscription of all Filipino males but was hardly a guarantee of proficiency. MacArthur's determination to build an armed force using draftees ignored the many obstacles faced by the indigenous population, namely poverty, illiteracy, and any number of dialects making communication—so vital in military maneuvers—almost impossible. But MacArthur blurred fact and fiction. He would raise an army of four hundred thousand Filipinos, he vowed, and boasted that it would take the Japanese half a million men and five billion dollars to take the Philippines, a cost, he reasoned, they were not willing to pay.[6]

But MacArthur's plan would take years to complete; by mid-year 1941, only eighty thousand Filipinos had been inducted on Luzon, and most of those were poorly trained. Even clothing was lacking. Most Filipino units were reservists with a minimum of infantry schooling and equipment. Marksmanship was sorely lacking. Many had never shot a weapon and, in the opinion of some American officers, hardly knew muzzle from breech. Only the Philippine scouts were crack soldiers, highly motivated, disciplined, and skilled. MacArthur also faced a disinterested US government, immersed in financial woes of the Great Depression and beleaguered by shouts of anticolonialists and paranoid isolationists. It was only with the Japanese incursion into China and militaristic posturing throughout Southeast Asia that General Marshall and Secretary of War Henry Stimson realized the importance of preserving the Philippines as a vital outpost in the Far East. In MacArthur's estimation, this was all too little too late, "an eleventh-hour struggle to build up enough force to repel an enemy."[7] Marshall's augmentation of Philippine forces was not authorized until July 31, 1941. By December 1941, MacArthur commanded a force of over one hundred thousand troops, including about twenty-two thousand Americans, only a fraction of whom, roughly 1,800 men, were army infantry—the 31st Infantry Regiment, part of the Philippine Division. The remaining Americans were attached to coastal and antiaircraft artillery batteries or tank units. By the first week of December, MacArthur's air force, under Major General Lewis Brereton, had 207 aircraft, seventy-four of which were the new B-17 heavy bombers, half of them parked exposed at Clark Airfield on Luzon, well within range of Japanese air strikes.

What probably pricked the Japanese into moving on the Philippines were MacArthur's widely publicized plans to build up his Far East Air Force by adding bombers and fighters across Luzon's airfields, a direct threat to Japanese shipping and communication in the South China Sea. His rantings about a base for the powerful Pacific Fleet certainly compounded their worries. MacArthur was, in essence, waving a red cape at an angry bull. Indeed the Japanese overestimated America's Asiatic Fleet, commanded by Admiral Thomas Hart. His ships hardly represented a threat, but their moorings in Manila Bay were uncomfortably close to Tokyo's trade routes. The navy base at Cavite, a bony digit sticking into Manila Bay, would be a prime target. But at the time of the Japanese invasion, the Asiatic Fleet at Cavite was a paper tiger numbering only four destroyers, twenty-seven submarines—many with outdated torpedoes that would thump harmlessly on the sides of Japanese troopships—three submarine tenders, five minesweepers, two tankers, and one seaplane tender. The only capital ships, the cruisers USS *Houston* and USS *Boise*, were hundreds of mile away in the Visayas.[8]

Filipino history is replete with invasion, occupation, and extortion. The islands were "discovered" by the Portuguese explorer Ferneo de Magalhaes, the anglicized Ferdinand Magellan, on his voyage around the world in search of a westward approach to the Orient and its riches of spices. He dedicated the islands to Charles V, the new king of Spain, in 1521. One month later, in April 1521, Magellan was killed in the islands he found, covering the retreat of his men caught up in tribal rivalry. Not until 1542 did the Spanish explorer Ruy Lopez de Villalobos name the islands Las Islas Felipinas, after Philip, the crown prince of Spain and regent of New Spain, present-day Mexico. The Philippine Islands continued as a Spanish colony for close to four more centuries. Millennia before, the islands had been populated by a diverse group of Asian migrants: Mongols, Chinese, and Annamites. However, the dominant ethnic influence were the Malays from Indonesia, a tribe called the Tagala, found predominately on the large, northernmost island of Luzon. Catholic Spaniards, swarming to the islands after Magellan's posthumous dedication, made concentrated attempts to westernize the Filipino people, focusing on two primary goals: reaping profits and saving souls. Their rule was brutal—absolute obedience—and the religious were especially fervent on the recruitment of minds and souls for the holy church. While native Filipinos accepted their plight, a sullen resentment gradually brewed, as so often happens to the colonized masses, easily aware of their second-class status. In the words of seventeenth-century voyager Antonio de Morga: "The great point in which Manila has been a success, is the fact that the original inhabitants have not disappeared before the Europeans, and that they have been civilized, and brought into a closer union with the dominant race."[9]

This gradually fomented into active resistance, an armed and philosophical movement for reformation and even independence from their Spanish overlords. Much of it was aimed at the clergy, who functioned as Spain's enforcers. In 1892, the *New York Times* ran a story with the headline "Worst-Governed People—The Inhabitants of the Philippine Islands—Priest Rule of the Dark Ages Rampant." The article portrayed the corrupted rule of Spanish clergy—Dominican monks it seemed—and colonial governors who seized land, burned dwellings, and displaced families.[10] The revolutionary Jose Rizal y Mercado gained immortality with his public execution in 1896 on trumped-up charges. He forever became a symbol of Philippine national pride and independence. Rizal called his homeland the "Pearl of the Orient Seas" in his last poem, written on the eve of his death, "Mi ultimo adios" (My Last Farewell). The fortuitous occurrence of Spanish conflict with the United States in Cuba that quickly spilled over to the Philippines toward the close of the nineteenth century led Filipino reformers and revolutionaries to imagine their hopes would be realized. But they simply traded one set of masters for another. The Spanish relinquished control of the Philippines not to the Filipinos but to the United States, the first, and only, colony of the new empire. This frustration soon led to armed conflict, not with the Spanish now but with soldiers from America. Bloodshed abounded, with atrocities on both sides abhorrent to natives and Americans alike, until guerrilla actions were slowly squelched and the United States became the colonizers, holding onto its Philippine territory as insurance of a presence in the Far East. The territories were vital to Asian trade. To be fair, America was a benevolent overlord, establishing schools and investing millions in the islands, creating a commonwealth with the eventual plan for total Philippine independence and self-governance by 1946. And the United States was their protectorate as Asian empires suddenly coveted this flanking fortress on the edge of their emerging economies.

Yet the colonies were indefensible. While grabbing the Philippines removed any temptation by Great Britain or Germany to snatch them up, the American possession was at the end of an extremely long tether of supply and reinforcement, and that through a gauntlet of potentially hostile island possessions from Hawaii to Manila. A quick rescue of garrison forces in the Philippines was out of the question despite delusional plans concocted by army and navy chiefs. It would take months, if not years, for sustaining help to arrive, and no garrison force, no matter how well prepared, could hold off an Asian aggressor for that long. And Japan was to be that aggressor. Eager for Asian domination, the island nation was impatient for the raw materials needed to fuel its economic and military engines, especially the materials found to the south, in Indonesia and Borneo. And what could be more threatening to this tenuous supply chain than an American force on its flanks, strategically poised in the Philippine Islands to monitor, harass, and interdict. It was elimination of this presence that preoccupied Japanese planners—and the destruction of the naval presence that could rush to their aid, the American Pacific Fleet based at Pearl Harbor.

2

A Trembling Leaf

WARFARE PLANNING BY THE US MILITARY BECAME A FULL-TIME obsession following the Spanish-American War. The realization that they now had an island empire almost seven thousand miles from the West Coast alarmed army and navy strategists. In 1903, the Joint Army-Navy Board was formed to develop contingency plans, primarily for an Asian war, particularly after Japan's stunning victory over Russia in 1905. From this joint board the "color" plans were developed. Each nation was assigned a color code, and war plans, codenamed Rainbow, were drawn up for the eventuality of conflict with any of them. Japan's color was orange. The original Orange plan, war with Japan, was developed, revised, and revised again so that by 1913 it had matured into a statement of principles that would be followed in such an eventuality. Basically, the plan assumed that Japan's first priority in a war with the United States would be occupation of the Philippine Islands. Such a move would guard Japan's sea lanes through the South China Sea to Indonesia. By 1938, and after countless revisions and philosophical disagreements between army and navy members, the Orange plan still held that the Philippines would be defended. This strategy hinged on a beefed up navy and army that would bang their way across the Pacific to come to the aid of a beleaguered Philippine garrison. Yet skepticism prevailed whether such delusional planning would ever rescue a besieged American force.[1] Rainbow plans were modified in the late 1930s with German incursions into Poland and Czechoslovakia. The United States might be squaring off against a number of enemy nations with or without the help of its allies. However, even with introduction of the Rainbow plans and the eventual decision to implement the Rainbow-5 plan, Japan remained at the forefront as a probable combatant in any scenario.

Rainbow-5, the latest iteration approved by President Roosevelt on November 19, 1941, provided for a Europe-first approach with action in the Pacific confined to defensive tactics to protect Allied possessions, even with Japan as a possible key adversary. The only offensive action would be raids from the sea and through the air. Troop movements would be at a minimum. A major flaw, though, was the assumption that war with Japan would be preceded by problematic relations during which the United States would have time—years, it was hoped—to mobilize and prepare for the defense of the Philippines. "There will be a period of strained relations preceding the outbreak of war with Orange during which period preparatory measures prior to mobilization can be taken."[2]

Admiral William Leahy, chief of naval operations, had reported to the Naval Affairs Committee that defense of the Philippines would be dependent on local resistance capabilities and the ability of a superior navy to keep open lines of supply—in short, sea power. Whether or not the navy had sufficient resources to meet that challenge was a debated topic. In fact, Admiral James Richardson, assistant chief of naval operations prior to 1941, had told the congressional committee investigating the Pearl Harbor debacle in 1945 that the president told him in 1940, "if they even attacked the Philippines he [the president] doubted whether we would enter the war." Considering a reduced presence of the Asiatic Fleet, based in Manila, navy commanders, now a bit frustrated by Douglas MacArthur, who seemed in no mood to cooperate with the navy, were in a quandary as to "how far we should go in maintaining our position in the Philippines."[3]

For the Allied garrison there, the Orange plan and Rainbow-5 called for a retreat to the Bataan Peninsula forming the western boundary of Manila Bay and thus deny the bay and harbor to any invader. Manila was felt to be the prize of the Philippines, the center of civilization, and a reasonably good sanctuary for warships. It would almost certainly be the prime objective of an invasion of Luzon. Colonial troops—American and Filipino—would hole up in the jungle across the bay and on the island of Corregidor at its entrance, harass the enemy with artillery, and wait for reinforcements. It was all a ridiculous scheme to address a hopelessly entrapped garrison. The only salvation was the arrival of overwhelming navy and air forces within months of attack, an event that had no chance of happening. With all the permutations of the Orange plan over the years, each equation spelled siege, encirclement, and capitulation. Furthermore, with Germany's invasion of Poland in 1939 and its quick succession of victories in the Netherlands and France, and with Great Britain facing an almost inevitable invasion, the United States knew its battle with Japan, should it engage, would rest solely on the shoulders of Uncle Sam. Yet in Rainbow-5, the German *blitzkrieg*, not the Far East, would command his attention. The Philippines, its stranded infantry, infantile air force, and gunboat navy would have to hold on. America's firm western line of defense would not be there, but farther to the east in an arc that included Alaska, the Hawaiian Islands, and the Panama Canal Zone. For those outside that rim, rescue would be a fading dream. One must count on nothing less than heroic deeds of desperate men. "Show me a hero and I will write you a tragedy," F. Scott Fitzgerald had said.[4] None so true as the heroes of Bataan.

MacArthur knew Bataan well. At his first posting, he had contracted malaria while surveying the region, and on his return as an infantry officer he continued his work of mapping forty square miles of the rugged, forbidding peninsula that flanked Manila Bay. Bataan, according to war plan Orange, figured prominently in defense of Manila and Luzon. Why a general as astute and informed as MacArthur thought Orange had any hope of succeeding was never explained, but he had told Commonwealth president Quezon, on his visit to Washington, DC, in 1934, when asked if the Philippines could be defended, that any place could be defended with enough men, munitions, and money. And when offered, in a megalomaniacal gesture, he gladly accepted the task. Perhaps MacArthur, like many of his compatriots, felt time was on his side, that congressional appropriations, even with the slumping economy, would provide necessary troops, planes, and ships that would afford a bulwark for defense of American interests in the Far East. Or maybe he felt, as would happen again in Korea, that his supreme strategy and force of character would actually make it happen; that he willed the Japanese to be an inferior force and his Filipino conscripts hardened combat infantry; that the outdated weapons, ineffectual artillery and mortar shells, and flimsy aircraft would transform into an unbeatable combination of armed resistance. Only a realistic Major Dwight Eisenhower, MacArthur's hand-picked implementer of the Filipino army, told the straight story to President Quezon, informing him that plan Orange was bunk and that the only way to stop an invading force was to halt it at the shoreline. And at the eleventh hour, convinced that the Philippine archipelago could be defended with renewed promises of men and material from War Secretary Stimson, MacArthur, maybe recalling Eisenhower's predictions, managed to persuade Washington to swap the traditional Orange plan of retreat to Bataan with a new scheme of defense. The entire archipelago would be held with a fantasy army of over two hundred thousand men, including a phantom air force. In a letter detailing his thoughts to the War Department, he wrote that a landing anywhere by hostile forces in the Philippines would be a springboard for invasion of Luzon. Forget delaying tactics—there would be stout resistance beginning right on the landing beaches. "The strength and composition of the defense forces projected here," MacArthur contended, "are believed to be sufficient to accomplish such a mission."

With approval from General Marshall on October 18, 1941, MacArthur organized his Philippine defense into a Northern and Southern Luzon Force and a Visayan-Mindanao Force.[5] For Luzon, the in-depth defense would begin at the beachhead, stockpiling food, ammunition, and medical supplies at prearranged points along northern Luzon. Outside the main depot in Quezon City, just south of Manila, there were medical subdepots at Tarlac, in central Luzon, Los Banos, on the shores of Lake Taal in southern Luzon, and Cebu. The distribution of resources thus deprived Bataan of a valuable reserve to feed, clothe, arm, and care for the garrison troops who were supposed to subsist for months in that godforsaken wilderness until help arrived. Of course, in MacArthur's way of thinking, this would be unlikely. Well before that, he might have reasoned, his army of mostly half-hearted but well-meaning Filipino reservists with little, if any, infantry training, would be responsible for driving Japanese troops, seasoned by combat in China, back into the ocean. However, MacArthur had no inkling of the imminence of war with Japan—or chose not to embrace it—and felt he had, at a minimum, until April 1942 to perfect his plan. Had he truly had two hundred thousand troops, modern weapons, and an air armada of planes equal in speed and agility to the Japanese aircraft, his preparations might have held together. Yet to any knowledgeable tactician, his beach defense was absurd. There were thousands of miles of coastline to defend, diluting his forces to an absolute trickle. But MacArthur was a master of self-deception. Once put on paper, his strategy was as good as true.

For the average serviceman and servicewoman, the Philippines were an attractive duty station. That was also true for members of the medical profession—the medical and nursing officers' corps—sent to care for army and navy personnel forming the garrison forces. War was a distant, muffled drum to most folks, the posting a romance, an adventure. Manila, capital city of Luzon, was truly Rizal's "Pearl of the Orient Seas," the finest port of the Far East, a tropical paradise of lazy contrasts with small-town America, from which many of these young men and women hailed. Manila, Americanized since Dewey's momentous victory over Spain in 1898 and the influx of American troops in the years following.

Manila, enfolding the bay and bisected by the Pasig River, was actually three cities. The old district of Tondo, the native city north of the Pasig, contained its crooked streets and open air markets—the bodegas. Along Calle Carriedo with its crusty street vendors hawking delicate *baluts* (duck embryos about ready to hatch, boiled in water and eaten whole), arcaded streets, and fashionable tourist attractions like the Astoria Tea Room. Streets were lined with stalls—cloth merchants, furniture, candles, and thousands of pairs of shoes piled high. And all avenues teemed with ubiquitous *caromata*, the two-wheeled, horse-drawn Filipino taxi, and *carabao*—ungainly water buffalo, the local beast of burden—patiently lumbering with cargo and led by equally patient masters. Intramuros, the Spanish walled city constructed in 1590, was called the "City of Churches"—San Agustin, Santo Domingo, San Francisco, and San Ignacio, reflecting the country's Spanish, Roman Catholic influence, enduring the passage of centuries—and of earthquakes. Down the narrow streets, the projecting balconies and grilled windows of the *bahay na bato*—stone, squared colonial structures—were reminiscent of old Spain. In the iron-grilled courtyards with majestic fountains and gardens were squatters, beneath steps and in doorways. Just outside the walls were filled-in moats of the Spaniards that had become drilling grounds for military and manicured golf courses for all Americans. Last, and most recent, was the American district—modern Manila. The Ermita area, envisioned by Daniel Burnham as a new District of Columbia and built on land reclaimed from Manila Bay, housed palatial residences ensconced in massive wrought-iron fences and graced by elegant palm trees, directly across from wide Dewey Boulevard, which skirted the bay.

The crown jewel was the Manila Hotel, designed by William Parsons, the New York architect. Built of white cement and red-tiled roof, the five-story structure played host to notables such as Somerset Maugham and Noel Coward, secluding them in carved mahogany four-poster beds and pampering them in marble bathrooms and wicker furniture. The Manila Hotel was where Douglas MacArthur, having been denied residence at the Royal Palace, decided to hold court. Not far away, visible from the balconies of the Manila Hotel was Pier 7, the "Million Dollar Pier," reputed to be the longest pier in the world, home to the luxurious cruise liners, the SS *President Hoover* and SS *President Coolidge*, which leisurely plowed the Pacific from San Francisco.

For American troops duty in the Philippines had been a cushy assignment: training only until noon because of the heat, marksmanship practice one two-week period per year, spacious accommodations (for officers) with Filipino servants, chefs, and doormen, golf and whiskey. Yes, the Philippines, where the mangoes were sweetest, the music the swingingest, the girls the lushest, and the sunsets the grandest.[6]

And for those young, adventurous officers there was the Army Navy Club just off the shore and down from Rizal Park, built on some of that reclaimed land, right next door to the Elks Club. The Army Navy Club was a three-story structure of white arches and decorated with palm and acacia trees. Inside were bowling alleys, a swimming pool, courts for tennis and squash, and an expansive bar with soft, cushy lounge chairs and generous tumblers of British gin. The club was exclusive: only white Americans allowed. "Brownskins" were prohibited, except, of course, the servants. Even President Quezon was not allowed in, a policy to which an enlightened touring US senator Hiram Bingham of Connecticut responded, after an invitation to visit the club was extended on his voyage to Manila in 1927, "Then I am sorry, gentlemen, but I shall not be able to accept your invitation."[7] And for sport—and gambling—there was the art deco Jai Alai Club on Taft Avenue, designed by Los Angeles architects Welton Becket and Walter Wurdeman, whose expansive Sky Room was the place to see and be seen. For those so inclined, Filipino cooks could be employed for forty pesos a month, houseboys for half of that. Colonel James Gillespie, the new chief of medicine at Sternberg General Hospital, arrived in Manila in May 1940, with his wife and two sons. They rented a spacious house in the suburb of Paranaque, six miles from Sternberg. For about $25 a month, he could afford a houseboy, cook, and *lavendera* (wash girl). With a liberal amount of free time, the family toured the sights of Manila, Intramuros, the Chinese Cemetery with its ornate Chong Hock Tong Temple, and life along the Pasig River.

They visited the country escape of Baguio, located at five thousand feet of elevation in the midst of pine forests in northern Luzon, a cool mountain retreat from the stifling heat of Manila, and even sampled the local Igorote delicacy: roast dog with its stomach packed with rice. But one year later, in May 1941, Gillespie's wife and sons boarded the steamship SS *George Washington* along with 570 other families, 1,200 people in all, departing the Philippines amid rumors of war. It was the last farewell for many of them.

Army first lieutenant Ralph Hibbs, a recent graduate of the University of Iowa School of Medicine, departed the SS *President Coolidge* at the Manila pier on June 20, 1941. He was assigned to the 2nd Battalion, 31st Infantry, the all-American regiment, and responsibility for the health of seven hundred soldiers. His duty station was the Quartel de Espana in Fort Santiago inside Intramuros. Work was more than comfortable, mostly dispensing medicine and sick call. Done each day by 11:00 AM, he was off to lunch at the Polo Club or golf at the fashionable Wack Wack course. Drinks were de rigueur at the Army Navy Club, followed by a late dinner down the street at the Jai Alai Club, dressed to the nines in a white, double-breasted, sharkskin dinner jacket. "Dear Mom and Dad," he wrote in late November, "Things are peaceful here. Life in the Orient is easygoing with emphasis on the *manana* and *siesta* ethic. . . . There's nothing going to happen here."[8] On December 5, the 31st Infantry was put on "red alert." Yet there was little care among its officers. Sunday, December 7, found them around a table at the Bamboo Bar of the Manila Hotel, crimson bougainvillea tumbling from the broad overhang, drinks served by a somewhat slinky Filipino *mestiza*.[9] The festivities continued well into the night. The next morning they were at war.

First Lieutenant John Bumgarner, an officer in the US Army Medical Corps, walked off the USS *U. S. Grant* at Manila Harbor on February 20, 1941. He was glad to be rid of the steel-hulled steamer. The ship was big but the Pacific Ocean bigger, and the constant rise and fall and side-to-side shifting made for a low level of queasiness that never quite left. His voyage of one month and seven thousand miles had taken him from San Francisco to Honolulu to Guam and finally to Manila. He was escorted to what was to be his place of residence at the old six-story Luneta Hotel, just off the waterfront and facing the flat, Bermuda plain of Luneta Park. Although Bumgarner thought it was "hardly luxurious," Dwight Eisenhower, then a lieutenant colonel and assistant military adviser to the Philippine government, felt differently. The Luneta Hotel held a coveted place with him. In 1960, he would reminisce: "To this day it [the Luneta Hotel] lives in memory as one of the most pleasant, indeed even one of the most romantic spots, I have known in this entire world. . . . From here [the hotel], looking across the peaceful waters of Manila Bay, I could see the gorgeous sunsets over Miraveles."[10]

Bumgarner had graduated from the Medical College of Virginia in 1939. Having completed a rotating internship at the Erlanger Hospital in Chattanooga, he had just begun a pediatrics residency when, as a reservist, he was abruptly called to active duty in December 1940. To his group of fellow officers a request was made for a volunteer for the Philippines. The volunteer had to be a medical officer, a reservist, and single. Bumgarner was the only one to fill that bill, and he took the bait. Now here he was in Manila, brashly asking for a position at the main station hospital on Luzon, Sternberg General. Even though war was not too distant from the Philippines—the Japanese had already occupied Manchuria, tangled with the Chinese, and slithered into Indochina—little concern was expressed by officers and men of the American army on the golf courses and polo grounds and cocktail lounges of this tropical paradise. Workdays lasted until noon and were followed by languid afternoons of indoor or outdoor activities. War was indeed a far distant rumor.

Sternberg General Hospital, named after Brigadier General George Sternberg, founder of the Army Medical Corps, was one of the five station hospitals scattered across Luzon developed by the army to care for American and Filipino troops and their dependents. The hospital was in the heart of Manila, just outside Intramuros, near the east bank of the Pasig River at the corner of Calle Arroceros and Calle Concepcion. On a four-acre plot of land sat a number of separate, Spanish-type, two-story wooden buildings, open air but screened, and connected, built around a central courtyard.[11] Each building housed a wardful of patients segregated either by disease (a tuberculosis ward) or age (a pediatric ward for dependents) or class (an officer's ward and a ward for retired military, Filipino and American). The grounds were carefully manicured, and walkways were lined with trees—a bucolic setting in the midst of an earthy city. Sternberg was the cornerstone of the military hospital system. Four hundred fifty beds awaited the ill of Luzon's garrison forces, but rarely were there more than three hundred patients at any one time. Notable army medical officers had passed through Sternberg as commanders, such as Norman Kirk, future surgeon general of the army; Oliver Niess, future surgeon general of the air force; and Patrick Madigan, the father of army neuropsychiatry, for whom Madigan Army Medical Center at Fort Lewis, Washington, would be named. In December 1941, the commander of the hospital was Colonel Percy Carroll, who had served in the Philippines as chief of the surgical service on Corregidor. He returned to the Philippines in 1939, first as post surgeon at Fort Stotsenberg and then as hospital commander at Sternberg. Dr. Carroll had attended Saint Louis University Medical School, graduating in 1913. During his internship, he was persuaded to join the army, reassured that it would be highly unlikely the country would go to war. Not long after that, he was on horseback with the 7th Cavalry roaming Mexico in search of Pancho Villa. There he met a young captain with two big pistols tucked into his belt—George Patton was his name. "Lieutenant," Patton said once to Carroll at reveille, "every time I see that flag lowered or raised, I love it more and more." Then Carroll was off to France during World War I to supervise a hospital train transporting wounded from the front. After that came a number of duty stations: Tennessee, Fort Sheridan, back to Saint Louis University, Walter Reed, New York, China, and then, as he approached fifty, back to the Philippines and Sternberg.

But there were other station hospitals as well. About sixty miles north of Manila was Fort Stotsenberg, a former cavalry post in Pampanga Province in the foothills of the Cabusilan Mountains, occupying over one hundred fifty thousand acres, and the Fort Stotsenberg Station Hospital. It now primarily served the Army Air Corps. Nearby Clark Airfield was built in 1919 and expanded in the 1930s to accommodate medium and heavy bombers as well as fighter aircraft. The climate there was distinctly cooler than in Manila, the lifestyle even more laid back. Swimming, golf, polo, and tennis were in abundance, and there was plenty of time to do any. "The bringing of American servants is discouraged and this practice has been found very unsatisfactory due to their lack of friends and the availability of experienced native servants," the Officer's Guide to Service in the Philippines for 1941 advised. The station hospital consisted of wooden buildings with the typical metal roofs to dissipate heat, except for the operating room, which was made of concrete. There were 350 beds with an average daily census of 175 before December 8, 1941. Stotsenberg Hospital was commanded by fifty-seven-year-old Colonel Carlton Vanderboget from upstate New York, a 1910 graduate of the University of Buffalo. He had assumed his new posting on November 20, 1941. His staff included six regular army and twelve army reservist medical officers. Also attached to Stotsenberg were flight surgeons for the Army Air Corps, medical officers attached to ground units such as the 803rd Engineer Battalion, the 192nd Tank Battalion, the 194th Tank Battalion, and the 200th Cavalry.[12]

Eugene Jacobs earned his medical degree from the University of Michigan in 1929. Now an army officer, he and his young bride, Judy, arrived in Manila after a honeymoon voyage from San Francisco to Hawaii to Guam on July 20, 1940. He was now a regular army officer. He was initially stationed at Fort McKinley just outside Manila but was transferred to the small, thirty-five-bed station hospital at Camp John Hay in Baguio, the only medical officer there and "the nearest U.S. doctor to Japan." Baguio was a mountain resort, nestled at five thousand feet among the pine trees in the northern Luzon highlands but only twenty miles from the white sands and palm trees of Lingayen Gulf. "Discovered" by Dean Worcester in 1900, it was a "wonderful region of pine parks" and "a magnificent spring of crystal-clear water." Realizing the tourist potential, a road was quickly cut from Baguio to Manila and the retreat developed by the Philippine Commission, which contracted with architect Daniel Burnham of Manila fame. It was soon touted as the Adirondacks of the Philippines, "taking away the necessity for long vacations spent in America," the commission reported.[13] For Europeans, it was to be the "Switzerland of the Far East." On the grounds of the old sanitarium was built a premier hotel, The Pines, on a sloping hill overlooking the small urban community and an expansive outdoor area called Burnham Park. By the 1930s, with the mining boom in the Philippines and the influx of wealthy American and European speculators, Baguio and The Pines were in full swing. Drinks, dinner, and tangos were the nightly routine, surrounded by cool evening air and a hint of frost even. "You haven't seen the Philippines if you haven't seen Baguio," an advertisement read. And for the military stationed in the Philippines, it truly was a "Rest and Recreation Center," a relief from the heat and humidity that smothered most of the islands. Camp Hay had been set aside by President Theodore Roosevelt for the military as a resort adjacent to the spa and was set up as the summer capital of the Philippines. There were no fortifications, only wooden barracks, an infantry detachment for housekeeping duties, some outdated World War I rifles, and only one cannon for raising and lowering the flag. Indeed, Eugene Jacobs won a prize duty station. Days were short, with plenty of time for Rotary Club dinners and rubbing elbows with wealthy American executives of nearby gold mines and lumber companies. Even after wives were sent home in May 1941, Camp Hay was a safe haven; it held absolutely no real military value, commanders would say.[14] The Japanese would feel differently.

The skinny, fingerlike projection into Manila Bay just south of Manila was the Canacao Peninsula. On the eastern side of the peninsula was a sheltered anchorage, a bay within a bay. It was recognized by the Spanish in the sixteenth and seventeenth centuries as an ideal haven for bulky galleons and was used as the main port of Manila for centuries. The anchorage was enclosed by pincers consisting of the peninsula and a splinter off of it where the Americans would build their naval base, the prime location for the Asiatic Fleet, on the wreckage of the old Spanish port of Fort San Felipe. With an American presence following the Spanish-American War, the port was further developed and renamed Cavite Naval Yard. At the tip of Canacao Peninsula, a naval air station was constructed called Sangley Point ("pure" Chinese were called Sangleys by the Spaniards and allowed to sell their wares on this tiny peninsula during the colonial period). In 1871, just down from Sangley Point, the Spanish built a naval hospital run by the Sisters of Charity. The hospital was remodeled and eventually rebuilt as a modern, three-story cement structure by Americans throughout the first two decades of the twentieth century and was renamed the Navy Hospital at Canacao.

Tactically, MacArthur had divided his USAFFE on Luzon into a North Luzon Force under Major General Jonathan Wainwright and a South Luzon Force under Brigadier General George Parker. The Philippine Division that included the American 31st Infantry and two regiments of crack Philippine scouts, the 45th and 57th Infantries, led by American officers, was to be held in reserve. The balance of army forces were inexperienced, ill-equipped Filipino army divisions, composed of and led by native Filipinos with only sporadic American "advisers," making up a total of nine divisions. But what was worse, there was a woeful lack of leadership. Some American junior officers were scattered among Filipino units as "advisers," but experienced commissioned and noncommissioned officers were rare. Mobilization of these reservists had only begun in September. They were issued outdated World War I-era, .30-caliber Enfield bolt action rifles, a meager number of light and heavy machine guns, few mortars, little ammunition, and almost no organic transportation. Even their uniforms were spartan: they had no steel helmets, and their flimsy canvas shoes with rubber soles wore out in about two weeks. Many were later found in combat barefoot. No entrenching tools, raincoats, or gas masks made it into their ranks either.

While discipline and equipment for American troops was better, assignment in the Philippines was still cushy. Training stopped at noon, the afternoon sun and heat unbearable. Marksmanship practice was held only one two-week period per year. Everyone carried the new M-1 Garand rifle, and both light and heavy machine guns were amply supplied. Yet ammunition was limited, mortar rounds were outdated—only two thousand 81-mm rounds existed in the Philippines—grenades were scarce, and motorized transportation was extremely primitive, mostly native conveyance. Much of the heavy artillery, though promised by Marshall, had not arrived by December. But accommodations were luxurious. Many officers had spacious housing with Filipino servants, chefs, and doormen. Recreation, indoors and out, was lavish. Golf and whiskey were mainstays—a lifestyle similar to British colonial troops in India.[15] The US 4th Marine Regiment, fresh from duty on mainland China, arrived on Luzon in late November 1941. They were deployed at Olongapo, guarding Subic Bay on the western coast of the Bataan Peninsula and at Mariveles at the tip of the peninsula, but eventually defended Corregidor once the Japanese invasion began.

At the time of the Japanese attack, the medical department supporting the USAFFE was headed by Colonel Wibb Cooper, Army Medical Corps. Dr. Cooper had spent time in the Philippines as a young medical officer, served in Mexico with Pershing, and commanded Base Hospital No. 8 in Savenay, France, during World War I. He took over from Colonel Adam Schlanser, another World War I veteran, who moved to Fort Riley, Kansas. It was Cooper's task to develop a medical plan in support of USAFFE in the defense of the Philippines. There were five station hospitals under his command: Sternberg General Hospital in Manila, Fort William McKinley Hospital south of Manila, Fort Stotsenberg Hospital near Clark Airfield, Fort John Hay Hospital in the hill country of Baguio, and a station hospital at Fort Mills across from Mariveles on the island of Corregidor. If war came, plans called for a consolidation of casualties to Sternberg and nearby "annexes," collectively referred to as the Manila Hospital Center. This, in effect, vastly expanded bed capacity and composed Annex A, the Jai Alai Building; Annex B, the dilapidated Estado Mayor Barracks near the Quezon Bridge; Annex C, the Spanish Club and Girls' Dormitory; Annex D, the Philippine Women's College; Annex E, the Santa Scholastica College;

Annex G, the Holy Ghost Convent and College south in Quezon City; Annex H, the La Salle Extension University; and Annex F, Fort William McKinley station hospital; as a last resort. Almost four thousand five hundred beds would be made available. Each annex—some primarily surgical and others convalescent centers—had been stocked with medical supplies and would be staffed by physicians and nurses from Sternberg and Canacao.

Such a sprawling medical effort required a stockpile of material. The repository for medical supplies, known as the Medical Supply Depot, was located in a group of buildings and warehouses at 92 Panderos Street in the Santa Ana district of Manila. Supplies for almost two thousand hospital beds were housed there. It was hoped that being near the Pasig River, additional material could be floated down by barge directly from the harbor. Equipment for two general hospitals began arriving in November 1941, and some had already been sent to Limay, Bataan, in anticipation of a general hospital there in case war plan Orange was activated. The remainder of the material was slated for the consolidated Manila Hospital Center under Orange specifications. Of course, the evacuation of Manila would change all that, and the best laid plans went awry.[16]

Field medical services for the Philippine forces centered primarily on the 12th Medical Regiment. That regiment was converted to the 12th Medical Battalion in August 1941, as the Philippine Division reorganized to the new triangular formation: three infantry regiments instead of four. Lieutenant Colonel James Duckworth had commanded the regiment before he was transferred to head up General Hospital No. 1 on Bataan. His replacement was Major Harold Glattly (soon to be promoted to lieutenant colonel), a Minnesotan and a graduate of the University of Iowa. A career military man, Dr. Glattly had previously commanded Brooke Army Hospital in San Antonio and had spent time at Walter Reed General Hospital. His medical battalion was formed into three collecting companies, responsible for casualty evacuation from aid stations, and one clearing company, a field hospital where some so-called resuscitative surgery could be done—life-saving procedures. It was left to Glattly to organize his resupply base and survey the Bataan Peninsula for suitable collecting and clearing station sites. The battalion had an educational mission as well: responsibility for training Filipino litter bearers, medics, and medical officers. According to war plan Orange, casualties on Bataan would flow from aid stations to clearing companies by way of collecting personnel and then on to general hospitals. The clearing company for the 12th Medical Regiment (soon to be re-configured as the 12th Medical Battalion)—Glattly's field hospital—eventually ended up near the town on Balanga on the east coast of the peninsula.[17]

THE BATAAN PENINSULA WAS A BRUTAL, unforgiving wasteland. It only held tactical value for the Allies, and then only for harassment and interdiction. It borders on Manila Bay, and its proximity to the city of Manila allowed menacing artillery positions to lob shells onto any occupying force there. Otherwise, the peninsula was essentially 450 square miles of dormant volcano, punctuated by two silent cones: 4,111-foot Mount Natib to the north and 4,554-foot Mount Mariveles to the south. A smaller, parasitic cone of Mount Mariveles, Mount Samat, about seven miles northeast of Mariveles's caldera, at 1,787 feet, loomed over the major east-west passageway from Orion on the east coast to Bagac on the west. It was mountainous terrain dominated by the lava-rich uplands covering over 80 percent of the entire area. To the northeast, heights receded into a sloping coastal plain favorable for agriculture. But for the most part, Bataan was jungled ground rich in acacia, coconut, bamboo, and mahogany. The tangled underbrush of ipil-ipil and molave plants were interwoven with rattan vines and creeper ferns that made passage almost impossible. Thirty- to fifty-foot ravines splendid in cogon and talahib grass up to three feet high spread down from the slopes of Mount Samat. In many areas, forests were so dense that visibility was measured in feet, and their canopies almost blocked out sunlight. Huge *balete* trees sunk flying buttress roots big enough to hide three or four men, and the swaying bamboo sang a soft sound in the breeze, almost melodious, like nature's wooden flutes. In this botanical opulence, snakes, insects—particularly mosquitoes—were in abundance, ready to bedevil anyone who ventured forth. Over one hundred rivers and streams emanated from the mountains, running into the bay and the South China Sea. In those rapidly moving streams, among the roots of bamboo and bankside vegetation, were the larvae of the *Anopheles minimus flavirostris* mosquito, the chief vector of malaria in the Philippines. It was a disease of the foothills and of those seasons when rainfall was not too brisk or too scarce. January, February, and March were perfect months for breeding and, for visitors, perfect months for transmission, and the Bataan Peninsula the perfect place.[18]

Intruders were unwelcome. It was real estate not meant for human beings. For those foolish enough to transgress, mere travel up and down the peninsula, especially the western half, was particularly arduous, as there were few mountain trails. Interminable steep ravines and numerous Anopheles-infested streams provided a challenge to even the fittest. Ill equipped for nature's exuberance and at the same time its heartlessness, trespassers paid penalties. Forget their warring tendencies, humans suffered a thousand indignities, some of their own design and some of Bataan's. In spite of its travails, MacArthur had picked the place. Perhaps it spoke of natural entanglements far surpassing anything man-made, that the jungles would surround and shield his troops, an impenetrable barrier for any pursuer. He perhaps surmised Bataan would be the great neutralizer, as layers of forest roofing rose to heights that barred all view from above. Air superiority became irrelevant, artillery marginally so. It would be an infantryman's battle, mano-a-mano. Yet a faithless paramour would Bataan be. Pitiless and impartial, she would devour even the best prepared. And once one was entrapped—once stricken—the jungle closed in, paralyzing escape. Transports, extractions, rescues were impossible tasks. Sick and wounded paid the dearest price. Passage through interminable vines, trees, and brush compounded suffering, delayed treatment, and weakened already disturbed physiology.

Indeed, MacArthur's legions were trapped on Bataan. They were cornered, surrounded, and harassed by nature and by a mounting Japanese force that sooner or later rode roughshod over defenders. Instead of a flanking threat to Manila Bay or a supreme natural fortification, Bataan proved to be a squalid, disease-ridden ordeal of sweltering temperatures, insufficient food, dysentery, malaria, malnutrition, and a suffocating vulnerability that pervaded all. Completely cut off, supplies, food, morale, and medical care dwindled. Rescue? Almost certainly not. In a communique to the army chief of staff dated January 3, 1942, summarizing resources needed for "Relief of the Philippines" Brigadier General Leonard Gerow, acting head of the War Plans Division, concluded "That the forces required for the relief of the Philippines cannot be placed in the Far East area within the time available," indicating that such an effort would divert precious assets designated for the "principal theater—the Atlantic." And that "operations for the relief of the Philippines be not undertaken."[19] Did MacArthur know? He seemed oblivious when on January 15, 1942, in supreme folly, the following message was issued to his troops on Bataan: "Help is on the way from the United States. Thousands of troops and hundreds of planes are being dispatched. . . . No further retreat is possible . . . it is a question now of courage and of determination. . . . This is the only road to salvation."[20]

For medical teams, challenges of casualty care (and care of nonbattle illnesses) was immense. Doctors and nurses had an equally despairing task as stricken troops and civilians consumed material in staggering amounts. Vital medical stockpiles—literally heaps of equipment—had been abandoned in Manila, warehouses of the Medical Depot left bulging for the Japanese. Along routes of retreat from north and south Luzon, stores redistributed with MacArthur's revamped defense were left behind by panicking Filipino troops. They had once been earmarked for Bataan. Care of the infirm consisted of the most rudimentary measures: cleansings, bandagings, and amputations. Among the congregations of besieged, sickness rose to overtake all thoughts and hopes, crushing resolve and shattering perseverance. In the end it was simple comfort that was a mainstay of treatment, delivered by a medical staff as ill as all the others, in the swamp of MacArthur's fantasies. Lieutenant Ruth Straub, an army nurse, told a reporter from the *Chicago Tribune* in September 1942: "It was hope that kept them fighting. Hope that help would come. That was what we lived for. It was hope that kept us all there. . . . We hadn't dreamed it would ever be war out there."[21]

Twenty-seven-year-old First Lieutenant Henry Lee, fresh from one year of training with the 31st Infantry, walked off the gangway of the SS *President Pierce* in June 1941 and onto the Manila docks. He was assigned to the Philippine Scouts Headquarters Company. Awed by the scenery, he soon wrote to his parents about the Manila Hotel ("It is said to be the most modern and all around best hotel in the Orient"), sat in the bamboo bar and "rubbed shoulders with Japs, Germans, English, and many other nationalities". In late November he scribbled another note, this time a bit darker, sensing the vulnerability of all those Americans so far from home: "You've probably been wondering how we really feel over here about our situation and our chances. Truthfully, we are in a pretty bad spot over here—or will be if hostilities ever begin."

Even at his junior level, Lee was aware of the lack of weapons, planes, air defense, and training of Filipinos, and of the *hara-kiri* philosophy of the Japanese who would rather commit suicide than capitulate. He realized his country and Japan were on a collision course, much "like two little boys who really don't want to fight but who, by threats and bluffs," cannot back down. "We all worry at times about our situation . . . and we never discuss it among ourselves. . . . We have no control over the situation, so we sit tight and don't worry too much."

Henry Lee soon echoed the feelings of many soldiers past and present who are about to embark on the uncertainties of war and of their own personal fate—one last hedonistic binge that might never happen again: "Englishman, Dutchman, Spaniard, and Jew / Soldierman, Sailorman, and pioneer / Get yourself a girl and a bottle too, / Blind yourself, hide yourself, the storm is near."[22]

Navy nurse Ann Bernatitus had never heard of Bataan, not even up to two days before her departure from a ravaged Manila on Christmas Eve 1941. In fact, she had stepped off the USS *Chaumont* onto Manila's dock eighteen months before, in July 1940, her first overseas assignment to the U.S. Naval Hospital Canacao. It had been a rough, sea-sickening trip from Norfolk, Virginia, through the Panama Canal to Pearl Harbor, then to Guam and finally the Philippines. There she stood, a Pennsylvania girl from Exeter, half a world away from home. She had done nurse's training at the Wyoming Valley Homeopathic Hospital in nearby Wilkes-Barre. Despite her nursing skills, jobs were scarce, even in the medical profession. That is what attracted her to the military, the simple reason that it was hiring. As a navy nurse, Bernatitus's stateside duties had been agreeable: Chelsea Naval Hospital on the tranquil banks of the Mystic River, just outside Boston, and the Naval Health Clinic on Hospital Point, Annapolis, Maryland (teeming with young midshipmen)—nothing that would prepare her for the teeming tropics. She loved the operating room and had done special training in Philadelphia prior to joining the navy.

On the trip from Manila's docks to Canacao Naval Hospital her first impression was the smell of copra, the native nipa huts perched on stilts, meandering *carabao*, and naked kids running in the streets. And life was good then, usually half-days of working, then bicycling and swimming. Scenes were reminiscent of a Somerset Maugham novel of British colonial life in the Far East, tennis or golf after four, a change to dinner attire, collecting around the bar, gin and tonics, smoking, gossiping, sumptuous dinners, and occasional ragtime. For a few bucks a month shoes could be shined, laundry washed and folded, or an evening dress hand-tailored. There was a Chinese man from Hong Kong who would visit the nurses' quarters, open his valise and spread out exotic silks and linens, all to be had with just a signature—pay later. Of course, there were those rumors of war. In November 1941, Bernatitus was advised by her Chief Nurse

Laura Cobb to get rid of any valuables. "I would suggest that anything you have, you pack up and ship back." And, dutifully, if somewhat dismayed, she packed up a chest and sent it back on the next steamer. Still, that shadowy stretch of land across the bay had never been mentioned, and anyway, like other days on this wild, glamorous adventure, it would be time for cocktails soon.

On observing the fate of empires, the French literary critic Charles-Augustine Sainte-Beuve once commented, "Extreme happiness [is] only separated from extreme despair by a trembling leaf—isn't this life."[23] The margin of safety was slim here in the tropics of Rizal and Joaquin. James Hopper, called "the Kipling of the Philippines," wrote in his 1906 book *Caybigan*: "always when you think you have at last mastered the problem of this life and evolved a system that promises smooth going . . . that the skies tumble down on you."[24]

Only too soon would American reverie tumble and fall victim to Japan's trembling leaf.

3

Invasion

WAR CAME WITH A STUNNING SUDDENNESS. IT WAS ALREADY AFTER midnight, Monday, December 8, in the Philippines when word sifted down: Pearl Harbor had been attacked by the Japanese. At first rumors were that the attack was unsuccessful, that the Japanese had been annihilated. But soon the ugly truth was known: the Pacific fleet had been decimated, thousands had been killed. The first to know was the commander of the Asiatic Fleet, based in Manila, Admiral Hart. His counterpart in Hawaii, Admiral Husband Kimmel, had radioed that famous message: "AIR RAID ON PEARL HARBOR. THIS IS NO DRILL." As a reflection of the chilly relationship between Hart and MacArthur, the admiral failed to share the information with the general, who heard about it via an enlisted army signalman listening to a California radio station and relaying the information through his superiors. MacArthur's aides meekly called him in his penthouse in the wee hours of the morning.

Percy Carroll, promoted from colonel to brigadier general since his move from Stotsenberg, had just seen the movie *Sergeant York* the previous Saturday night. At 4:30 AM, his telephone rang with the message about Pearl Harbor. For the rest of that morning, he toured Manila and all the annexes that could accommodate wounded soldiers. For his surgical teams he decided on the Jai Alai Building, that spacious streamlined modernist arena not far from the waterfront on Taft Avenue across from Luneta Park, the large playing court and four gaming rooms serving as hospital and morgue. The Keg Room and restaurant were outfitted with X-ray and surgery. Fronton Pavilion, that highly polished wooden playing floor, would now be crowded with hundreds of surgical cots. The building had already been supplied with enough food—including sumptuous Australian beef—to last a year and outfitted with quarters for doctors and nurses. Carroll expected to be inundated with casualties after reports of the carnage at nearby Clark and Nichols Airfields. The hums of airplane engines propelled him outside, and he was expecting a major bombing run over the city. There they were, flights of dozens, their fuselages sparkling in the sunlight. But Manila was spared. The Japanese apparently wanted to preserve the city to use as their headquarters. Instead, Nichols Field and the Cavite Navy Yard at Sangley Point were targets. And casualties poured in from Stotsenberg and Canacao, more dead than living. Bombs were terribly effective—and indiscriminate. Soldiers and civilians alike fell victim. The Jai Alai Building became an expanding morgue.

Captain Robert Davis, director of the Canacao Navy Hospital, had already implemented war plans for the hospital with the first notification of hostilities on December 8. Located at the end of Canacao Boulevard, the hospital was bound to be caught up in any strikes at the Navy Yard itself. Two days later, Davis had fifty tons of supplies delivered, including cots and mattresses to Annex E, Santa Scholastica College in Manila, and Sternberg. At the Navy Hospital, forty-eight caskets were taken from the Supply Depot to a garage and replaced with cots—six hundred of them. Davis would only too soon need a wealth of both. Sandbags were stacked all around in preparation for what would most certainly be a hefty aerial bombardment, considering the military prominence of the Naval Yard. Cavite and the Canacao district had to be high priority for the Japanese. Davis stripped the hospital of any nonessential personnel, making it, in effect, little more than a field dressing station, to be staffed by five doctors and twenty corpsmen. As soon as they were treated, all patients were to be quickly shipped to Sternberg or one of the medical center annexes, either Santa Scholastica College or the Philippine Women's College, which had been designated for navy casualties. In fact, the aerial bombardment on the Navy Yard would generate over four hundred wounded and flood the deserted hospital with critical, mangled men.

At 3:00 AM Tuesday, December 9, Davis was awakened by the bombing of Nichols Field only a few miles away. By early afternoon, he had transferred 154 patients to Sternberg. His hospital was emptied and prepared for a sure onslaught of desperate casualties. By the following day, four hundred patients had filled empty cots, one hundred were sent to surgery. As soon as they were treated and stabilized, motor launches took them and a number of dead to the San Roque docks and near the Army Navy Club. At Davis's hospital, darkness reigned. All lights had been extinguished, the elevator was dead, but a 50-kW unit illuminated the operating room. For good reason, the space was never empty. The chief of surgery, Lieutenant Commander Thomas Hayes, recalled that casualties were "brought up to us and dumped like piles of human offal, all guts and brains and bones."[1]

Ann Bernatitus was told by nurse Bertha Evans St. Pierre at six in the morning on December 8 that war had been declared after the debacle at Pearl Harbor. St. Pierre had been given the news in a call from her boyfriend, a navy officer at Cavite. The next morning, Japanese planes were overhead. Bernatitus was coming off work early when Nichols Field was bombed. All suspected the navy base would be next. Anyone who could be discharged was sent off, Filipinos were sent home, and those too sick to leave were put in a subbasement under the hospital. The three-story wooden structure was thought to be a potential tinderbox. The sandbagging started, slim protection against aerial bombs. The decision was soon made to transfer the hospitalized patients to the army's Sternberg General Hospital. Bernatitus was picked to accompany them.

And indeed, the day after she arrived at Sternberg, the navy base at Sangley Point was obliterated by Japanese bombers. The entire naval operation on Cavite and Canacao was systematically leveled. She and the other nurses watched the whole spectacle from their foxholes at the nursing barracks. From Sternberg, she was moved to the makeshift hospital at Santa Scholastica, commandeered as an emergency surgery center and overflow from the Philippine Women's College. On December 22, Bernatitus was informed that Lieutenant Commander Carey Smith, a navy surgeon, had handpicked her as one of the surgical nurses to go into the Bataan Peninsula as part of plan Orange. With little delay, her convoy left from the Jai Alai building, now a bustling, one-hundred-bed infirmary, on Christmas Eve. It was an odyssey of sorts. On their way around Manila Bay, the buses crawled through villages awash in natives cheering on their American saviors, the trip punctuated by overflights of Japanese planes, forcing all out of the vehicles and into ditches for safety. In contrast, the stark, tropical lushness of Bataan struck her as somehow incongruous with the noise, fire, and explosions of this new war. Her destination was General Hospital No. 1 at Camp Limay on the eastern coast of Bataan.

Forty-four-year-old Captain Carey Miller Smith arrived with his family on a trans-Pacific steamer in Manila's harbor on October 2, 1940, after a month at sea, sailing from San Francisco through Honolulu, on to Shanghai, then Hong Kong and finally Manila.[2] He had been a navy surgeon thirteen years and brought his wife and three children, ages fourteen, eighteen, and twenty, with him. He was chief of surgical service at the Canacao Naval Hospital. One month later, his family left for the States, and Dr. Smith found himself in bachelor's quarters instead of the comfortable, cozy house he had shared with his family. A little over one year later, he was told, while eating breakfast, that Pearl Harbor had been attacked. He knew the Philippines would be next. Two days after that news, huddled under the navy hospital's concrete and steel floor, he watched the Cavite Navy Yard across the bay being bombed and destroyed by waves of Japanese planes coming frightfully close to the Navy Hospital Reservation. Some fifty-four planes, according to historian Samuel Eliot Morison, "flew back and forth at leisurely tempo and in graceful curves, at 20,000 feet elevation beyond range of the 3-inch antiaircraft guns, the bombers releasing at will."[3] It was like bombing practice, a flyover picking out targets, banking, and then a run in to drop their load. The blitz was amazingly accurate, almost all ordnance falling within the Navy Yard. The power plant, dispensary, torpedo repair shop, supply office and warehouses, signal station, commissary, receiving station, barracks and officers' quarters were all hit. Over two hundred torpedoes, stacked on the dock and slated for use on navy submarines, were lost. Filipino workers, running from cover in fright, were cut to ribbons by shrapnel. Corpses cluttered the ground, some missing heads, limbs. A sailor handed off what he thought was a baby covered in blood, but the blood was his, his left arm had been completely severed at the shoulder—he was completely unaware.

Casualties from the attack rolled in by the dozens: mangled, broken, and in pieces. "They were lying on boards, old doors, corrugated roofing material, or just anything a patient could be moved on," said nurse Dorothy Still.[4] For the next twelve hours Smith and two teams of surgeons worked on bombing victims. The noise of the generator and smell of blood were thick in the air. Dr. Fred Berley, a young navy lieutenant, assisted Smith for a while. He had been bored, working at the Cavite dispensary before the war broke out. Since then it had been continuous action, narrowly escaping the bombings on Cavite and near the navy hospital. He had asked if they needed help. Now, surgery was nonstop, doctors not even changing their gowns between cases. "You'd amputate a leg, you'd amputate an arm. It was just horrible," Berley later recalled. "Someone would die on the table. It was just a nightmare, when I think back on it." When they finished at one or two in the morning, Berley's shirt and trousers were soaked in blood. Berley himself had cut off a Filipino workman's hand the day before because it was barely attached, dangling by a thin strip of skin, all in the dim glow of a flashlight. Electricity went out early.[5] This was nothing like medical school at Northwestern University or the mundane peacetime activities of a medical officer dispensing drugs for the Asiatic Fleet.

After a day and night of nonstop operating, doctors and nurses collapsed and slept in that dingy hospital subbasement, the only reinforced concrete shelter available. What remained of the night was fitful for most, the memory of so many damaged kids, the danger of further raids, and God knew what else a constant interruption to sleep. The following day Smith and his surgical team were ordered to evacuate and report to Sternberg. Canacao was ablaze, cratered, and being evacuated. The Japanese had delivered an ultimatum to Canacao to evacuate, that the hospital would be targeted as a military objective. Already, the streets of Cavite were packed with refugees streaming out of the area. All sensed the inevitable. But where to put them at Sternberg? After days of continued bombings and torrents of wounded, beds ran short. The hospital had become a heaving, noisy mixture of walking wounded mixed with bed-ridden and moribund patients as doctors fumed on how to distribute casualties.

At Sternberg, Lt. John Bumgarner found staff scrambling and patients littered about. One wounded man in particular stuck in his memory. A young lieutenant commander was brought in after the bombing of the Cavite Navy Yard. He was on a stretcher with a gaping, sucking wound of his chest. "We were no more prepared to care for him, than we were to orbit the moon," Bumgarner recalled. There was not even a bed to put him in. The young man's stretcher was placed in a hallway, and he was given injections of morphine. Bumgarner checked on him often, asking if there was anything he could do. No, the young officer replied, "There's nothing you can do." On a return visit some time later, Bumgarner found him lifeless, his eyes staring "10,000 miles away: home."[6] Streams of casualties were brought in those first few days with nowhere to put them. The halls and floors were packed with injured. Surgeons lacked training for chest and head injuries, and most of the equipment was outdated. And then the quartermaster laundry was hit in collateral damage, liberating scalding steam from fractured pipes. Dozens of Chinese laborers who worked there were taken to Sternberg with ghastly burns, skin literally falling away from blisters covering 60 to 70 percent of the body surface of some victims. There was no room inside by that time. These horribly burned and suffering men were laid out in the grass in front of the surgical pavilion and treated with what intravenous fluids could be found—and liberal amounts of morphine. Many soon died of burn shock and sepsis. Operating room activity never let up. Doctors and nurses were working eighteen to twenty hours a day, catching sleep when they could, an hour or two of napping right on the operating tables.

Far to the north at tranquil Camp John Hay, Eugene Jacobs was roused from sleep before dawn on that Monday by the ringing of his phone. "We are at war with Japan! Pearl Harbor is being bombed! Report to Headquarters at once!" Jacobs was the closest doctor to Japan, a country with which the United States was now in a mortal struggle. Just minutes after eight in the morning, war had arrived in the Philippines. Camp John Hay, that remote mountain retreat that surely no one cared about, took Japan's first thrashing. Eighteen Japanese bombers languidly circled overhead and dropped seventy-two 250-kg bombs in and around the camp, hitting barracks, parade ground, and even family dwellings. Each blast, like an earthquake, jarred everything; in fact, some hit so close as to bounce around President Quezon, then in residence at the summer presidential palace. In short order, wounded arrived at Jacobs's small infirmary. A doctor rarely faced with even civilian trauma, he was swamped with mutilative explosive injuries. Shattered men filled corridors, and their puddles of blood made footing treacherous. Sounds of moaning and screaming, pleas for mercy from hopelessly broken men, pierced his equanimity almost worse than the sights. Jacobs was "shaking and woozy" but managed to find composure and began organizing his teams. "Everybody! Listen to me! These patients are bleeding. We've got to stop the bleeding quickly. . . . Elevate extremities! Use anything you can get to stop the bleeding! Tourniquets! Compression bandages! Hemostats! Even your fingers!" The doctor quickly learned what every trauma surgeon knows: stop the bleeding. A retired surgeon, the wife of the post's quartermaster, Dr. Beulah Allen, ran to assist him.

In missionary spirit, Allen had been in practice for years at the Mary J. Johnston Methodist Hospital in Manila, serving the poor of that community, a mission in concert with her Mormon upbringing. Allen was a graduate of the University of California at San Francisco School of Medicine in 1932, one of only a handful of female graduates each year in the country, and had interned at Women's and Children's Hospital of San Francisco. Her career then took her to the Philippines, where she spent two years in training at Saint Luke's Hospital, a Spanish stone edifice in the impoverished Tondo district of Manila. There she honed her surgical skills. After meeting and marrying Colonel Sam Allen, she became a contract surgeon for the army, accompanying him eventually to Baguio, where, on December 8, all their belongings were packed and at the dock ready to be shipped home. His tour was coming to an end. But now there was no returning home. Beulah Allen found herself in the operating room amid all the ruin of the day and in the middle of a war that would not end for her for over three years.

Extensive tissue trauma taxed both doctors. Arms and legs came off, wounds were explored, bleeding points ligated; the dead were moved aside into the garage area for later identification. Jacobs was so preoccupied with caring for injuries the likes of which he had never seen that only later did he realize the imminence of danger. Thirty-foot bomb craters pocketed the camp grounds. Over the next several days bombing runs continued. Jacobs and Allen operated, ran for cover during air raids, and then hurried back to their patients who were often left on the table, towels covering exposed wounds from falling debris.

Japanese general Masaharu Homma's 14th Army first landed at Lamon Bay, east of Manila, on December 22. This task force might have been successfully contained had not Homma landed a second large contingent at Lingayen two days later. At first green Philippine recruits held up well. But the Filipino forces were soon outflanked by a third prong of Japanese infantry which landed farther to the north at Vigan.[7] Some Filipino troops, spooked by enemy fervor, put down their weapons and ran. From Camp Hay, soundless puffs of antiaircraft fire could be seen, resembling, some thought, Japanese parachutists drifting nearby. Before long, the enemy filled the roads south, some even pedaling bicycles as if on holiday. An occasional Philippine scout would pick one or two off, but not enough. Realizing Camp Hay would soon be overrun—rifle fire like corn popping could easily be heard in the distance—doctors and nurses began evacuating patients to civilian hospitals in Baguio. In fact, it was time for all American military forces to "bug out." Jacobs entrusted his two nurses to a detachment of scouts, destroyed his vehicles loaded with medical supplies, put what equipment he could salvage on litters, and headed out on foot across mountain trails. The Japanese now controlled both roads out of Baguio. It was on this trail that Jacobs ran into Clark Lee, an Associated Press correspondent wandering Luzon in search of the war. All were fleeing Baguio, he said, except a handful of foreign nationals. There was one German doctor who stood out. Completely disinterested, Herr Doctor sipped a cocktail at The Pines Hotel and listened to Manila radio, confident the Japanese would not bother Baguio. "After all," he said in accented English, "there is nothing here for them." He and other guests then dined on cold turkey, goose liver, salads, and wine, served by an apologetic Filipino manager sorry that only a buffet supper was set out. Baguio soon became an occupied town. As for Jacobs, cut off from Bataan and roaming the mountains of Luzon on horseback, "Each night I thanked God for sparing my life."[8]

Transplanted Bostonian Alfred Weinstein was on duty at the station hospital at Fort William McKinley, located south of the Pasig River about seven miles outside Manila and adjacent to Nichols Field. Weinstein had been educated at Harvard University but moved to a surgical practice and teaching position at Emory University in Atlanta. He joined the army in 1940 and volunteered for service overseas. His duty station, Fort McKinley, was the home of the Philippine Division, the Carabao Division. Nichols Field was bombed late in the day December 8. Weinstein and his buddies hit the deck in their quarters as antiaircraft shrapnel tore through the roof. Once the explosions were over, they grabbed helmets and gas masks and ran to the hospital, just as ambulance sirens were heard coming through the south Carabao Gate. The hospital was a two-story structure in that ornate Spanish architecture with wide, sweeping vistas, so characteristic of many buildings in and around Manila. It ordinarily housed mostly medical patients, recipients of amorous but infectious couplings endemic around military posts.

In the airless operating room with humidity as thick as the flies, Weinstein partnered with another surgeon, Lieutenant Frank Adamo, the son of Sicilian immigrants. Slender in build, a bit graying at the temples, he was a native of Tampa, Florida. An unlikely prospect for medicine, as a youth Adamo attended school for only a few years, went to work rolling cigars, and spoke little English. He finally made his way to Chicago, finished grammar school at eighteen, worked through a high school curriculum, attended one year of college, and then entered the Chicago College of Medicine, where he graduated in 1919. He became a surgeon at Tampa General Hospital, returned to Chicago for some pick-up surgical training, and went back to Tampa. Adamo joined the army reserves in 1923 and found himself on active duty by 1941. That summer, fortunes brought him to Fort McKinley. And now, fortunes would embroil him in the Second World War.

Their first patient brought in was a young Filipino soldier struck in the abdomen by a dollar-size piece of bomb fragment. A quick laparotomy incision was made and blood and feces scooped out. On further exposure, Weinstein found the intestine and colon riddled with holes, through which a huge, pale *ascaris* worm slithered. The worm was removed and holes closed with catgut, all with the nonchalance of an appendectomy. Then it was on to the next patient.[9] Weinstein and Adamo worked until three in the morning. The stream of wounded, some with devastating injuries beyond repair, seemed endless. Army nurse Lucy Wilson recalled, "We worked around the clock. It was pure hell, seeing all those patients with limbs and parts of bodies missing, and all sorts of hideous wounds, having to wait in line to get into surgery."[10] At times, frantic attempts and unfaltering concentration could not put off the inevitable outcome; spiraling blood pressure and pulse until there was nothing but a lifeless corpse. The misery of these cases soon took its toll. After the last patient, Weinstein "physically weary and mentally unstrung," went to the toilet and threw up.[11]

North of Manila, at Fort Stotsenburg, newly arrived Colonel Carlton Vanderboget had received the announcement of the bombing of Pearl Harbor that Monday morning. Knowing Clark Field was a likely target, he assembled his staff and designated surgical teams for casualty care. Despite the immediacy of war, he then returned to his quarters and took a short nap, "which everybody does in the Tropics."[12] Nor were routines broken elsewhere at the fort. Almost everyone was enjoying their usual Monday lunch. That is, until the first bombing stopped the clock at exactly 12:43 PM. Indeed, Clark Airfield was the target. It was defended by the 200th Coastal Artillery, an antiaircraft unit from New Mexico, three battalions of 37-mm, .50-caliber, and 3-inch guns spread out to cover the fields. This might have been formidable if not for the fact that, the unit having just arrived in November, not all weapons had been set up, and many were outmoded and defective. Powder-train fuses could not reach high-altitude bombers, ammunition was old and corroded, and most shells were duds. The results were predictable. The Japanese bombed and strafed with impunity. What was worse was the wingtip-to-wingtip parking of planes of the Far East Air Force. They had just arrived that morning after searching for Japanese. Thinking saboteurs were a bigger threat, officers crowded the planes together for easier surveillance. They turned out to be so many sitting ducks. Thorough aerial bombing left hardly one intact. Amid the explosions, Vanderboget was shaken from his nap and ran to the hospital. It was not fifteen minutes before the first wounded arrived. In the confusion, many had been thrown into private cars and dumped off. Ambulances followed a short time later. The parade of casualties was so prodigious that Vanderboget soon lost count. He estimated over one hundred. Almost all were surgical cases, and many died. "I don't remember the number of deaths," he later wrote.[13] Others *were* counting. Eighty dead littered the grounds. Most were aerial bomb fragmentation wounds, some were bullet wounds from strafing Japanese fighters. And as Japanese aircraft winged away, twelve B-17s and thirty P-40 fighters burned and lay in twisted ruins. Five more B-17s were severely damaged. The Far East Air Force ceased to exist as a threat.

Major William Fairfield remembered that day. He was an engineering officer for the 19th Bombardment Group stationed at Clark Field. Just as lunch was finished, the Japanese came over. Running out the door to the slit trenches for cover, he saw Buck Davis fall and not move, and another pal, Bill Cocke, hit. Running to his aid, Fairfield was struck as well; his left leg gave way, punched full of holes, and then his right collapsed. Finally, stumbling into a trench, he spied two medical corps officers, Luther Heidger and Roy Day. Both were scurrying from body to body, out in the open—no helmets, no regard for safety. Heidger earned a Distinguished Service Cross that day, but he never saw it. Captured later that day, he would die as a prisoner of war. Fairfield and his friend Bill Cocke were picked up by one of those "goon" cars carrying injured. "Bill Cocke had his back and chest blown out and was in bad shape," Fairfield later recalled. "I put my arm around him and pressed his back up against my shirt front, hoping to stem some of the bleeding." At the station hospital they were unloaded, and Fairfield heard the nurses say about Cocke, "Mark him 'killed in action.'"

Fairfield will never forget his hospital experience. "I was pushed in to the operating room where they had two tables going; the chief nurse, Miss MacDonald was giving the anesthetic and the doctors were working there from one table to the other. The usual operating room aroma, plus sweat and blood, was rather unpleasant."[14] He ended up with a pin through his knee, strung up in traction with weights hanging off the end of his bed. During bombing raids, of which there were many, he recalled that nurses were supposed to leave and take cover. But none of them ever left. They stayed with the men, had a smoke, and acted as if nothing was wrong. The next Sunday, he and other casualties were put on a train to Sternberg General Hospital, some in coaches, he and a few others in a boxcar. Fearful that he was going to get his leg amputated—the feeling was he would be a more pleasing prisoner of war to the Japanese than if he were strung up in traction—he eventually was put in a hip spica cast. Little did he know, but Bill Fairfield would be selected for evacuation out of Manila on New Year's Eve.[15]

The number of wounded had overwhelmed the available staff, and Vanderboget put out an urgent call to Sternberg to send more nurses and doctors.[16] That Monday evening, a bus carrying two doctors, five army nurses, fifteen Filipino nurses, and some enlisted personnel arrived, finding the fort in ruins and the Far East Air Force in pieces. Lights were out, and the only way the new arrivals could find the hospital was by the moans and cries of the wounded. Nurse Helen Cassiani was one of those volunteers. She recalled her first impression of Stotsenburg Hospital the evening of December 8: "so many broken bones, so much scorched flesh."[17] Doctors and nurses were put to work, and were up throughout the night. Nurse Ruth Straub was another volunteer. That night and her inauguration to all the broken, hopeless men were seared into memory. She wrote in her diary:

> The hospital was bedlam—amputations, dressings, intravenouses, blood transfusions, shock, death. . . . Worked all night, hopped over bannisters and slid under the hospital during raids. It was remarkable to see the medical staff at work. One doctor, a flight surgeon, had a head injury, but during the night he got up and went to the operating room to help with the other patients.[18]

The flight surgeon was Major William Kennard, born in Cuba but the son of American citizens. He graduated from medical school at the University of Pennsylvania in 1930. Kennard entered the army immediately and served his internship at Walter Reed in Washington. Finishing Medical Field Service School, he was assigned to the 2nd Medical Regiment at Fort Sam Houston and finally sent to the Philippines as senior flight surgeon of the Philippines Department, stationed at Clark Field. A bomb fragment struck him in the right temple that day, but he continued to work. Somehow Kennard escaped captivity—one of a lucky few—and returned to the United States in August 1942. That head wound earned him a Purple Heart and Silver Star.

Over the next two weeks, until the hospital closed as Japanese troops advanced, Vanderboget and his staff cared for well over 750 casualties, practically all surgical in nature. For several days, the fort and adjacent Clark Field were regularly pounded by Japanese air raids. The hospital overflowed with wounded, now placed in corridors, lobbies, and verandas. On December 24, Vanderboget received orders to abandon the grounds. All patients were to be shipped by train miles into Manila, and all medical supplies were to be left behind. The tired senior surgeon and his executive officer were the last to go, dismayed at leaving so much valuable material for the enemy. As the two motored toward Manila, Stotsenberg receded into the background along with tropical savannahs, crisp air, and afternoon naps. Not for a long time—over three years—did Carlton Vanderboget feel the freedom of that evening drive and the open road that was now leading to war.

Lieutenant Paul Ashton could have been at Walter Reed General Hospital taking care of high-profile politicians and their wives. He could have been rubbing elbows with his mentor at Letterman General Hospital in San Francisco, future Surgeon General of the Army Colonel Norman Kirk, entertaining dignitaries and sipping champagne in dress blues. He could have been on the fast track to promotion. And he could have been with his young bride, Yvonne, with whom he had eloped that spring of 1940. But here he was in the Pearl of the Orient Seas, his destination for "excitement, color, and adventure" (as he had seen it advertised). Here he was at Fort McKinley, a ward surgeon caring for one hundred patients, part of the Philippine Division's 12th Medical Battalion, Headquarters Company, also based at Fort McKinley. Ashton was no warrior, at least not yet. Nor did he have much appreciation for the intrigues of battle or the desperation of battle wounds. He had been a peacetime surgeon more concerned with the complexities of acid peptic disease or consequences of tuberculosis than the resurrection of damaged men. Nevertheless, the regimentation, the discipline, the starch and polish of army life resonated with him. Nor did he shy from the rumor of war, in his mind as distant in Manila as it had been in San Francisco. He had watched the oceangoing tubs full of scrap metal sail under the Golden Gate Bridge on their way to Japan, to him a sign of cooperation and mutual interests—surely not warlike behavior. To be sure, there had

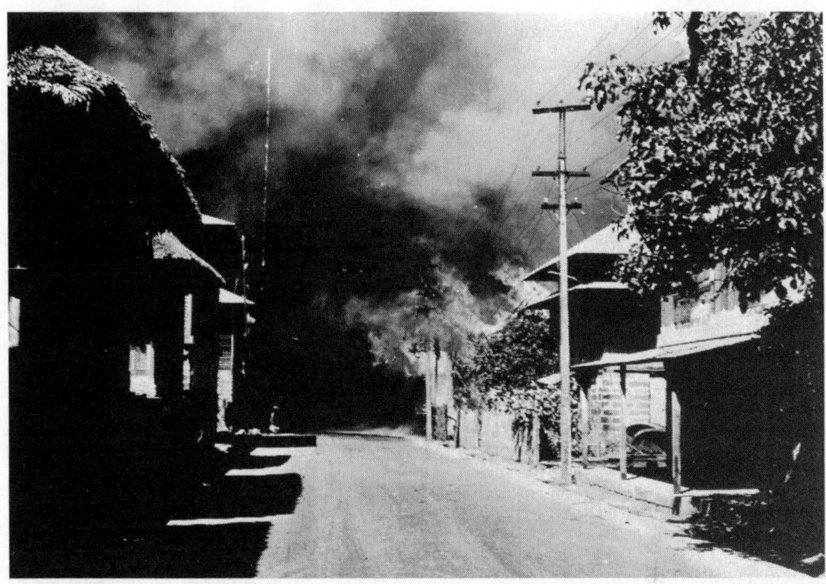

A town in Bataan burning following a Japanese bombing raid. (*Library of Congress*)

been practice and drill as of late, but all was harmonious, and the gentleman's life of officer privileges far surpassed the grit of soldierly duties.

There were frequent letters home to his wife; the last one was dated December 7, 1941, and went out by *China Clipper* the next day, the day of war. In it he told of his travels that Sunday south of Manila to the Tagaytay highlands, a picturesque venue overlooking Lake Taal to the south and the tablecloth of Manila spread to the north, on down into Batangas Province, then west to the coast of the South China Sea and the sandy beaches of Wawa and Nasugbu with their quaint *nipa* huts and clumps of fishing boats. They sailed in outriggers with native fishermen up the shore and had lunch in a paradise of tall cliffs, dense jungle, and gentle, crystal-clear surf, to an overture of chattering monkeys. "It was truly a most wonderful trip . . . I'd love to show you all these things," he wrote that night, and turned in for bed at Quarters No. 65.[19] It was his last night indoors. It was the last letter he wrote for three years. The next morning, his civilian life, his books and clothes and Chinese ivory, were packed away in a steamer trunk and taken to storage. There were quick goodbyes to his roommates and household help. Almost in a blur, he was out the door and over to headquarters. "Not even a disordered mind could have predicted the events about to befall us," he scratched in his diary. "It was the end of an existence on a very pleasant planet."[20]

Ashton's battalion provided the bulk of medical support for the Philippine Division, and senior members acted as advisers to other Filipino divisions. It was largely field training: first aid, collection and transport of wounded, clearing station activities. On December 8, drills turned into action. MacArthur ordered his combat units to deploy. A Japanese invasion was expected at any time. Ashton and the 12th Medical Battalion packed up and followed suit. MacArthur would hold his Philippine Division, arguably the best equipped and trained, in reserve—including the 12th Med. As a member of Headquarters Company, Lieutenant Ashton was tasked as an observer. He was to learn "the military features of the countryside" and where placement of medical stations would be most effective. Peculiarities of the battle zone were crucial to combat care: recesses, ravines, depressions, anything to provide line-of-sight shelter for soldier and medic. It would be vital information for all combat units, American and Filipino. His journeys took him from Manila around the bay and into Bataan's interior, looking for fordable streams, hills for defilade, trees that would obscure view from the air, and proximity to trails, roads, and streams for water.

THE JUNGLE BECAME A DUALITY OF EXISTENCE, at once a kingdom of nature's exuberance, all smells, and sights, and colors, an entwining of brilliant hues and utter darkness as the sky only seeped through a ceiling interdigitating with vines and branches and blades as thick as thatch. And for those toiling underneath a sauna, humidity not only felt but seen, literal steam seething from each bush, each copse, each clump of sweating brush. Man was the alien, unwelcome and quickly alone as the forest closed in, almost on purpose separating and assaulting until solitude engulfed as surely as creepers, and isolation rivaled the panic of unseen human enemies. It all oozed a loathsome dankness.

By 6:30 AM on December 8, Lieutenant Ralph Hibbs was headed to his battalion's bivouac area at Nichols Field, just outside Manila, not quite a mile from the end of the runway. News had already spread that Clark Field to the north had been demolished. They were to be on the lookout for Japanese paratroopers. There would be no fifty-foot buffet at the Army Navy Club's Baroque Bar tonight, he sensed, as he dug his foxhole. Yes, the Army Navy Club, where drinks were twenty cents and the bartender poured until told to stop. At two the next morning, the bombs arrived, whistling as they fell, a flash, then the ear-splitting roar of an explosion. The runway was cratered, hangers ruined, and the Pan-American beacon station brought down. Raids continued on Nichols Airfield throughout the early morning, and the fires burned incessantly. Almost miraculously, there were few casualties. Most personnel had vacated the field and dug in. Hibbs's unit, the Second Battalion, though, was flushed from its foxholes by the relentless bone-jarring cadence of explosions, and fled to the safety of a high ridge just below Fort McKinley—or so they thought. The scurrying figures on the ground were soon spotted by Zero pilots who came after them with a vengeance, lacing the dirt with .30-caliber wing rounds. Once again, luck prevailed. Only one soldier was wounded. By December 11, Hibbs and his men had been pulled back to Manila standing guard in Luneta Park, thought to be a perfect spot for a parachute drop, they were told. Hibbs had grabbed a .38-caliber revolver, gas mask, and steel helmet and settled in for the night, a far cry from sharkskin suits and premium gin.

Their stay in the city was short lived. War plan Orange had been activated. Off to Bataan. Finding transportation was a challenge. The unit had no vehicles. Hibbs's medical detachment was given two decrepit taxicabs, both of which broke down just outside Manila. A school bus was finally commandeered, and they were on their way down the dark, blacked-out, single-lane National Highway, jammed with bumper-to-bumper cars and crowds of refugees. At Layac Junction, near the town of Dinalupihan, they faced the Bataan Peninsula. Their first bivouac was farther south along the Pilar-Bagac road that ran across the peninsula to guard against a landing in Bagac Bay on the western coast. Shortly after New Year's Day, they moved back up to Layac Junction, that tiny crossroads of a town at the mouth of the Bataan Peninsula and dug in; the ground was so hard that it even defied solid swings of a pick-ax. Some soldiers tried urinating on the dirt to soften it up. Others hardly cared. The 1st Battalion, short on weapons and discipline, was put in reserve, and Company B promptly took advantage of the "rest and relaxation" to ice down and consume a washtub full of San Miguel beers brought up by Filipino troops. But by January 5, battalions had regrouped and rearmed. There were no more beers; the regiment was in position at Layac Junction directly in the path of advancing Japanese streaming south down Route 7 from Lingayen Gulf. Hibbs's battalion, the 2nd, was on the left, the 1st Battalion was on the right, and the 3rd Battalion was held in reserve. They were to be a speed bump; slow down the Japanese, force them to pause, deploy their infantry, bring up artillery—buy time. The Filipinos and Americans, in the meantime, would pull back to new positions farther south—tactics employed ever since the Japanese landed at Lingayen Gulf. It was here at Layac Junction that Lieutenant Hibbs's life changed, from treating sprained ankles and urethral discharges to combat surgeon; from a man of leisure and exotic adventure to a warrior fighting for his life.

4

Into Bataan

By Christmas Day the decision had been reached to abandon Manila and the Manila Hospital Center. Manila would be declared an open city, "In order to spare the metropolitan area from the possible ravages of attack."[1] General MacArthur realized the city was indefensible and would probably be destroyed in the process. His war plan Orange, withdrawal to Bataan, was the only option left. It would be a delaying action: bottle Japanese troops up on the peninsula for weeks, maybe months, and avoid a disastrous building-to-building battle in Manila. Acting USAFFE surgeon Colonel Wibb Cooper was directed to coordinate medical efforts in support of Orange and the defense of Bataan. Troops were already moving to Bataan or Corregidor and along with them medical officers and nurses. Casualties would be handled there in makeshift field hospitals—plans had already been drawn. Those still hospitalized, too ill to transfer to Bataan, had to be evacuated. Occupying Japanese troops, even now closing in, would have little time for the infirm; as an expediency, execution would be the probable outcome. Colonel Percy Carroll got the word from Major General Basilio Valdes, commanding general of the Filipino army, that the American Red Cross would undertake evacuation of all badly wounded from Sternberg Hospital to Australia. He and a group of Filipino doctors and nurses were to select those in serious condition to be ferried out. A makeshift hospital ship was found, the SS *Mactan*, a dumpy old interisland steamer launched in 1898. It had been used to send army troops to Corregidor, but with the unfolding crisis in Manila it was released to evacuate Sternberg's casualties.

The *Mactan* dutifully arrived at Pier N-1 at five in the morning December 30. One hundred painters immediately doused its hull and superstructure in white and adorned its sides with brilliant red crosses. By late the next afternoon, the job was finished, and it was ready to take patients. On cue, a steady procession of ambulances roared down to Pier 1 alongside the moored ship. For the next three hours, they disgorged their fill of stretchers. American and Filipino casualties sporting bandaged heads, splints, casts, and clanking plasma bottles were hustled up gangplanks and stored away. Some ended up bedded on open decks right up to the railing. As for the paperwork, a charter agreement was scribbled out between the American Red Cross and the ship's owners. The *Mactan* was hurriedly commissioned in the name of the president of the United States, and the Japanese government was notified of its status as a noncombatant. That was all well and good, perhaps, but it did not erase the anxiety of simply leaving Manila Harbor. The waters were mined, and without maps, disaster was almost assured. Captain Julian Tomayo, now piloting the *Mactan*, knew better and demanded charts. He refused to leave without them. At the last minute, some were found on the SS *Don Estabon*, an army transport ship that had taken MacArthur and his staff to Corregidor on Christmas Eve. Not the right ones, Tomayo muttered, too general. Yet Manila was now ablaze as the army dynamited gasoline storage tanks. There was no turning back. Tomayo gave a less-than-inspiring "I think so" when asked if he could make it out of the bay without charts, and, with a corvette leading the way, the *Mactan* cast off mooring lines, throttled up, and set off.[2] Manila Bay, too, was on fire, or so it seemed, its waters blazing in the reflection of its burning city.[3]

Major Fairfield had been hoisted aboard the *Mactan* with 223 other wounded and strapped into a bunk. He chose not to listen to rumors that the ship was hardly seaworthy. "You can't put them on that because it's suicide, the ship has been condemned!" Colonel Carlos Romalo reportedly told MacArthur. MacArthur is said to have replied, "It's suicide to leave them here; put them on!" The trip out was understandably nerve-wracking. All expected to either hit a mine or be torpedoed by the Japanese. Feelings of helplessness were overwhelming; most of the wounded were strapped into bunks or so weighed down with casts as to make survival highly improbable should the boat be struck. "I can't see," Fairfield lamented. "The porthole is way over my head and I'm locked in this bunk." Among men enfeebled with broken limbs, amputation stumps, bleeding remnants of arms, hips ruined by bomb fragments,

Fairchild took his place, watching the daily rituals of doctor visits, pill passing, and chaplain's calls. He listened to his bunkmates moan and gasp, heard of others buried at sea, and kept track of the "Cockroach Derby" as they scurried up walls and across ceilings. Finally, on January 25, the unseaworthy *Mactan* arrived at Brisbane and then, on the twenty-seventh, at Sidney. For Fairfield it would be the 113th Australian General Hospital, thirty-five pounds lighter than when it all began. By the grace of Neptune, the *Mactan*, Colonel Carroll, the crew, and most of the patients had made it through.[4]

Nightfall on December 23 found a convoy of thirty trucks full of medical equipment leaving the Medical Supply Depot in Manila bound for Bataan. A second installment of seventy trucks left the following day. A Field Medical Supply Depot was set up at kilometer post 162.5 on the Bataan-Mariveles Road. A second supply depot was placed farther north, at Orion, on the eastern coast, to furnish front-line troops with medical supplies. For the next week, trucks shuttled to and from Manila, dodging bombing raids to supply the hospitals of Bataan. Not a single truck was lost. Crate upon crate was off-loaded at the depots with supplies essential for running two general hospitals. It would never be enough.

Major Alfred Weinstein had made the best of his time at the Jai Alai Club. In between cases, he dined on turkey and filet mignon, onion and mushroom soup, broiled lobster, and Viennese pastries. There were literally tons of fine food sitting in the cold-storage plant at the club. Spirits were high, casualties light. Hearing rumors of a retreat to Bataan, he wondered what would happen to all the gourmet food in storage. In fact, it all would be abandoned and left to the Japanese. And on December 23, the ominous news arrived: pack up for Bataan. All too soon, Weinstein and his Chrysler were headed out Dewey Boulevard, across the Pampanga River, and, at the crossroads at San Fernando City, he turned left and headed into the foreboding Bataan Peninsula.

On December 24, Carey Smith's surgical team, including nurse Ann Bernatitus, climbed aboard buses for their freakish journey into Bataan. The National Highway was a sea of humanity, mixtures of buses, carts, cars, military vehicles, refugees piled high with belongings, and troops, all heading in the same direction, all in one sluggish caravan. The sight of soldiers mixed with civilians did not escape the attention of Japanese pilots, who, now and then, banked their Zeros and screamed in at treetop level for strafing runs. For Smith and his team, their first destination was the coastal barrio of Limay and a former Filipino army training camp.

The compound, their future hospital, was between the main eastern coastal highway and the ocean. This was General Hospital No. 1. Sixteen wooden buildings with steep, pitched, nipa roofs covered an area of about four city blocks. Each hut was raised three feet off the ground with rough lumber for the floor and a corrugated sheet-iron roof for cover. Measuring twenty-five by seventy-five feet, they were ideal dimensions for hospital wards. Other buildings on the compound were used for officers' quarters and officers' mess. Adjacent were four warehouses and shops for offices and receiving wards—large enough to put new arrivals in for examination and triage. General Hospital No. 1 had been planned as the surgical hospital. Combat wounded were sent there, much like an army evacuation hospital. The former Post Exchange, because it was almost twice the size of the hospital ward buildings, was the surgical space, big enough for several operating tables. Eight surgical teams were formed. Each had an operating surgeon, an assistant surgeon, an instrument ("scrub") nurse, and two hospital corpsmen. The surgical building needed ventilation, though. If it was closed up, people would cook in the Philippine heat and humidity. Windows remained unceremoniously propped open—a portal of entry for all kinds of airborne visitors; flies and mosquitoes found the invitation irresistible. For supplies, gauze and linen were sterilized in kerosene-driven pressure cookers and instruments in a tub of Lysol, then rinsed in alcohol. But expediency was key. According to nurse Bernatitus "the period of sterilization depended on how fast they were needed."

In keeping with the Geneva Convention roofs of three warehouses were painted with large white crosses, and three red crosses about forty-five feet in diameter were made from sheets and other cloth. And for good reason. Japanese planes buzzed the hospital compound almost daily, but no bombs were dropped nor did they interfere with operations at Limay compound.[5] Colonel James Duckworth was appointed commander. He was a regular army man, former chief at Fort McKinley and of the 12th Medical Regiment. This was his third tour of duty in the Philippines. Duckworth was an imposing figure, six feet tall and weighing over 280 pounds. Subordinates told of his "cool" nature, "always speaking in a low, well-modulated voice and never perceptibly ruffled in any crisis."[6]

On December 25, nurse Ruth Straub recorded in her diary: "Christmas. We hardly realized it. Sent more nurses out today to Bataan and Corregidor. Only 14 left now. Orders say we are all to evacuate by the first."[7]

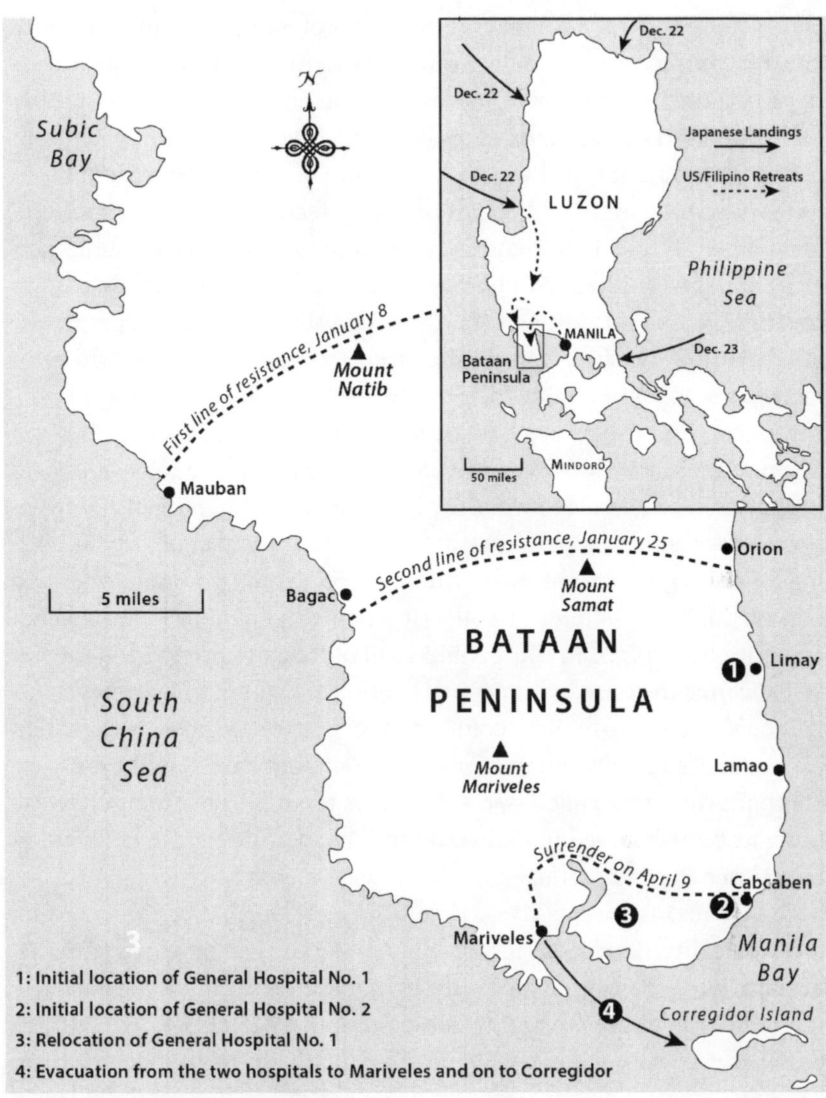

Map 1. The Bataan Peninsula, 1941–42.

By December 26, all crates had been unpacked, including scrub gowns from 1917. And young Bernatitus, now embedded with General Hospital No. 1 on godforsaken Bataan Peninsula, became Dr. Smith's personal scrub nurse. They were the standouts—the navy team, swabbies among doughboys. All other crews were army. But the routine was the same. Jovial rivalries of the peacetime military evaporated with the monumental tasks at hand: processing a sea of khaki-colored casualties. For Smith and his people, once combat started, patients came in a continuous stream; those first few days, they operated an entire weekend, from early Saturday morning straight through until Sunday afternoon without pause. The casualty load was so heavy that all eight teams were busy.[8] On January 16 alone, 182 operations were recorded.[9] Smith vividly remembered his first days of combat surgery at General No. 1. Eight operating tables were filled with hemorrhaging and shattered bodies, clumps of congealed blood on the floor, discarded suture and bandages in the mix. Outside the surgery building, often in open air, another thirty or forty patients waited, saline dripping into their veins, wounds hurriedly bandaged. And the rest of January was little different. Even at night, it was not unusual to see four or five surgical teams at the tables, surgical lights casting an eerie glow in the place, the hum of mumbled conversations background noise. Smith was struck by the number of dirty wounds in casualties not brought in for thirty-six or forty-eight hours, who had lain on the battlefield or at collecting points, unable to be evacuated. Their injuries coated in the fertilized soil of Bataan's rice fields—human feces were often used. Many such wounds had already turned gangrenous—that bluish-gray color of stubby gram-positive rods called *Clostridia*. As a result, amputations were commonplace. "Guillotine" amputations they were called—straight across the limb, no attempt to close it up; just a stump, red muscle and tan bone. Closure came later, when infection had passed. Nurse Bernatitus witnessed it firsthand, brutal but necessary efforts to save lives. Before long, a separate operating room and surgical team were designated just to handle gas gangrene patients. Segregation was essential, many thought, because the microorganism responsible was felt to be highly contagious and a danger to every fresh postoperative patient. It was depressing duty, with the odors of rotting flesh almost overwhelming, men in various stages of disassembly, all fearing loss of limbs. There was little middle ground with this problem, though. Less-aggressive treatment, avoiding amputation, might result in loss of life. Better to be radical, Smith felt, than watch patients spiral into sepsis and perish before his eyes. With January's bitter engagements, General Hospital No. 1 filled quickly. Postoperative patients, those needing convalescence, were moved to General Hospital No. 2 farther south, near the tip of Bataan, to make room for new arrivals. Despite a burgeoning patient population, every attempt was made to keep General Hospital No. 1 a surgical focus.

On Christmas, forty-five-year-old Lieutenant Colonel William "Riney" Craig, a graduate of Vanderbilt University Medical School, was ordered to collect his fellow medical officers—seventeen in total—twenty-three nurses, and thirty enlisted men to board the harbor freighter SS *McHyde*, depart Manila, and set up a second general hospital on Bataan. In this group was John Bumgarner (the former lieutenant was now a captain—most men received an almost immediate battlefield promotion). The ship, thought by some to be hardly seaworthy, chugged to Corregidor first, spent the night, and early the next day made the brief trip to Bataan, mooring at Lamao, toward the eastern tip of the peninsula. Personnel and supplies were ferried ashore, where they spent a restless day and night uncertain where exactly their hospital was to be. Eventually, a site a little over a mile west of the town of Cabcaben and the Cabcaben airfield, on the banks of the Real River was chosen, an area of roughly one and a half square miles. It was just eight miles from Limay and General Hospital No. 1. This location had been scouted months earlier by Major Harold Glattly, now Luzon Force surgeon. He felt it ideal for proximity to a medical supply depot that had been placed in a mango grove less than a mile away, just off the coastal road. Ordinarily, the Real River—a swiftly moving stream of clear, cool water—would seem idyllic. But on Bataan, it was also a perfect breeding ground for *Anopheles* mosquitoes. Still, the river, about twelve to fifteen feet wide, served as the primary source of water for drinking, bathing, and cooking. Glattly's site was heavily wooded, covered with bamboo and various trees and vines, providing excellent concealment from the air. In fact, the isolation was so complete that there were no roads leading to it, only one narrow carabao trail. Engineers quickly bulldozed a path connecting to the National Highway, a kilometer to the south.[10]

Trees were selectively felled, with care taken not to disrupt the protective canopy above. Stumps and underbrush were cleared, mostly by hand, Filipino laborers swinging their long *bolos*, carving out spaces for soon to be hospital wards. No enclosed units here; all patient areas were exposed to the elements. Wards were designated and numbered by signs nailed to trees, and they contained a spread of iron beds or wobbly cots under shielding copses. With over a square mile of hospital grounds, cots stretched as far as the eye could see. Staff quarters became a patchwork of hanging sheets, ponchos, and tent canvas with no rhyme or reason. Personal items and clothing were either stashed under cots or hung from branches, with scenes resembling shanty towns from the Depression—

hobo camps, they were called. Sometimes animals wandered in: wild pigs, monkeys, rats, carabao, and the ever-present geckos.[11] Shelter halves, which were standard issue to troops, were scavenged for some cover for the patients but never matched the need. By April, only three thousand were in use, not nearly enough for the huge numbers of patients crowding in. Downpours could spell disaster, but fortunately, only one light shower occurred during the entire service of the camp in January, February, March, and April. Perhaps at first bucolic, the setting had become a bizarre—and pitiful—outdoor dormitory by April. Of her first days there, nurse Straub wrote in her diary: "This is a place of another world. The only covering is the sky. It is jungle land and everyone lives under the trees. . . . It is eerie and fantastic. I found a cot, no mattress, beside a brook, but not far from the latrine. Can look up from my cot and watch the moon and stars."[12]

On December 30, Colonel Carlton Vanderboget, former chief surgeon at Fort Stotsenberg and, following the outbreak of war, surgeon of field forces, was sent to General Hospital No. 2 as commanding officer, a post he held until the end of February. It was his job to make the camp accessible and operational. The first order of business was accessibility. By January 1, engineers had cleared and leveled a passable road so ambulances could skirt into the compound with relative ease.

In contrast to the open wards, surgery spaces at General Hospital No. 2 were enclosed. Overflow from General Hospital No. 1 was almost certain, and surgical services at General Hospital No. 2 were essential. More room was hacked out of the jungle, and within six days there stood an operating tent—basically a ward tent on a wooden frame—with two operating tables (a second tent was put up within days to handle four more operating tables). At first, a receiving tent was set up at the end of that one-lane road, right next to the operating tent. Patients were brought there by ambulance, evaluated, and triaged. Those needing surgery were taken a short distance to the operating area—those, that is, without signs of gangrene. Gangrenous cases were housed in a separate tent a distance from the main operating suite. This ward was the place for putrefied flesh—the place for slicing and carving and amputations to somehow stay ahead of bullae and crepitance and creeping rot. These cases were identified on admission in a selection process casting them to the realm of the quarantined, the "unclean."

One of the characters under Vanderboget's command was Lieutenant Colonel William "Uncle Willie" North. North had been put in charge

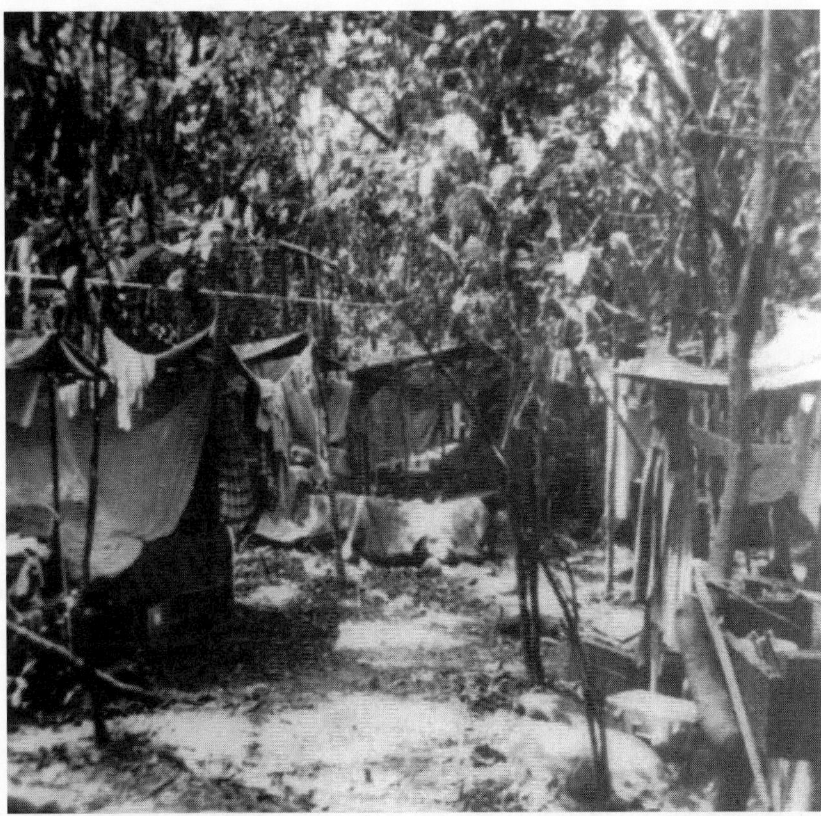

Outdoor ward of General Hospital No. 2, Bataan Peninsula. (*Courtesy of American Defenders of Bataan and Corregidor*)

of the receiving areas. As intrepid as they come, Uncle Willie knew the importance of stashing medical supplies. Manila would soon be cut off, he surmised. Without notice, he was off to the city on December 29, careening through throngs heading the other way, dodging occasional Japanese air sorties. That foray brought back four truckloads of supplies from the Medical Depot. A second trip on December 30 was more hazardous—the two trucks sent were bombed going and coming, but North arrived untarnished at the hospital with loads of surgical supplies from Sternberg: ten thousand blankets and sheets, three thousand five hundred beds and mattresses, pajamas, pillows, and all the creature comforts for sick men. Not stopping there, Uncle Willie found a much needed sterilizer, essential for a surgical unit, at Fort Stotsenberg in a last-minute raid through territory by then thick with enemy. He himself drove the deuce-and-a-half through country roads way too fast for his own good, sterilizer in hand.[13]

Eventually, because of traffic, dust, and noise, a new, larger operating pavilion that could hold several operating tables was built off to the side of the hospital site beneath several towering trees for concealment. Engineers constructed a building of wood with a tin roof forty feet by twenty feet. At first three operating tables were set up for all types of surgery, including a skeletal table for orthopedics. All surgical supplies, sterilizers, and radiology equipment were stored there. On December 30, Colonel Vanderboget arrived and took command. General Hospital No. 2 opened its doors the following day. On New Year's Day, 150 patients arrived, evacuated from the hospital at the Philippine Women's University in Manila. Colonel Cooper, now on Corregidor, sent Colonel Gillespie, former chief of medicine at Sternberg, on an inspection tour of the two general hospitals set up on the Bataan Peninsula. Gillespie arrived at General Hospital No. 2 on January 3 and was quickly impressed. Eight hundred patients were already housed and bedded. Electric lights were functioning in the operating rooms and staff offices, and the field water purification unit held a full four-thousand-gallon reservoir, diverted from the Real River. A pharmacy and medical supply depot were operating smoothly and, for the time being, all beds were covered with shelter halves and mosquito netting. "Morale was excellent," Gillespie added.[14]

Dr. Gillespie had been in the Philippines for almost seventeen months. His appointment as chief of medicine at Sternberg General Hospital was intended to be a Pacific adventure for his wife, Ila, and children, James and Ronald. Like other medical officers and their families, they had enjoyed a lavish tropical life in and around Manila, occupying a spacious, two-story home overlooking Manila Bay in the suburb of Paranaque near Nichols Airfield. Cooks, houseboys, and washing girls were de rigueur, so easy to procure and afford in Manila, and the Gillespies had all of them. The family traveled widely, visiting sites around Luzon and even making forays to other islands such as Cebu, Negros, and Mindanao. Gillespie's professional interest was infectious diseases, particularly those of the tropics: malaria, dengue fever, dysentery, leprosy, amebiasis, and the common worm infestations. However, their adventure came to an end in May 1941. Like other military dependents, Ila Gillespie and the children departed for home, evacuated because of the heightening tension between Japan and the United States.

Nevertheless, that morning of December 8 caught Gillespie by surprise. "What a sickening feeling in the pit of my stomach," he recalled. His first duty was to empty Sternberg of all but the most seriously ill patients to make room for casualties sure to come.[15] After the evacuation of Manila, Colonel Gillespie was sent to Corregidor, where he was responsible for overseeing development of Bataan's medical depot and the workings of both general hospitals. On his first visit to General Hospital No. 2, he was struck by the idyllic yet primeval scenery. A tropical paradise it was not. The place seethed with *Anopheles* mosquitoes and malaria. His soldiers would be in an area of "high malarial endemicity," almost certain to be infected. In contrast, when he visited General Hospital No. 1, he found "a radically different situation . . . very adequate surgery, bakery, mess halls, laundry, latrines . . . all the equipment was new, having been just unpacked." Next were as many field units as he could get to, considering unfriendly terrain and enemy movements. What bothered him most was the undisciplined rush of refugees into Bataan, mind boggling on the scale he witnessed. Besides the seventy-eight thousand military and six thousand civilian employees, incalculable numbers of destitute exiles tagged along—many times that anticipated by war plan Orange. All depended on the military—especially for foodstuffs—to subsist. All had to be housed, fed, and treated—an impossible task considering the dwindling supplies of food, shelter, and medicines, and considering the close, untamed tangle of the Bataan interior. The possibility of malarial outbreaks posed an even bleaker picture. Unless relief came from across the Pacific, Gillespie knew their situation on Bataan was untenable.

For surgical teams—there would be five in all—headed by Major Jack Schwartz, the first serious casualty arrived January 5. Colonel Eddie Mock had suffered shrapnel wounds to his left chest and abdomen. A tense, tight belly foretold heavy bleeding. He was quickly taken to the new operating room, where Schwartz opened him up to find blood welling from a lacerated liver. The fractured liver was packed and compressed to stop the bleeding. Suture after suture dug into flimsy tissue finally curbed the hemorrhage. Colonel Mock made an uneventful recovery. But their first death came soon afterward, the body buried in a nearby rice paddy. There would be no caskets on Bataan; the dead were covered—barely—by a layer of damp earth, incompletely expunging smells of decomposition. Before long, surgery was almost an assembly-line production. As soon as one patient was finished, another was brought in, moved to the table, swabbed with antiseptic, and anesthetized. Work began again. Sometimes there was such determination to keep up with the flow of cases that nurses stepped in to stop surgeons from cutting. The Novocain had not yet taken hold, and the screaming from patients was too much to stand. With the feverish activity, surgical supplies were constantly running short. Rubber gloves, rectal tubes, and urinary catheters were cleaned and reused. Major Schwartz himself made frequent expeditions to scavenge equipment from General Hospital No. 1. Still, some provisions were almost nonexistent. Colostomy bags—essential for colon injuries—and tracheostomy sets became sought-after items.[16]

Sanitation was a parallel issue. Crowding in soon were Filipino refugees fleeing to Bataan to escape the Japanese. The peninsula eventually had almost twenty-five thousand Filipinos by some estimates.[17] Most of the civilians had little familiarity with basic sanitation. Even some Filipino military were poorly versed in field hygiene. The digging of open-pit latrines—slit trenches—was taught, but tilling below four feet in the sandy loam of Bataan broke the water table, and trenches quickly flooded. Burning human waste became impractical, and soon makeshift toilets were nothing but breeding grounds for flies that carried minute excrement—the microbes of dysentery—to anyone around. *Shigella* and *E. coli* found new homes in the food lines and mess kits and bread and rice and meat. Flies were so thick that people ate with one hand while sweeping them away with the other. It was not until the arrival of Major Wilbur Berry, a South Dakota native and son of a physician, that any change occurred. He had been assigned to Sternberg and took on the role of a sanitary medical officer. His single achievement on Bataan at General Hospital No. 2 was to convert the open-trench latrines into wooden, box toilets with removable seats that closed off the contents between usages. This simple measure effectively curtailed the accumulation of flies and spread of bacillary dysentery. The plague of diarrhea subsided—at least for a while.[18]

Proximity to nearby military installations posed a constant threat. The Cabcaben airfield, less than a mile away, was home to the few P-40s that were still operational and a frequent target for Japanese raids. Antiaircraft fire directed overhead sent flak fragments falling within hospital grounds, as deadly as direct artillery fire. On January 14, while relaxing in his bed, twenty-three-year-old Private Frank Pigg from Beatrice, Nebraska, was struck by a dud antiaircraft shell launched at Japanese planes. The shell landed midchest, passed clean through, and buried itself in the ground below his cot. He died instantly, his midsection nothing but a bloody hole. On February 13, an incendiary bombing raid killed forty-four Filipino civilians and wounded an equal number who were under treatment in the hospital. Another death occurred February 17 when a civilian employee was struck and killed by a falling piece of antiaircraft flak. Collateral damage spared no one. A ten-year-old Filipino boy had both feet shattered from a phosphorus fragment, tissue still burning when he was found.[19]

LIEUTENANT HIBBS HAD FOLLOWED HIS DOUGHBOYS, the 2nd Battalion, into battle at Layac Junction on January 6, his first taste of combat. Elements of the 31st Regiment, positioned to intercept Japanese columns marching down Route 110—more commonly referred to as the East Road—into Bataan, were to delay enemy advances and buy time for repositioning of Allied units farther south.[20] American and Filipino forces opened up on the marching Japanese with their short-range, 75-mm howitzers. The Japanese, with unencumbered aerial reconnaissance, answered with sleek, split-tail, 10-cm cannon spitting fire out of range of the Allied field guns, exacting brutal retribution. With pinpoint precision, they dropped rounds right on top of Allied gunners. What high explosives did not do, raging grass fires did, driving artillerymen from their positions and torching their World War I-era field pieces. There was nothing the Allies could do to answer back; longer-range 155-mm howitzers had been placed too far in the rear to be useful. Soon the enemy barrage turned on Allied infantry, the noise and flying debris unnerving many virgin Allied soldiers. Infantry attacks shortly followed—charging, bayonet-wielding fanatical troops—and it was only the bravery and fortitude of American and Filipino troops that prevented a complete rout. Lines held, but under cover of darkness all units successfully pulled back down the East Road to their new defenses. Hibbs saw the withdrawal as a "tragic and painful sight of men and equipment clogging the road."[21] Layac Junction proved to be a very costly delaying move. Fortunately, his team was able to carry their footlockers of bandages, splints, medicines, syringes, and needles out with them. Injured soldiers discarded by the roadside still needed first aid. Hibbs's 2nd Battalion was assigned a position on the outskirts of a little town named Abucay farther south.

It was a day Lieutenant Hibbs would not soon forget. A valuable lesson in battlefield medicine had registered. "There were two things to do," he wrote later, "tell the soldier he was not going to die . . . and secondly, ease his pain." His most useful of meager medical supplies was the morphine syrette, a slug of one-half grain (32 mg) of morphine tartrate shot via hypodermic needle into any body part available, an arm or thigh, just under the skin. Within half a minute, the pain-relieving and sedative effects were impressive. The danger was respiratory depression, particularly with repeated injections. But its narcosis swept away pain—and anxiety. After the battle, when sound and fury had subsided, "a profound exhaustion" came over him. Outpourings of primal fight or flight hormones had sapped all energy. In fact, he spent more time clutching the earth than doctoring—at least in his mind. "I personally had done nothing except to panic in my foxhole, cowering like a rat burdened with the helplessness of our situation." In reality, his only mistake was locating the aid station too close to artillery. Enemy shells fell with irrational violence. The explosions were deafening—a white noise that drove out all other sounds. And the concussive effects of blasts literally knocked the wind out of you. Soldiers thought of nothing but an immediate need to breathe. Even more than rifle fire, artillery overpowered men physically and mentally. Those stupendous barrages of the First World War brought about a twitching, weeping, paralyzing terror called shell shock. Troops never knew where the next shell would hit but understood their deadly effects, wiping out men only feet away. Survival became an irrational uncertainty. This was what rattled Hibbs and his men. But they were lucky. His team suffered only three "light" shrapnel injuries and one nonvenomous snakebite. However, all acquired "a fundamental dislike for artillery barrages."[22]

The Japanese did not pursue but plodded down the East Road and found the Allied front—the so-called Main Line of Resistance—by dawn January 8. There, two armies bristled for a decisive engagement. General Akira Nara, one of General Homma's most trusted commanders, was given the simple order "destroy the enemy."[23] On January 9, a thunderous artillery barrage signaled the opening of their offensive against II Corps. Infantry attacks followed, breaching American-Filipino lines and forcing commitment of all reserve units to barely forestall a rout. That evening a banzai charge by wild-eyed Japanese troops pushed hard on Allied lines, with wave after wave of enemy soldiers throwing themselves on barbed-wire entanglements as human bridges, pressing on despite frightfully effective, point-blank cannister fire. Singing volleys burst among their ranks, fracturing bodies like ripe watermelons. Yet they kept com-

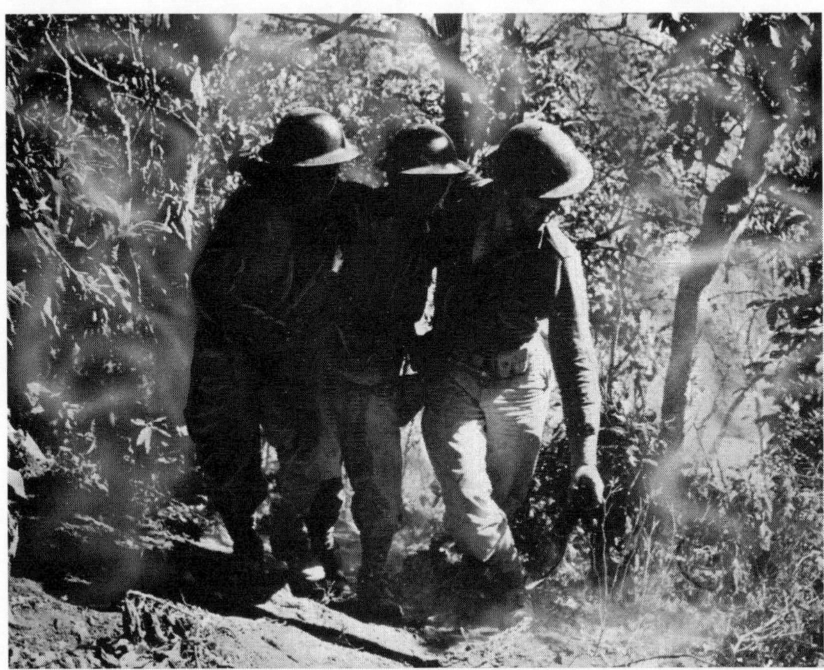

A Filipino soldier injured in the fighting on Bataan, being brought back to a first aid station. (*Library of Congress*)

ing. Allied infantry wavered but held, and the night and next day were filled with attack and counterattack in both I and II Corps, often in bloody, hand-to-hand combat. General Homma was surprised at the tenacity of the Allied resistance yet managed to send a terse message to General MacArthur on January 10: "You are well aware that you are doomed. The end is near. . . . The question is how long you will be able to resist . . . you are advised to surrender. . . . Our offensive will be continued with inexorable force which will bring upon you only disaster."[24]

Prophetic, perhaps, but premature. MacArthur declined to respond. He let his cannon in II Corps answer. True to his word, Homma fired his own cannon tubes until they glowed and ordered his legions forward.

The Main Line of Resistance for the Bataan defenders extended from Mabatang just north of the town of Abucay on the bay across Mount Natib to Mauban on the west coast, a line that extended about twenty miles up and over the mountain. The front of II Corps was held by the 57th Infantry on the east, the untried 41st Philippine Division in the middle, and the 51st Philippine Division on the west. Near Abucay was a large plantation, the Abucay Hacienda, expanding up the gentle slopes of Mount Natib. Terrain was reasonably flat, however, allowing for maneuvering of infantry and armor units. The plantation was partially wooded but also contained fields of rice and sugarcane. As the ground rose toward the mountain, the landscape became decidely more rugged, wooded, and covered with cogan grass, mango groves, and more sugarcane fields. Here scouts, bearing the brunt of the enemy onslaught, leveled their Springfields and Garands and Brownings and cut into ranks of screaming banzai troops, only to find them replaced with others, equally fanatical. By Sunday, January 11, rabid assaults had pushed back the scouts, forcing them across the Calaguiman River several kilometers north of Abucay to the banks of the Balantay River. Casualties were dragged from the battlefield and somehow made their way back to the aid station located in a quiet *convento* (convent) next to a majestic, sixteenth-century Spanish church in Abucay. On the scouts' left flank, the 41st Infantry's medical battalion put its casualty-collecting area and aid station even farther back. Another stone church in the town of Balanga had been commandeered and the Provincial Hospital taken over. At both stations, ambulances loaded up and drove all but those with the most minor of wounds back to the general hospitals at Limay and Cabcaben; speed was of the essence for the critically wounded.

Relentless Japanese attacks pounded Allied lines. Weary elements of the 51st Division began to crumble and give way, bowing back the left flank of II Corps. Some Filipino troops, undone by Japanese savagery, simply turned and ran, leaving gaps between I and II Corps in what was already a thinly held skirmish line. As Allied lines faltered, distances from the front shrank for medical units, and concerns for safety magnified. The 31st Infantry, ensconced in a fallback line to the south, hurriedly mobilized to plug a major leak near the hacienda. On Saturday, January 17, it clashed head on with advancing Japanese. The bucolic setting was shattered by booming artillery. Caught in the open, Hibbs, heeding previous experience, put his aid station in a shielded mango grove along a footpath east of the hacienda. There he quickly learned another combat lesson: trees and artillery shells do not mix. High branches detonated falling rounds, showering the area with shrapnel and wooden shards and forcing his unit out of the grove and onto exposed ground—that damned artillery yet again a dark cloud hounding him. Now, in the open, there was little semblance of shelter, and the skirmish line was painfully close.

Major Calvin Jackson had also been part of Headquarters Company of the 12th Medical Battalion. He was a thirty-seven-year-old native of Mercer County, Ohio, educated at Ohio Northern University and then medical school at Ohio State University. He had completed an internship and one year of surgical residency at the medical center there and began a practice in Kenton. It wasn't long before active duty called, and he left from Fort Mason, San Francisco, aboard the SS *President Cleveland* bound for Manila. In late August 1941, he walked onto the dock in Manila and received his orders for Fort McKinley. He and Paul Ashton became fast friends, dining at the Army Navy Club, swimming in the bay, renting *bancas*, the Philippine outrigger, for lazy afternoon sails. Like many medical officers of the 12th Med, he was assigned to Philippine Army divisions—his was the 51st Division. As an advisor, he was there to bolster medical capabilities and train Filipino medics. But like other advisors, Jackson found supplies meager, motivation erratic, and ambulances scarce. With evacuation from Manila, he landed in II Corps, somewhere behind the Abucay front. There he spent his thirty-eighth birthday supervising the transport of wounded to Limay. It was no easy task. Footpaths were few and hardly passable, being jammed with traffic. Getting wounded out was torment—slow litter carries, maybe now and then an available ambulance, and always running a gauntlet of enemy artillery. With intensifying combat—Japanese inching perilously close—his Filipino medics were not inclined to stay. In one particularly hot sector, an entire litter company bugged out—gone—leaving him alone with two wounded and one dead soldier. A hail of automatic fire overhead flattened him to the ground. Spotted motionless by Filipino soldiers, he was reported "killed in action." Jackson somehow managed to collect himself, pull the wounded with him, and make it back to headquarters. There he thoroughly spooked his friend Colonel John Boatwright of the 53rd Infantry. "My God he's walking in," said the startled commander, who had just been notified of his demise. Nights were no less "hellish." Constant cannonading kept everyone awake, and shrapnel shredded anything in its way. Jackson took one in his chest on January 18 while getting into one of his ambulances. "I guess I blacked out," he remembered, and woke up catawampus half in and half out of the ambulance. Bloodied but intact, he roused himself and "got the hell out of there."[25]

It was near Abucay that fellow battalion surgeon Captain Jim Brennan distinguished himself. A fragment, maybe from one of those 150-mm howitzers (each shell weighed seventy pounds) caught M Company commander Captain Tom Bell in the left leg, slicing through and amputating it at midthigh. The liberated femoral artery sprang open like a firehose until Brennan, frantic to find the end, finally pinched it off with his fingers and with the other hand fumbled in his first-aid pack until he found a hemostat to clamp off the artery. There was nothing sterile about this action—the wound was coated in fertilized soil—but Brennan's efforts were life saving. An army reservist, Brennan, who had attended Creighton University in Omaha, Nebraska, had only a year of a surgical internship under his belt when he was called up to active duty. Nothing singled him out as particularly brave or adventurous; he was just an ordinary medical officer wanting to do his job—a formidable task this time. Brennan faced a wound the texture of raw hamburger, the air buzzing with ordnance and pungent with explosives. Laser focus was the key. Tune out all else for the sake of stanching the bleeding. To fail at that would cost a life. Yes, he had done a good thing.

It was here also in a green sea of waving cogon grass that Lieutenant Hibbs lost his first team member, hit in the chest by a sniper's bullet. One would likely remember that, the first personal death—details kept alive by a memory that would surely want to forget. Blood poured out—way too much. Others in the detachment picked him up, still alive and still bleeding, and carried him back until they found an ambulance. Hibbs soon knew the blank stares and pallid color of those about to die. And so it was for his comrade. Sometime during that Philippine night he passed away.

Gentle slopes around the hacienda roared with gunfire, leveling grasslands and humans without distinction. Hibbs finally found a location for his aid station—in a ravine that also held the 31st Infantry's command post. Good place for an aid station, he reckoned. Skirmishing just to the front had turned vicious. Soldiers fell with regularity, and litter teams braved intense automatic fire to retrieve slumped battlefield forms. Peering over the edge of the embankment, Hibbs was so close to the front that he could hear the cries of Japanese after each mortar explosion. Before long his aid station was filled with casualties. Yet there was so little he could do: treat shock by controlling hemorrhage—hemostats, pressure dressings—relieve pain, get the patients out. There was no blood, no intravenous saline. And Hibbs would wonder: did the army really need to have doctors on the front lines? Surely corpsmen could do just as good a job. It was merely a morale booster, he concluded. Physician presence comforted the combat soldier, much like ancient soothsayers.[26]

And evacuation posed real risk for his litter bearers: a slow carry across open meadows in the face of enemy fire, four men hunched over, each assigned a corner of a stretcher. And then another corpsman went down, struck in the head by a bullet—killed instantly, the man he was helping along uninjured but splattered with blood and brain. These were simple feats of heroism, selfless efforts to bring wounded to safety. Medics were more exposed than infantry, out in the open. Prime targets.

At collecting points across the front, casualties were again inspected. Triage was straightforward: no chest or belly wound and able to walk—head for the rear tagged with medication given and wounds cataloged; more serious chest or belly cases were littered out, sometimes by two bamboo poles tied together with vines and covered with a blanket, one end dragging on the ground, the other secured to a calesa pony, just like Native American travois. Lucky ones found an ambulance, were tossed in, and began a worried journey back. Moving vehicles were prey for roving Japanese aircraft or bands of renegade enemy who had slipped through Allied lines.

What would be known as the First Battle of Bataan—clashes around Abucay Hacienda—continued for several days. Hibbs's 31st Infantry and attached units of Filipino troops assaulted and were repulsed and assaulted again. Each side was equally determined; it was a seesaw engagement of dug in and determined Americans and Filipinos battling a zealous enemy. But blanketing Japanese howitzer fire and total aerial domination bent the left flank of Allied forces. There, embattled Filipino troops began falling back and turning in, endangering all of II Corps. Once again gaps opened and Japanese troops spilled through. By January 22, MacArthur, from his Corregidor command post, surmised that further efforts to hold might catch his forces surrounded. The Japanese were already in the Allied rear, sniping at unsuspecting Filipino troops. He and his staff began working on contingency plans to move the Main Line of Resistance farther south in an effort to pull together disjointed units and consolidate his military capital. Meanwhile, Arisaka long rifles and Nambu machine guns bit into the Allies, racking up alarming numbers of wounded who tumbled into General Hospitals No. 1 and No. 2 in record numbers. At No. 1 on January 16 alone, 187 major surgical procedures were performed, the eight operating tables and one orthopedic table rarely unoccupied. Hospital beds were kept full, even with the evacuation policy to General Hospital No. 2. By the end of January, General Hospital No. 2 housed 2,160 patients filling fourteen of its open-air wards. Six hundred eighty-two of these had come directly from General Hospital No. 1 in a single night. Herculean efforts were needed to keep beds open at both hospitals. And the Japanese pressure on American and Filipino troops was bringing the action disturbingly close to General Hospital No. 1, now coming within range of Japanese cannon.

Meanwhile the horrors of war multiplied. Lieutenant Ashton came face-to-face with them. A battalion of the 23rd Infantry of the Philippine Army was caught in the open by Japanese air and artillery near the Abucay front. "The terrible sight of a bomb-plowed field, covered with dead and fragmented bodies, interspersed with horribly wounded, screaming men, haunts me still," he later wrote. Ashton and his men unloaded their medical chest and began giving first aid—tourniquets, pressure dressings, morphine injections—and sent many off to the collecting station at the Abucay church. They dragged others to positions of cover from the sun and enemy fire and did what they could. Eventually those who were movable were carried away, over fifty in all, he estimated. The dead, many unidentifiable, were simply buried almost where they fell. "The stench of the dead Nips was overpowering," he recalled—no doubt intermingled with Allied dead. Corpsmen were left with the "improbables" for comfort care—there was just no room in the ambulances for any who might die on the way. Few of those left behind survived until morning.[27]

And on this same battlefield, as MacArthur had feared, Americans of the 31st Infantry began to weaken. The Japanese were pushing hard on their front, and lines were beginning to sag. Troops took an awful beating from mortars and artillery, and their numbers were cut down with small-arms fire. The wounded who clustered in that stone Abucay church were a sorry lot. The boisterous, confident crowd who launched into battle weeks before were now sullen, depressed, dirty, sweaty, and drained, Ashton observed. With meager diets of mostly sugar cane and constant enemy harassment—artillery and air raids during the day, infiltration and stealthy killing at night—soldiers were worn, defeated, and scared. Suffering days of continuous combat, they had now been forced to reduce their diet by half, to about two thousand calories per day. In normal combat, with the physical strain of crawling, sprinting, and diving for cover, all in stifling heat, and the tremendous catecholamine outpouring of fight or flight, a soldier might consume four thousand calories in one day. There was simply not enough food stockpiled on the Bataan Peninsula to feed over eighty thousand troops and civilians at that level. Maddeningly, much food and supplies that had been left in Manila or in depots around Luzon fell into civilian or enemy hands. Some incidents were unfathomable. Two thousand cases of canned fish and corned beef was left at Tarlac and demolished as part of a retreating Allied scorched earth policy. The quartermaster was forbidden by MacArthur's headquarters to move it. From now on, enough to eat would be a constant concern of the fighting man.

Captain William Donovan, assigned to Fort McKinley before December 8, had been briefly transferred to Sternberg General Hospital with the onset of war and then ordered to join the 2nd Battalion of the 45th Infantry, one of the regiments of Philippine scouts. His men were crack troops led by American officers, an elite outfit. The 2nd Battalion was moved to General Wainwright's I Corps, occupying the western half of Bataan, the rugged coastal areas around Bagac. They, like other battalions of the scouts, were to be held in reserve. In mid-January, as the battle around Abucay Hacienda raged, the regiment was ordered to move over to Bani, in II Corps sector. The Japanese were threatening a breakthrough. Here terrain was especially brutal, deep gorges covered by dense jungle—nearly impenetrable vegetation of brush, plants, and entwining vines. An organized defense was almost impossible; security would be maintained by frequent foot patrols. In moving to II Corps, Donovan's medical detachment somehow separated from its parent unit and was lost in the chartless wilderness of Bataan. They ran into men of the 3rd Battalion, so they set up their aid station with them.

Here it was jungle warfare: hot, dense, primitive. Tall cane and bamboo, hardwood trees seventy feet tall, and innumerable vines and creepers limited visibility to maybe ten yards. Roaming groups of enemy could be anywhere, not seen until the last moment. Then came sharp clashes—brutal firefights at short range. In between, when there was a chance to sleep, all slept on dank, bug-infested ground along with beetles, vermin, and snakes. Being a doctor, Donovan had the luxury of snatching a litter and using it for a bed, his leather sidearm belt a pillow. At work or rest, though, everyone had to be vigilant. Japanese sharpshooters were always a danger. Lashing themselves to tall trees, clad in black, supplied with a bag of rice, they stayed there for days waiting for an unsuspecting American or Filipino soldier to amble down a trail. One clean shot through the helmet—that Brodie "doughboy" helmet of World War I—was usually the result. Fighting in this maze was close and personal. Wounding came with a suddenness few expected, sometimes at the tip of a bayonet. Just after he arrived, Donovan saw forty-five men in quick succession. Most had bullet wounds, the weapons of choice being rifles and handguns. Grenades and mortars were too dangerous; tree trunks and tree branches were impediments that might prematurely trigger an explosion. Nights were particularly treacherous. Most men, after the cut in rations, became vitamin deficient, and, lacking vitamin A, blind in the total blackness of Bataan. Of course, triple canopies cut any light regardless—even moonlight. It was so bad that at one point, Donovan was summoned to care for a man who had been hit. In the dark, he crawled forward by feel, found the casualty, felt for a shoulder, then a head, and discovered there was no head, it had been shot away.[28] Jungles were horrid places, Donovan concluded. No country for sane men. Some days later, his battalion scrambled back into II Corps, almost civilization, to the south of Abucay, with the rest of his Philippine scout regiment.

Toward the end of January, American and Filipino lines had weakened and begun to buckle. As they sagged, General Hospital No. 1 was only six or seven miles from the battle and now well within reach of even short-range artillery—too close for safety. In fact, by January 23, the hospital was almost three miles closer to the front than one of the clearing companies serving it. Colonel Duckworth decided to move to a new location, half way between Cabcaben and Mariveles near the tip of the Bataan Peninsula, twenty miles from Limay. The hospital would be just down the road from General Hospital No. 2, close enough for rapid movement of patients—postoperative patients from No. 1 to No. 2. The new No. 1 would be on a five-hundred-foot rise, conjuring images of the resort-like retreat of Baguio in northern Luzon. The new location, "Little Baguio," was a former campsite used by the 14th Engineer Regiment. There were three large wooden buildings roofed with strong, galvanized iron. One was used as the main operating room, measuring forty by forty feet and, unlike the wards, was totally enclosed. Two large, open-air garages, 30 by 120 feet and running parallel to each other, were made into six wards. A smaller operating room was set up to the rear of the camp for quarantined gas gangrene cases. The spaces could comfortably accommodate 250 patients, but the casualties soon filled those. Expansion would be needed—up instead of out. Triple decker bamboo beds were constructed in one of the wards, and the open space between the two garages was covered so that additional triple decker bunks could be placed there, expanding capacity to well over two thousand patients. By January 25, the hospital was open for business. Its primary role remained a surgical hospital. Doctors and nurses had accumulated vast experience. While at Limay, over one thousand two hundred battle casualties had undergone major surgery.[29]

What was lacking in all this wizardry was expertise in orthopedic trauma. None of General Hospital No. 1's surgeons had any specialized training in fixing bones or joints. Dr. Smith petitioned the commander of the 16th Naval District (overseeing the Philippine Islands), Vice Admiral Francis Rockwell on Corregidor, to release Lieutenant Edward Nelson. Dr. Nelson had a reputation as a highly skilled orthopedic surgeon but now was doing routine dispensary duties on "The Rock." Smith's request was granted. Nelson, a graduate of Johns Hopkins University, suddenly found himself in the sizzling jungle of Bataan plowing through crushed limbs, aligning fractures, fixing traction, and applying plaster. During lulls in the fighting, he found time to court and marry nurse Rita Palmer from New Hampshire, using a jade ring he had bought for his mother in Hong Kong. Nurses were ordinarily forbidden to marry, but now who cared? Everyone knew the situation was desperate. But she returned from the war a widow. Her husband, that talented thirty-six-year-old surgeon from Huntington, West Virginia, died a prisoner of war, trapped in the hold of a Japanese transport as it was torpedoed and sunk by American submarines.

Traffic shifted to Little Baguio without missing a beat. How could it not? The Japanese, their guns and planes, generated a roller coaster of casualties—some days only a few, many days scores. Four, five, or six operating tables were in constant use in sunlight, and even one or two throughout the night. Neglected, festering wounds were now seen more often. Delays in evacuation, lack of supplies, and sanitation issues contributed. Simple cleansing was improbable at the front, maybe a slapped-on field dressing if anything. Waiting for ambulances or litter teams could take hours, and circuitous routes back to general hospitals were an overnight adventure. Navy surgeon Carey Smith estimated that over 10 percent of the wounded showed signs of gas gangrene and a fraction of those full-blown *Clostridium* myositis.[30] To compound matters, non-battle-related admissions slowly multiplied. Malaria and dysentery were now epidemic. All were beginning to suffer the effects of privations and illness.

But morale was still high, Smith felt, fueled by battlefield successes and the prospect of imminent Allied relief from MacArthur's phantom reinforcements. Upbeat conversations spurred optimism. Journalist Sebastian Junger proposed a theory about the oppressed and besieged: they all become a "community of sufferers." The evolutionary clock is turned back thousands of years to a time when there was no survival outside of group survival. As one survivor of the siege of Sarajevo in the 1990s reported to him, "We were animals. It's insane—but that's basic human instinct, to help another human being who is sitting or standing or lying close to you."[31] Smith's optimistic reports on Bataan, however, may have been more groupspeak than individual conviction. While most hoped for rescue, clinging to rumors of "help on the way," at the same time they grew to acknowledge the improbability of that occurrence. "We knew it was only a matter of time," Smith wrote, belying his own positivity. At more cynical moments some felt they were part of a "sacrifice force" whose primary function was to delay Japanese occupation as long as possible. Yet a strong spirit of charity prevailed, all more concerned for the less fortunate than even their own miserable plight.[32]

5

Jungles of Despair

BY MID-JANUARY, AL WEINSTEIN KNEW THE HONEYMOON WAS OVER. At General Hospital No. 1, casualties were arriving with frightful regularity. There was an endless process of sterilization—operating gowns, linen, gauze, towels, and surgical instruments—to keep pace with incoming wounded. The surgical suite was primitive but functional. Spotlights were on stands rather than overhead. Between the eight operating tables were sawhorses of unequal height so that critically wounded men in shock could be positioned with elevated legs—the Trendelenburg position—to encourage blood from the lower limbs to flow to the heart. Surgical teams consisted of a surgeon, a nurse, and a medic. And the operating tables were never empty. Weinstein teamed up with his friend Frank Adamo. They were to focus on cases with brain, bladder, chest, or belly injuries. For all those men needing anesthesia and pain control, there were only two experienced anesthetists: one whom Weinstein admired and another "short, loud-mouthed, cocky, cigar-smoking wise guy" who detested being an anesthetist. This character had already tried his hand at surgery, apparently botching a number of complex cases and earning a reassignment to a frontline unit. Like a bad penny he was back, so thoroughly spooked by combat that he was willing to take any role to avoid field duty—a true "wash-out," as Weinstein called him. And so here he was, their new gas passer, but never at a loss for obnoxious behavior.[1]

Over the next inhuman weeks, lines of beaten and sick appeared as if ushered in by some demonic purveyor of misery: bleeding, shaking with malarial fever, weak, hungry, and helpless. The call to triage came all too often; sleep was a remote luxury. Of the wounded, some injuries were hopeless: head gouges with skull blown open, pinkish brain matter, like cottage cheese, rolling out; faces split open by machine-gun bursts; smashed legs—muscle, skin, and skeletal pieces one unrecognizable heap. A background sound in the operating room was the rasping of saws cutting through bone, freeing a patient from his mangled limb. Hours upon hours of tedious debridement, with scalpel and scissors paring away devitalized tissue, plucking out clothing, dirt, grass, metal, and bone chips from the raw depths of cavities ripped open by high explosives consumed their energy—and compassion. Before long, doctors moved through casualties mechanically, focusing only on legs and arms and bellies, the faces now indistinguishable; all were suffering a white noise that no longer could be heard. Instead, it was a search for survivability so that hours spent in surgery would account for something. Others, those glassy-eyed ones, were left to the chaplains. Minds numb with fatigue quickly filled with self-doubt. Did that leg really need to come off? Should I have taken more contused bowel? Why didn't I find that bleeder sooner, the poor guy bled to death while I fumbled. Nights became days and days became nights without the slightest notice.

As January came to a close, American and Filipino positions along their first defensive line—the Main Line of Resistance—all across the Abucay-Moron parallel, were no longer tenable. Pockets of enemy were now already in the rear, and guerrilla tactics—raids, sniping, nighttime throat slitting—had seized troops with fear and foreboding. Further breakthroughs by the Japanese would jeopardize the integrity of the entire defense and threaten encirclement. General MacArthur estimated that his losses had been exorbitant, perhaps over a third of his troops. Some divisions had lost "as high as sixty percent," he reported to the War Department.[2] The commander was sufficiently alarmed that he assigned the highest priority to his staff in developing alternate defensive positions, a place for his final stand. General Wainwright and his aides determined that consolidation of forces farther to the south, around the high point, Mount Samat, with thick jungle and deep gorges, would afford excellent observation over the entire corps' front and provide dense, almost impenetrable vegetation to retard enemy advances. To the east was flat terrain with excellent fields of fire—good defensive spots. During the nights of January 24 and 25, a general withdrawal commenced to the new position. It was called the Second Defense Position, a line

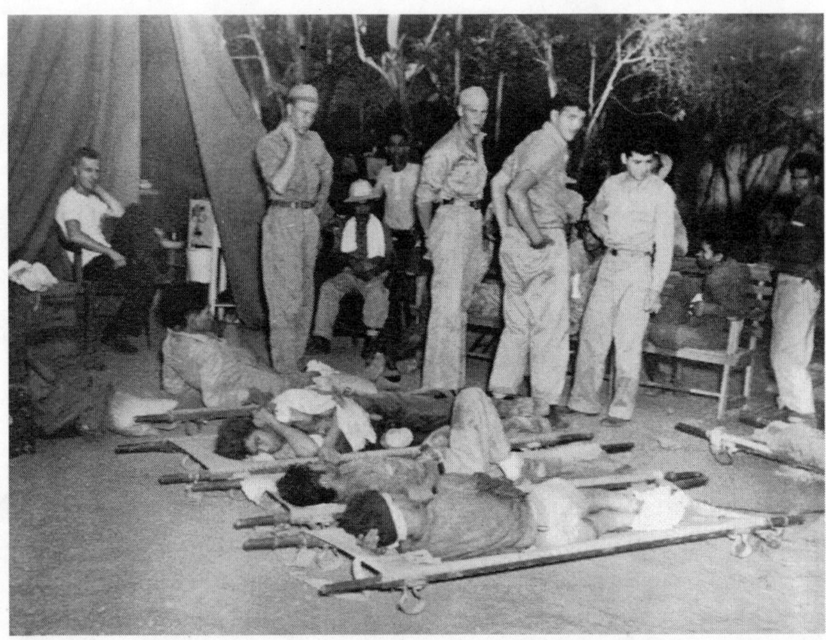

Aid station somewhere in Bataan. (*Courtesy of American Defenders of Bataan and Corregidor*)

roughly defined by the Bagac–Pilar–Orion road. The Allies dug in just south of this road, more or less traversing the saddle of Mount Samat and Mount Mariveles and connecting the West and East roads. At one thousand eight hundred feet, Mount Samat, an offshoot cone of Mount Mariveles, gave a commanding view of Bataan, Corregidor, and even Manila; it was a convenient lookout post.[3]

But it meant forfeiting a vital east-west passage. Movement of casualties was immensely more difficult, now confined to coastal trails, which, on the west side, were little more than winding footpaths. In between lay a luxuriant maze of forest, foliage, ravines, and rapidly flowing mountain streams providing unlimited concealment but also ideal breeding grounds for the *Anopheles* mosquito. In the interior of I Corps sector, which was devoid of walkable tracks, medical and surgical care would have to be done in clearing company hospitals—thick jungle made evacuation almost impossible. There was an old logging trail; known as Trail 17, it was barely passable. Here three medical units set up in hewn-out clearings; no better place could be found, but it was well within range of Japanese artillery. In the interior of II Corps, engineers bulldozed a primitive road along Trail 2 as far as the San Vicente River. Medical battalions from the 41st and 21st Divisions (Philippine Army) constructed four-hundred-bed field hospitals after clearing away underbrush and building bamboo frames on which to set patients. No tentage was available. To stave off the elements, dense, triple-canopy forest had to do. First-aid now meant surgery. Transport to the surgical hospitals, totally by hand carry, was slow, exasperating, and dangerous. Doctors with a modicum of surgical training were forced to intervene as best they could on the spot. Almost nothing could be done for abdominal or chest injuries, but on-site (usually out in the open) probing, cleaning, splinting, and suturing to preserve limbs and restore manpower were critical. But those with life-threatening conditions were not abandoned. Patients were bundled up and carried out, with little regard for the carriers' personal safety. Neither did this intrepidness escape notice. A letter of commendation on March 5 to the surgeons of the 21st and 41st Divisions from Brigadier General Maxon Lough, commander of the Philippine Division, read:

> Your officers and men are deserving of the highest praise and commendation for the speed and efficiency with which the wounded have been evacuated by hand litter over difficult trails and under fire from almost inaccessible areas of the Out Post Line. The work of the medical personnel accompanying patrols has been an exhibition of the highest courage and a major morale factor in the operation of these patrols.[4]

MacArthur's tactical withdrawal was supposed to be an orderly military repositioning, each battalion providing a shell force covering their retreat. All units were expected to be behind the new line of resistance by the morning of January 26. Tanks would cover all movements to the rear. In reality, it turned into a punishing exercise. Exhausted, poorly disciplined and trained troops staggered along like zombies, some so weak they were loaded onto buses for the trip to Orion.[5] With only one road available for traffic—the east coastal road—the scene quickly came to resemble a jammed up herd of human sheep. Colonel Ernest Miller, commander of the 194th Tank Battalion, tried to shepherd withdrawing troops along a single corridor out of the Abucay battlefield but found total disorganization and confusion: "The result was a continual milling, sweating mass of humanity. . . . It was impossible to do anything else but keep the mass moving to the rear—praying—hoping—talking . . . trying to make yourself understood. It was a nightmare while it lasted."[6] Had there been even rudimentary Japanese surveillance of this gridlock, Miller noted, an artillery barrage would have produced mass slaughter.

Captain Donovan's unit, the 45th Infantry, was ordered to pull back that night, but not before one of its collecting stations located in an old Balanga church was shelled by Japanese artillery. The barrage produced a number of casualties among patients already housed there and wounded an American medical officer. The injured—and newly reinjured—were rounded up and carried out to their fresh positions in II Corps, almost twenty-five kilometers away. In pitch black, Donovan and his fellow soldiers force marched on trails barely wide enough for one man to walk, ground that was so uneven and rugged that men needed extraordinary ingenuity just to keep stretchers level. It was back-breaking work, the toiling with heavy litters and the dead weight of casualties enough to exhaust even the sturdy—and there were few, if any, of those. Knowing the privations affecting everyone now, particularly lack of food, Colonel Wibb Cooper was amazed that his medics could muster that kind of effort: "I am of the opinion . . . that never in the history of warfare have men of the medical profession been required to carry out their duties under more trying and disheartening circumstances. In some instances the terrain was such that wounded men on stretchers would have to be lowered from the steep cliff of a deep ravine by ropes improvised from vines cut from the jungle and then carried by litter back to the only road that penetrated the area."[7]

Everywhere along the route, American officers were stupefied by the mob scene. Captain Calvin Jackson was disgusted by the behavior of troops the night of January 24. The entire spectacle was disorganized, even chaotic. "MacArthur says we are withdrawing to 'previously prepared appropriate positions.' I say we have been 'routed,'" he wrote in his diary. For his part, the trip was made in relative comfort aboard a big Buick sedan loaded with beer and good cheer. His new location would be in I Corps on the shores of the South China Sea with the 1st and 91st Philippine Divisions, but the same problems abounded. "The outfits are in a mess here too," he quickly concluded.[8] There were no more flatlands, either. "Terrain is nothing but almost straight up, sided gullies, some 50 feet deep." And no ambulances: all evacuations would be walking, hand carry, or not at all.

Soldiers in Hibbs's detachment joined in the withdrawal. Though it was hailed as a tactical success on paper, Hibbs, too, found it often a jumbled, disorganized crowd of scared, retreating soldiers. He saw many wounded lying in ditches along the way, so fatigued they simply dropped out of the "march" and collapsed. Some wounded were only identified by a pair of legs sticking out of the jungle. Hibbs himself had not bathed in two weeks or even had his shoes off for ten or eleven days. Men of the 194th Tank Battalion provided covering fire for the frazzled soldiers who looked to Hibbs like walking dead men. But the tankers kept the Japanese in check, deterred from shelling the human logjam and causing near genocide.

Lack of nourishment was beginning to tell. Emaciated soldiers were so hungry they chewed on stalks of sugarcane for the glucose and to quench nagging thirst. It was the only option. Many watering holes were full of decomposing human corpses, polluted, and clearly unsafe to drink. The standard staple was rice; sometimes oatmeal, and small measures of evaporated milk were added. Protein was at a premium. Hunting game to eat was as intense as hunting the enemy. Anything with four legs was edible—carabao, lizards, and wild boar were all shot, cooked, and eaten—and even snakes were fair game. In turn, the beloved horses and mules of the 26th Cavalry fell victim: butchered and consumed. Even those sources soon evaporated. Lack of protein slowly weakened the men. Hibbs himself dropped from 178 to 140 pounds just during the Hacienda battle. And so appeared the ravages of malnutrition: the swollen legs of kwashiokor and beriberi, skin hemorrhages, and night blindness. It had a pervasive effect, not only weakening the frame but also the spirit. Apathy, lethargy, and a sense of doom began to eat at morale. But what hunger also did was rid men of the fear of death, whether by artillery, gunfire, or bayonet. Those gnawing pangs for food left them embittered and miserable, as if death would be a welcome respite. "To hell with them," Hibbs said of his enemy. There were few delusions. He knew their time was limited; his only wish was that his executioner be an enlightened college graduate and not "a dumb, uneducated Jap."[9] And they were all around it seemed, infiltrating past the front lines, hiding, waiting until nighttime when unsuspecting soldiers, catching a few hours of sleep, would fall prey to an enemy armed only with a knife or bayonet, found the next morning in their foxholes, throats slit, eyes sightless. For the rest, the living, each morning was a sober awareness of another day of hunger and fighting and surviving: Saved for hunger and wounds and heat / For slow exhaustion and grim retreat / For a wasted hope and sure defeat. . . .[10]

And those mercy trips to get the wounded out were especially notable, considering the languor brought on by reduced rations, now at a daily level of one thousand calories or less. Muscle wasting was obvious, the masculine tone of young physiques morphing into a decidedly scrawny appearance. On the trails, impediments loomed even larger for men with strength a fraction of their youth. Boulders; thick, entangling vines; streams; precipitous drop-offs—four men to a litter hoisting, lowering, slipping, and stumbling—quickly consumed whatever stamina remained. The Luzon Force surgeon, Lieutenant Colonel Harold Glattly, had estimated that the nature of the terrain on the Bataan Peninsula required from three thousand five hundred to four thousand calories per man per day, far more than was being taken in at that point.[11] Pack animals were too unsteady in that terrain—a tumble would have been disasterous for a critically wounded soldier—and before long most animals were eaten anyway.[12] For those on foot, it often took up to three hours to transport patients from the front to the first collecting station and another hour before arrival at some type of field hospital where doctors could operate. By now medical stores were meager—anywhere. Even intravenous needles were sometimes lacking. Fluid for resuscitation was often by hypodermoclysis—injecting saline under the skin and allowing for slow absorption into the bloodstream—painfully medieval and unreliable. Sterilizers were not always available, and surgical instruments were wanting, in disrepair, or dirty. Those few patients with internal injuries—chest or abdomen—waited, their fate decided by time. The luckier ones were suffused with morphine and rendered oblivious to Providence.

UNBEKNOWNST TO AMERICAN OFFICERS, the Japanese had been stymied by their inability to break through the Main Defensive Line. Granted, some of their troops, actually an entire division, had penetrated in pockets of resistance behind the Allied front, but at the present rate, General Homma knew, complete destruction of enemy forces was unlikely. The conquest of Luzon was not on schedule and was far from over. It would take more men and more equipment. His troops were equally beleaguered, hungry, and ill. Their rations had also been cut, and supplies of quinine were exhausted. In short, they were in little better shape than their Filipino and American counterparts. And the Japanese command had trivial regard for the rank-and-file soldiers, often treating them no better than they would Filipino and American prisoners of war. Health and welfare had always been petty considerations, with officers as likely to slash rations as throw their men recklessly into battle. But there was now a price to pay in efficiency. Homma, after conferring with his staff, decided to break off engagement, withdraw to a more secure position, and humbly request reinforcements from Tokyo. More *ashigaru-sha*—"cannon fodder." He was confident that Bataan had been completely encircled and blockaded and that eventually the Americans and Filipinos would be starved into submission—their supply line nonexistent. But he knew the timetable was vital to the success of Japan's Pacific offensive, and he was not going to wait. Homma was not a man of patience. There would be a pause but no retreat. Americans and their Filipino peons would inevitably capitulate.[13]

Yet a relative calm characterized February and March. Homma's respite was misinterpreted. For the Allies, there was celebration, a fleeting hope of victory even. President Roosevelt, perhaps goaded by falsely optimistic reports from MacArthur, wrote: "Congratulations on the magnificent stand that you and your men are making. We are watching with pride and understanding and are thinking of you."[14]

Once troops realized the Japanese were disengaging, there was a feeling of jubilance. Some American officers even pushed to return to the offensive and recapture the Abucay line. Seasoned staff, however, were wiser, their optimism tempered with the reality that they were resting on borrowed time, that the Japanese would be back, reinforced and rejuvenated. All felt the choke of Japanese blockade and air supremacy. Allied military resources were scarce, and supplies—ammunition and food—were getting scarcer. Soldiers on the defense required less of each, and a smaller amount of territory would be easier to defend. Any ideas for the offense were scrapped. Yes, Homma was still there, just out of sight. Sporadic artillery shellings and air raids were reminders of that. In the meantime, loathe to attack, the belligerents faced each other across an expanse of no-man's land that served no better purpose than foraging by intrepid patrols from either side, hunger now as much a threat as the guns of opposing forces. And the noose around Bataan would tighten still, cutting off what scant supplies were getting through from the Visayas. Homma fortified the southern coast of Manila Bay to discourage friendly Filipinos from sending food across and directed his troops to occupy the island of Mindoro, just off the southern point of Batangas Province, a way station for blockade runners. Those desperate runs across the Sulu Sea, up the South China Sea, to Bataan and Corregidor became fewer and fewer. And there was little doubt that Japanese transports were churning toward Luzon, packed with fresh troops. The only hope was a rescuing force of American navy and army, promised by MacArthur, but skepticism was rife that they would ever appear.

After moving back to Little Baguio with General Hospital No. 1, Al Weinstein noticed that incoming casualties wore gaunt, apathetic expressions. They showed the strain of combat and the inadequacies of care near the front. Muscle wasting was apparent, movements were sluggish, many men were dehydrated. It was not uncommon to hear that some had lain in foxholes for days waiting to be evacuated, only to endure hours of litter carry up and down treacherous terrain and across swollen streams. Their uniforms were in tatters, they stank, and rancid, gray wounds were invariably infested with fat maggots. Even worse, the sweet sickly smell of gas gangrene accompanied some. Dead—"devitalized" was the term—tissue was fertile ground for anaerobic *Closridia* organisms, especially the species *Clostridium perfringens*, an inhabitant of soil contaminated by human excrement. Specialized wards were set up, the feeling was that the *Clostridia* organisms were highly contagious—at least they were resilient, their tiny endospores resistant to many usual hygiene measures, able to survive decades without nutrition, a constant danger in large aggregations of sick. Dormant but not dead, they waited for a new host, resplendent in his putrid wound.

Treatment was straightforward: removal of all devitalized tissue, even if that meant amputation. A surgeon's scalpel was indeed the cure. Gangrene had been almost epidemic on the western front in World War I, death rates skyrocketing. French soil, where much of the fighting was done, was rich in human fertilization and was a breeding ground for the bacteria—*gangrene gazeuse*, it was called by the French. Not until techniques of tissue debridement were introduced—removal of any skin, muscle, or bone that would not survive—was any effect on mortality realized.[15] So notorious was the bacillus that it deserved special comment by Major James Coupal of the Army Medical Department in 1929. He described gas gangrene as: "a spreading, moist gangrene produced by gas-forming anaerobic bacteria in extensively traumatized tissues. It is characterized by a gaseous infiltration and edema of the part affected, and by changes in the color and contractility of the muscle . . . the onset and course are generally rapid and accompanied by profound toxemia and high mortality."[16]

The wonder antibiotic penicillin, scarce as it was in 1942, was ineffective. In vitro, it could certainly kill *Clostridia* organisms, but, unable to penetrate tissue deprived of blood flow, it was useless in clinical settings—surgery was still the mainstay. Involvement of the torso, if the infection had progressed that far, was by definition a death sentence. Weinstein saw a number of these patients, the gas creeping steadily onward, too far advanced to consider separating living and dead tissue, and the dilemma was whether to tell the hopeless cases the truth. Most chose not to, reluctant to make the last few hours or days even more agonizing for the dying, preferring to let them slip away in an opiate haze, gripping hope like the sides of their cots. Better to "lead them to the grave," as some physicians believed, let the patient come to the realization that he was not going to make it, which many often did. But some, smiling at the thought of survival and return home—those comforting words from doctors and nurses—simply fell asleep in a nostalgic reverie and were soon dead.

Among the trapped garrisons, lack of provisions was beginning to tell. General Wainwright had noted that by March 1, the troops were barely getting a one-fourth ration. "By 1 March," he recorded, "serious muscle wasting was evident and by the latter part of March the combat efficiency was rapidly decreasing."[17] Colonel Wibb Cooper noted that one can of salmon served fourteen men—and even that was gone by the end of February—and each soldier received only nine ounces of rice per day.[18] Dr. Gillespie's predictions on food rationing and medical supplies were coming to fruition. The extreme stress of combat, dwindling nutrition, disease, and demoralization were hitting soldiers hard, all combining to sap strength, endurance, and tenacity. A lassitude descended on all: movements slowed, conversations subdued, physical exertion was brief, sleep was excessive. For the most part, joy left faces and was replaced by a sober countenance that spoke neither of hope nor disgrace. Each day had become its own challenge, and expressions were set merely to surmount its obstacles and survive to tomorrow.

On Bataan, lack of food magnified all ills. War plan Orange had stipulated supplies for forty-three thousand men for six months. MacArthur's switch to defending the beaches erased that. Much of the 2,295,000 pounds of salmon and 152,000 pounds of fruits and vegetables had been moved forward—and lost from the peninsula.[19] Unbelievably, provincial regulations prevented the transport of ten million pounds of rice from Cabanatuan to Bataan. In any event, the number of mouths to be fed had swelled to over one hundred thousand, far too many for the food at hand. By March 15, all meat on the hoof had been consumed: carabao, pack mules, and horses. Major Achille Tisdelle, aide to Brigadier General Edward King who was now the commanding officer for the Bataan Peninsula,[20] announced that the last of the 26th Cavalry horses were gone; a total of one thousand three hundred tons of meat in all had been slaughtered and eaten.[21] But even as early as January reduced rations—basically a semi-starvation diet—began to tell on front line troops. In the ranks of the 31st Infantry daily rations consisted of four ounces of rice and less than two ounces of salmon per man per day. Weight losses of twenty to thirty pounds were not uncommon, and vitamin deficiencies such as beriberi (B1, thiamine) began to appear. Leg edema was common, portending lack of protein and calories. Gillespie appealed to USAFFE Surgeon Colonel Wibb Cooper to allow increases in beef, vegetables, milk, and native fruits, but the Japanese stranglehold had tightened, and little was getting through from Corregidor. Foraging by American troops hadn't turned up much wild game, other than vermin and snakes. Rice became a main staple, and even that was rancid.

What did get through the blockades from Cebu was poor quality red rice, the kind their Japanese captors would wryly comment later was not even fit for a horse to eat. Surprisingly, some rice continued to be harvested. While the Bataan Peninsula consisted mostly of mountains and forests, what little agricultural area there was could be used. A small strip of land bordering Manila Bay around Abucay *Hacienda* hosted two rice mills at Balanga and Orion. Despite hazards of working the fields in wide-open country—Japanese flyovers were frequent—ten thousand *cavanes* of palay were gathered in by Filipino workers.[22] Once Balanga and Orion were abandoned, the rice mills were disassembled and moved to the quartermaster depot near Little Baguio. But giving up the flat, rice-growing areas around Abucay meant an end to rice harvesting.[23]

It was a replay of Victor Hugo's candid comments during the siege of Paris: "It is not even horsemeat that we are eating. Maybe is it dog flesh? Maybe is it rat? I now suffer from stomach ache. We are eating the unknown."[24] What canned meat, salmon, tomatoes, beans, and fruits could be found were given to patients. By the end of March, the staff made do with boiled rice and a thin, watery gravy, a consumption of less than one thousand calories per day. The Filipino soldier was a bit more adept than his American counterpart in foraging for food. Chickens, pigs, bamboo shoots, mangoes, and bananas were found, along with dog and monkey meat, even innards of the iguana lizard and python meat, the python eggs considered a rare delicacy to the natives. American troops never quite savored local fare as easily as Filipinos. Paul Ashton recalled one encounter with a Filipino unit and its innovative cook. Bat was roasted over an open fire, fur and all. It seemed that bats, in hanging upside down all night, urinate liberally on themselves. Cooking in their fur allowed the stink to burn off. Still, bat meat resembled chewing on erasers, a texture hardly conducive to ingesting large quantities. A favorite of Ashton's was rat meat, particularly when served with mongo beans. For others, mule meat was decent, pony tougher—all gone too soon—and monkey meat tolerable, as long as recognizable parts did not show up on the plate. After sampling the inedible, many returned to a staple of rancid rice. Hardly conducive to appetites, the air around campsites and chow lines was rich with the smells of war, particularly dead, rotting things, providing a sickening overture to their meager meals.[25]

The stench of dead Japanese in the surrounding jungle hung everywhere. So did the straddle trenches, inadequate for the growing number of dysentery-plagued men. Bloated green flies spread diseases. Bodies in the streams polluted the water.[26]

On March 2, Colonel Gillespie took over as commander of General Hospital No. 2. Dr. Vanderboget moved as commander at General Hospital No. 1, and Colonel Duckworth was sent to set up a convalescent facility at Iloilo in the Visayas. Both men narrowly escaped death in the process, Vanderboget injured during a bombing raid on General Hospital No. 1 on March 26 (two other medical officers with him were killed) and Duckworth avoiding shrapnel from a raid at Little Baguio on March 30. At the time of Gillespie's arrival at General Hospital No. 2, infectious diseases, particularly dysentery and malaria, were epidemic. Some improvements were made through the efforts of Major Berry and his wooden-lid privies. But malaria spread almost unabated. Bucolic streams bred *Anopheles* in droves, and the indigenous population, ravaged by the disease, supplied the *Plasmodia*. It affected all.

Quinine was the mainstay of treatment in the first half of the twentieth century. Jesuits missionaries in Peru in the seventeenth century discovered that the bark of the local cinchona tree,[27] called *quina-quina* by natives, was helpful in alleviating symptoms. That substance was eventually isolated as the alkaloid quinine and was found to be cytotoxic to *Plasmodium* parasites. Clinical trials in the 1860s found that over 98 percent of treated individuals ceased their febrile episodes, and quinine subsequently became the backbone of treatment. Side effects were substantial and often referred to as cinchonism: impaired hearing, headache, nausea, diarrhea, and vertigo. It was a poor prophylactic agent, however, effective only after the protozoa had entered the red blood cell and, therefore, after infection had occurred.

When supplies of quinine dwindled, more of the besieged garrison became symptomatic. Soon doctors and nurses were felled by the effects of the disease as often as their patients. Surgeons, in the middle of a case, would start shaking in the throes of a malarial chill. In the midst of routine ward care, a nurse might collapse in a faint from malarial fever. One nurse, Sally Blaine, racked with fevers, set up her cot in the middle of her ward and directed nurses from there. Another, Lucy Wilson, braced herself in the operating room so she could remain upright during cases.

Yet through it all, everyone paid due diligence to hygiene and sanitary measures. Nurses washed their patients, scrubbing off battlefield grime, blood, and waste, changing dressings, even laundering piles of soiled garments and sheets, aided by Chinese volunteers from Corregidor. Linen was washed in the Real River, boiled, and hung to dry in huge quantities, the laundry workforce eventually expanded to include Filipino volunteers. Because by March many patients admitted were already showing signs of nutritional deficiencies, one and a half rations were issued for each patient, usually rice, and whatever meat product could be found: carabao, horse, or mule. It did not last. Already in March, vegetables were not to be had and meat would soon be gone, and by April, fruit juices and canned milk had vanished as well.

In the field, "healthy" men were not in much better shape. In fact, March saw a noticeable deterioration in their health. Soldiers were thin, weak, and listless. Despite occasional peppy comments, morale was never so low. Dysentery, fevers from malaria, and lack of food all played into a feeling of doom. And a number of the men were so depleted they no longer could function. It was not uncommon to see cots and beds filled with soldiers too shaky to stand. Lieutenant Colonel Glattly, Luzon Force surgeon, estimated that at least three thousand patients were being cared for in these small encampments. Rations had dropped to one thousand calories or less per day—starvation levels. On March 10, the influx of malaria patients from the front at General Hospital No. 2 was so critical that Colonel Gillespie sent a memo to Colonel Cooper on Corregidor that read:

> Malaria is rapidly increasing. . . . The admission rate is alarming, 260 patients arriving March 9th. Most of these are medical and a large proportion have malaria. . . . Quinine prophylaxis having stopped we anticipate additional hundreds or even thousands of cases. . . . It is my candid and conservative opinion that if we do not secure a sufficient supply of quinine for our troops from front to rear that all other supplies we may get, with the exception of rations, will be of little or no value.[28]

And now the insidious enemies, not the Japanese but disease and starvation, crept into foxholes and mango groves and forests. They permeated the ranks of both armies, but replenishment was not an option for Americans and Filipinos. No, the bleeding of calories and protein and energy—and the bleeding of mosquitoes—was as sure a crippler as artillery shells, aerial bombs, and machine-gun bullets. Soon, malaria became the chief cause of admission to clearing stations. In March, nearly five hundred cases were arriving per day. At the front, estimated rates of infection exceeded 50 percent. In fact, the day before Gillespie sent his memo to Cooper, he and his adjutant, Lieutenant Colonel Maupin, both developed signs of malaria, confirmed in both men by a hefty load of parasites seen on blood films. Gillespie tried to "tough it out," confining himself to his cot for a few days. Quinine seemed to help, and within days he was back to a full schedule. Still, the slightest effort was exhausting. Fevers and hunger had sapped his strength.[29]

6

Flickering Forlorn Hope

THE FATE OF BATAAN'S GARRISON AND ITS IMPOVERISHED REFUGEES came into clearer focus by April. Tens of thousands of troops and civilians vied for livable space, all existing on meager rations, all in the throes of malnutrition and disease. At General Hospital No. 1, Ann Bernatitus noticed a change in new arrivals. Her patients appeared more disheveled: whiskered, scrawny, and ill-kempt. By the time they had moved to Little Baguio, wounded came in caked in dust and grime, covered in lice, and suffering neglected wounds. The sight of those pitiful cases who now swelled Bataan's hospitals evoked outright sympathy. Among the wounded, gas gangrene was rampant, and amputations were the order of the day. Medical supplies were in deplorable shortage. Soiled dressings, almost black with dried blood and dirt, were washed, sterilized, and used again. Malaria and dysentery affected most. Despite the best sanitary efforts, overcrowding and contaminated food—even lack of hand washing—led to the spread of enteric disorders. Among the many culprits, *Shigella* species of bacilli were notorious agents for gastroenteritis. Found in human excrement and contaminated water and food, the bacilli elaborate an enterotoxin, invade intestinal lining cells, producing voluminous, at times even bloody, diarrhea.[1] Brown, feculent expulsions stained the jungle floor with the slime and mucous of liquid stool. Cramping, uncontrollable urges laid victims low, causing dehydration and inanition. In extreme cases, the condition could be lethal.[2]

As equipment and medical supplies were consumed, care of the patients switched from technology to compassion. What surgery could be done was carried out under the assumption of sterility—no one was truly convinced asepsis was attainable. Bedside care—*caritas* the Greeks called it—took preeminence. Nurses spent their time sitting with their patients, holding their hands, wiping their brows, calming frayed nerves. Doctors did the same. There was little healing now, not in any medical sense. Concerns about wounds, internal damage, infections had become academic—there was nothing with which to treat them. And by now, few were healthy. Doctors, nurses, and medics were all affected, each struggling with cramps, hurried trots to relieve explosive bowels, shaking chills and burning fevers. What next, they all wondered. Surrender? What then? Imprisonment or worse? Immediate execution for the men? Repeated raping for the women? And their charges? Likely massacred where they lay, images of the Nanking atrocities fresh. Was it magical thinking that kept them going? That rescue was just a step away? That their country, as MacArthur had promised, would at the last minute, like some giant, benevolent Santa Claus, appear and wipe clean the battlefield of this relentless enemy?

John Bumgarner had moved from General Hospital No. 1 to No. 2 in early January. He was assigned to Ward 2. His good friend, the ingenious "Uncle Willie" North, would be working beside him. In this space, a clearing amid shrubs and bamboo, he had up to one hundred patients, mostly medical problems—malaria and dysentery. In those early days, each patient was amply supplied with a cot and two blankets. As January passed to February and then to March, his admissions were noticeably more worn, thin, sick with fevers and dysentery—their effects much more disabling now. There were several cases of cerebral malaria, splitting headaches, fevers, chills, sometimes paralysis, then lethargy, somnolence, and finally coma. Equally feared was blackwater fever, a complication of malaria from release of hemoglobin into the bloodstream causing jaundice and kidney failure.[3] Those with dysentery were particularly pathetic. Filipinos would drink anything, even spring water, not realizing that upstream floated rotting corpses and human excrement. Men were so weak they could not make it to the latrines; the footpaths were slippery with watery expulsions. Medics and nurses busied themselves trailing these poor souls, scooping their waste off the ground; some cases were so shaky they almost fell into toilet pits trying to squat, a thousand flies their escorts. Some simply lay in bed too weak to even get up, soiling precious linen and mattresses. Doctors soon required those too sick to stand to sleep on the ground, stooling in dirt instead. By late

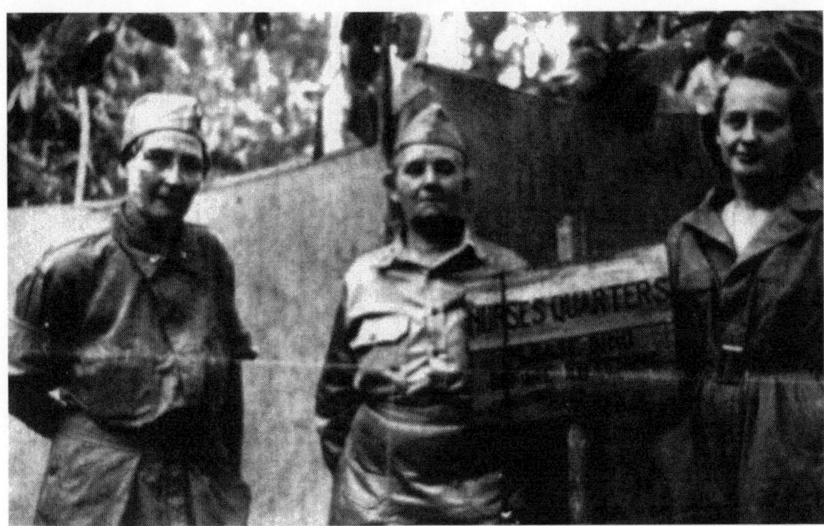

Nurses' quarters somewhere in Bataan. (*Courtesy of American Defenders of Bataan and Corregidor*)

March, Bumgarner's ward had swollen to four hundred, a ragtag mix of hollow-eyed soldiers and civilians. Even Bumgarner, like so many of the doctors and nurses, was stricken with malaria and dysentery. He could barely remain upright. The quinine was gone. Promised supplies from Mindanao were quickly consumed or simply failed to arrive. Ward rounds became a futile exercise. There was no medication, nothing to offer but kind words. Even the mosquito netting was gone, patients now at the total mercy of hungry *Anopheles*.

Lieutenant Hibbs was able to write one more letter to his family. Despite his now daily routine of hiding "in holes," and unable to sate the gnawing grip of hunger, he managed to fabricate a reassuring letter home in February: "Life is not too bad. I have a bamboo bed, a blanket, plenty of water, a few too many mosquitoes. The food is fair . . . everyone is content and in fairly good health [he lied]. No need to worry. We have plenty of room to maneuver and fight and we have plenty of it left in us. Turn the calf out to pasture."And then prophetically: "I'll be delayed awhile. Ralph."[4] The letter was delivered to Oskaloosa, Iowa, one month later. It was the last his family heard from him for a year.

Dr. Paul Ashton became a warrior. His journeys to the front, taking stock of medical units linked to the Philippine divisions, allowed him to see firsthand casualty care deep in the jungles of Bataan. He linked up with medics from the 33rd Infantry (Philippine Division) on the slopes of Mount Samat, not far from the Pantingan River. Day-to-day life hinged on patrols to scout for Japanese troops. Soldiers hacked through brush that was otherwise impenetrable. Few trails were to be found. Pack trains were the only access—or hand carry. Motor transport was laughable. It was a world of tall talisay trees and ipilipil plants, chatterings of dozens of monkeys, and squawkings of perturbed kingfishers. War? Only the infrequent rat-tat-tat of automatic rifle fire reminded Ashton of it. As for the wounded, any surgery would be done right then and there—or not at all.

But artillery and strafing planes were still a menace, even in March. Nighttime was the worst. The Japanese invariably penetrated, silent, waiting. They had perfected cover and concealment, the high trees a favorite location for ambush. Night brought on blackness, absolute blackness. "It was black as the inside of a cow," soldiers remarked.[5] Ashton learned to dig deep foxholes; they all did. But still the Japanese slithered, creeping silently like snakes, inches at a time until they tumbled into holes full of anxious men, afraid to sleep. Then it was life or death, kill or be killed. Knife against bayonet. Who could be trained for that? Who was ready to kill with bare hands, to plunge knives into flesh again and again, tearing, slashing, blinded by spurts of blood? Muffled grunts, curses, mumbling, groans, and once again silence. Only dawn showed who the victor was.

It was on such a night that Ashton became a warrior. Awakened, who knows why, he heard a scraping sound nearby. Was that someone breathing? He reached out, felt the muzzle of a rifle, and, slipping a hand under the barrel, grabbed it; with the other hand clutching his bayonet (yes, he had followed the sergeant's advice; keep a bayonet handy, razor sharp) he drove it deep into the neck of his enemy. Out and in, out and in, in a frenzied rush of adrenaline, the lip of his foxhole slippery with blood. Only then did he hear the gurgling and choking, and stillness. First light brought him his truth. A Japanese soldier, thick spectacles and all, lay dead close to his hole, his windpipe and carotid artery severed by Ashton's blade, the ground a slimy mess of mud and blood. He washed himself off, numb from the violence, and slogged up the mountain to breakfast. The life saver had become a life taker. Of course, he told not a word to his wife. Folks at home were not to know the truth about Bataan for a long time. In a letter on March 5, Ashton wrote to Yvonne:

"Dearest, I'm fine, well, and of course, very ready to return to you. As you know, things fall in my lap—more I can not say. Just know I'm well and safe and please don't worry. Be good and wait for me."[6]

Indeed, Yvonne would wait a long time. Now reinforced with fresh troops, General Homma was ready, eager for complete victory, to save face with his superiors in Tokyo. Embarrassed by the swift conquest of Malaysia while his forces sputtered, he desperately needed a decisive military solution. During most of February and throughout March, Japanese poured ashore on Luzon, revitalizing Homma's tired troops. All units then on Luzon were brought up to authorized strength. A new division, the 4th Division from Shanghai, and a crack unit of the 21st Division were diverted to Luzon along with artillery crews. No longer would there be rationing of food, ammunition, and allotments of basic equipment that had plagued Homma during January. Coffers were now full, war chests stocked. Rest and recuperation along with crisp, healthy troops had made his front-line elements combat ready. The major effort was to be launched April 3, advancing in three columns, preceded by a heavy artillery barrage and air bombardment. Homma's focus would be in II Corps sector, directly in the path of the two general hospitals. This would be "an all-out offensive in Bataan." Homma and his staff were confident. "There is no reason why this attack should not succeed," he said, despite tenacious resistance by Filipino and American troops."[7]

"I have not the slightest intention in the world of surrendering or capitulating the Filipino forces of my command. I intend to fight to destruction on Bataan and then do the same on Corregidor" was the fallacious rhetoric General MacArthur offered from his bunker on Corregidor. Then, on March 15, he departed "the Rock" for Australia on orders from President Roosevelt, turning command of the garrisons over to General Wainwright.[8] MacArthur had made only one trip to Bataan, on January 10, promising "help is definitely on the way. We must hold out until it comes," and knowing full well it would not—or maybe horribly misled by his superiors in Washington. His absence on the battlefield was noticed by almost every soldier, officer and enlisted alike. For that, his nickname was "Dugout Doug," referring to the solace of his command post buried in Corregidor's hardened lava core. But there is no question MacArthur was heartbroken to leave. The Philippines, in all their alien beauty, had become part of him, as if his child, to shepherd through adolescence and into adulthood and independence. The yielding of all that was so hopeful, the energy of the people, their vibrancy and, yes, naiveté, struck him like a crushing blow. Perhaps he was loathe to tour the battlefields because it pained him to see so much devastation wrought on his beloved people, and a country so close to death. He could sit deep in Corregidor's tunnels and dream the dreams of delusion. It was over, at least for now. Whether he truly believed he would return one can only speculate.

On Tuesday, March 24, Lieutenant Colonel Glattly, Luzon Force surgeon, fearing capitulation was approaching, issued a memorandum instructing all medical department personnel to wear numbered Red Cross brassards in accordance with the Geneva Convention. He hoped this would provide them some protection as non-combatants and allow them to continue to care for the sick and suffering.[9]

On Monday, March 30, Ruth Straub entered in her diary, "Many good rumors today . . . perhaps our convoy really is on its way."[10]

It was not to happen. That same day Japanese bombers took aim at General Hospital No. 1 and dropped clusters of bombs destroying the officers' quarters, mess hall, headquarters tent, and main operating room. There were over one hundred casualties, twenty-three of whom were killed. Private First Class Fred Lang, one of the hospital enlisted, died after being struck by shrapnel that pierced his left lung and heart. Four other noncommissioned officers were wounded. Al Weinstein's quarters were shattered. He stumbled out to see a scene of ruin and death. A pile of charred bodies greeted him, and two of his aides were fatally injured. Despite apologies by Japanese radio, Weinstein echoed a common belief: "We knew we were living on borrowed time."[11] On Easter, twin-engine bombers returned, and this time there could be no doubt. A bomb fell squarely on the big red cross in the hospital yard. More bombs fell on the hospital grounds, ten in all, killing 73 and wounding 117. Sixteen more died of their wounds over the next forty-eight hours. Only a small section of nurse Juanita Redmond's ward remained. She was knocked flat by a one-thousand-pound bomb. "My eyes were being gouged out of their sockets, my whole body was swollen and torn apart by the violent pressure," she recalled.[12] Redmond felt that several men who died did so from shock, being simply too weak to live through the shattering explosions.

Surgeon Carey Smith, in the middle of an operation, refused to stop. Despite the noise, smoke, and debris, he managed to keep focused on his patient. The surgery completed, nurse Bernititus, a little more unnerved, dove under a wooden bench just outside the operating room for safety. Other nurses and corpsmen ran through the wards cutting men out of traction so they could roll under the cots for protection. Some patients were so petrified with fright they refused to move. Convalescing soldiers helped the immobilized, even tending to their wounds, wrapping dressings. Others, in fright or panic, rolled out of their bunks onto the ground and crawled under anything that might give protection, some even falling from upper levels of the triple-decker beds. A Catholic chaplain, Father William Cummings, suddenly arrived, saw the panic, climbed onto a desk, and pleaded for silence. "All right, boys, everything's all right. Just stay quietly in bed, or lie still on the floor. Let us pray," he shouted above the din. With his words of the Lord's Prayer, people inexplicably quieted and prayed along, even though another wave of bombing quickly followed.[13] It was then that Cummings, in the middle of prayer, was struck by a bomb fragment, fracturing his arm and opening a sizable laceration. Taken to Weinstein's ward, he had a tourniquet applied. The bleeding slowed, Weinstein splinted his arm, and the father was back to his ministrations.

Meanwhile, Weinstein and Adamo had plenty of other work. Medics carried in almost "unrecognizable masses of human wreckage." There was no letup for over twenty hours, one casualty indistinguishable from the next; a flow of mashed arms, legs, and torsos. By now the work was mechanical, no wasted moves or wasted time, because there was always another case waiting. Truly profanity, they both thought. And what of their work? Were they thorough? Was it enough? Or was it simply to finish and get on with the next case, and the next? "Did these patients live? Did they die? To this day I have no idea," Weinstein later wrote.[14]

During the night of April 2, the 12th Medical Battalion began evacuating patients from three forward clearing stations in II Corps to the general hospitals. It was hardly a smooth process, but the enemy was closing in, and the clearing stations were in danger of being overrun. Seventy-five buses were commandeered to hold patients, traversing coastal roads clogged with fleeing troops and refugees and often caught between friendly and enemy fire. The buses joined a milieu of frightened civilians, weaponless Filipino soldiers, and armed military filling the East Road heading south toward Mariveles. Discipline among poorly trained Filipino troops was unraveling. Many were confused, aimless, and barefoot, some clad only in loincloths. Often they just disappeared into the bush, hoping to somehow make it home or fend for themselves in the mountains. Others, the scout units, and Americans tried to hold together, to maintain some decorum and fighting spirit. But tattered uniforms bespoke tattered fortitude. One officer remarked of his troops, "They had a blank stare in their eyes, their faces covered with beards lacked any semblance of expression." It was with robotic indifference that any could function at all. Ralph Hibbs was struck by it, too. "Hopelessness is the greatest personal enemy of a soldier," he wrote. "One is never more alone than when without hope."[15] It was in this mob that the ambulance-buses inched along, searching for the general hospitals; some wounded inside were near death. Japanese advances in I Corps prompted a similar evacuation, almost an impossibility there. Men struggled through barely passable footpaths carrying sick and injured, trying to beat the enemy back. Despite the improbabilities, almost seven thousand casualties had made it back to the general hospitals by April 8.[16]

On April 3, Good Friday of Holy Week for Christians and the anniversary of the death of the Seventh-Century Emperor Jimmu, the Japanese opened up mid-morning with a deafening artillery barrage that darkened the landscape in convulsions of earth and flying metal stupendous enough to rival those of the First World War. Close to 150 howitzers, cannon, and mortars fractured the lassitude of another hot, sunny spring day as if a new Jerusalem was once again suffering the wrath of a crucified Christ. Officers sensed a major Japanese offensive was unfolding and began mobilizing what troops were left. Hibbs's unit was ordered forward. Out of an authorized strength of seven hundred, a mere 128 men were able to muster and move out. Hibbs's medical detachment, now just sixteen men, went along, carrying almost nothing, as all medical supplies had been used up. Food consisted of sticks of sugarcane, which, when consumed, produced the expected Queen Isabella's revenge—tumultuous peristalsis from the sugar load that vented in uncontrollable diarrhea.

As they neared Mount Samat, the cannon fire intensified and the area was blanketed by high explosives. With little cover, Hibbs's doughboys were cut down as they inched forward, hoping somehow to engage an approaching enemy yet unable to avoid a rain of incoming shells. Jagged metal fragments cut with passionless ferocity into soft human flesh. Hibbs's first-aid dugout, not more than 40 feet square and three feet deep, soon filled with shrapnel casualties. One soldier stumbled in with blood flowing from his neck, gurgles and bubbles occurring with each breath. His trachea had been lacerated and opened. Hibbs leaned the poor fellow forward, hoping to forestall aspiration, and put pressure on both jugular viens. This stopped the bleeding. He bandaged the wound and pointed the soldier to the rear, a swarm of flies accompanying him (equally surprising, he survived and turned up as a prisoner of war, yapping away, his vocal cords miraculously spared). Another was given up for dead, barely conscious, with brain oozing from a wound to the head. Yet he was still breathing when Hibbs ordered him picked up and carried back, fully expecting the worst. He, too, somehow survived. It was triage at its essence, survival not by intervention but by fate. Before long, officers realized the situation was hopeless—it would be a piecemeal slaughter if fighting continued. Further advance was halted. Soldiers were ordered to fall back. Weeks earlier, the Luzon Force surgeon had noticed that some men were "becoming so weak from starvation that they could hardly carry their packs."[17] By now it was painfully obvious: Hibbs's men were absolutely depleted.

The barrage also filled Lieutenant Ashton's field hospital with a wasted mob. A steady stream of extremity wounds—those with a chance of survival—filled dressing tables. More serious injuries—abdominal, chest, and head wounds—were given morphine and set aside. There would be no laparotomy, no thoracotomy, no craniectomy for these men—there was no time and precious little equipment for that kind of surgery. In this setting, a man's chance of surviving now rested with the type of injury he suffered—medical intervention was unlikely to happen. With wounds of the limb, chances were good; to the chest, questionable; to the abdomen, very likely fatal; to the brain, probably fatal as well. The only practical treatments were controlling bleeding, giving intravenous fluids, and splinting for fractures. There were so many casualties that every available doctor was pressed into service. An obstetrician even found himself working among battle casualties. "This was the most frightful, noisy, dusty, fly-ridden, helpless, hopeless medical disaster I ever saw or conceived," Ashton later wrote. The few medical supplies on hand were quickly consumed—the hospital by then held several hundred wounded. It was a matter of "dispensing morphine to the hopeless, water to the bloodless, and reassurance to the restless."[18] And without warning, strolling into the open wards as if on a sight-seeing tour, was a string of Japanese soldiers. Uninterested in the injured, they wandered off in search of the healthy. Their prey, American and Filipino soldiers, were so weak and disoriented they simply staggered through the jungle and along the trails, hardly able any longer to mount a resistance.

Dr. Calvin Jackson, now assigned to General Hospital No. 2, spent Easter in the operating room. Here, too, wounded were coming in record numbers. Some were brought in by litter, but most hobbled in under their own power; no one could be spared, or had the strength, to carry a stretcher. Some never even made it, so incapacitated by their injuries or just plain sick they simply collapsed. With no gasoline or workable ambulances, these men sat abandoned. Six hundred were admitted that day. The sudden surge of fresh battle casualties taxed doctors. All beds were filled with malaria cases. Every niche, every balete tree—its huge flying buttress roots could hide three or four men—was used to shelter the wounded. For Jackson and his team there was maybe an hour's sleep that night and only morsels of food—some cracked wheat and a gruel of "awful" Australian hash, he remembered. In the background was the incessant thunder of artillery creeping closer; the sound of small-arms fire could be heard. The end was fast approaching.[19]

Casualties arrived now with dread in their eyes. These were men so weak they were barely able to lug weapons to the front—and then fighting artillery and planes with rifles and pistols. For nurse Ruth Straub, it took an effort to keep up her diary. She was on her feet continuously, exhausted. The work was endless. Only at night could she find a few minutes to scribble her thoughts. Her only light to write by was a kerosene lamp painted blue for blackout purposes. Always there were the sounds of tumbling bombs or incoming shells. And around her jungle cot, the scurrying of iguanas (and God knows what else). In fact, another nurse, Rita Palmer, had been bitten by a rat in her bed. But Straub saw the beaten men, too—their haunting look. On the evening of April 7, she wrote, "Our line had broken. . . . The 31st [Infantry, the American unit] had been forced to retreat. How serious the situation is we do not know. Morale is very low tonight."[20]

Lieutenant Hibbs's unit had been fighting steadily for seventy-two hours before the order came to pull back. Troops wounded by Japanese .25-caliber bullets and mortar fragments lined his open-pit aid station. They suffered silently. "How long have you been bleeding? Can you walk?" he would ask. Afraid to evacuate by daylight—they were sure to be picked off—he had urged those who could to wait until night before trying to make it to the rear. Now exhausted, men were told to shoulder heavy guns and ammunition up and down steep terrain around Trail No. 2 and through the canyons of Mount Mariveles. Impossible. One commander had commented, "Even if my troops were unopposed they couldn't crawl forward on their hands and knees." On their retreat, Hibbs could see bodies along the way, blackened feet protruding from the bush, flies and stink signaling another decomposing corpse. One dead American soldier had carried the book *Look Homeward, Angel.* It was found underneath his lifeless frame with an inscription inside:

> Janet dear
> I'm not going to make it home. I've looked homeward oh so long.
> All my love to you and the girls
>
> And below that:
>
> Whoever finds this book, please carry it on and hopefully Janet someday will get it.[21]

Somehow, by April 8, Hibbs and his men had reached General Hospital No. 2, now swollen to over eight thousand patients—there had been just three thousand five days earlier. The patient load was absolutely overwhelming for doctors and nurses; there was simply not enough time to care for them all. Each ward had only a couple of doctors, sometimes three, two or three nurses, and a few enlisted men for hundreds of patients.[22] Most arrivals were medical cases, feverish, prostrate, suffering the ravages of malaria, dysentery, malnutrition, and exhaustion. Very little food remained, only some boiled rice.

It was the same at General Hospital No. 1. Nurse Lucy Wilson remembered: "Men bled to death. We had no blood—nobody had any to donate. . . . We couldn't make any intravenous fluids, because we had no filter. So those with abdominal wounds . . . they just starved to death."[23]

On April 8, all nurses from General Hospital No. 1 were evacuated to Corregidor. The same imperative was soon issued by Colonel Gillespie at General Hospital No. 2. There had been discussion about this by Colonels Glattly, Duckworth, and Gillespie several times during the siege. Capture could mean torture, rape, and execution—much like what happened to thousands of Nanking women. Now there was little choice. Evacuation was essential. Nurses left in the midst of surgery, with their hair still in curlers and sick with dysentery, grabbing what personal belongings they could. Nurse Minnie Breese recalled, "I remember vomiting and running behind a bush with dysentery. I didn't care if I lived or died."[24] That evening, buses carried nurses to the Mariveles dock and then by launch across Manila Bay to Corregidor.[25] They left with the rumble of artillery and the staccato of gunfire drawing closer and closer; any organized defense by American and Filipino soldiers had vanished.

That very day, Brigadier General Edward King, commander of Philippine-American forces on Bataan, himself stricken with malaria, looked over the tactical situation with his staff. At each point, his troops were outnumbered, outgunned, and outflanked. Not one soldier could marshal the stamina to engage an enemy that seemed well fed, well equipped, and intent on conquest. He knew that further defense of the Bataan Peninsula was futile and likely to end in a massacre. The Japanese would soon reach Mariveles at the tip, and Bataan would be theirs. In direct disobedience of orders issued by General MacArthur and President Roosevelt, he contacted the Japanese to discuss surrender negotiations. Further killing of his gaunt, hungry men would accomplish nothing. Help would not arrive, rescue would not come. Bataan was not a fool's paradise. Once the nurses were gone, early in the morning of Thursday, April 9, King, in his last clean uniform, went forward to meet with Major General Kameichiro Nagano, commander of the 21st Infantry Division, who led him to a meeting with Colonel Nakayama, 14th Army senior operations officer. There was no listening to negotiations. Nakayama demanded, and received, an unconditional surrender of all Filipino and American forces on the Bataan Peninsula.

Doctors waited for the inevitable. After spending the night in his car, Calvin Jackson, with nothing to eat and a canteen of water, started toward Mariveles on April 9. Before long, he and his companion were met by two Japanese soldiers with fixed bayonets. They were herded into a fenced-in area with other soldiers, given a rice ball, and guarded by enemy troops. There was no latrine but there were plenty of flies to share the rice. Thus began Jackson's imprisonment. Early that same morning, Colonel Duckworth ordered Red Cross flags taken down at General Hospital No. 1 and replaced with white bed sheets, signaling surrender. At General Hospital No. 2, John Bumgarner and Jack Schwartz took to their cots the evening of April 9. Out came a bottle of champagne from Schwartz's duffel bag. Two others congregated to help drink it dry, a toast to the unknown, to forgetting for a few moments what might lie ahead. On that day of surrender, Lieutenant Hibbs parked himself beside the road leading from General Hospital No. 1, wracked by fevers of his own malaria. Before long, victory-crazed, bayonet-toting Japanese troops arrived "unshaven, dirty and smelly . . . sated with the belief of invincibility," wanting, like simple street thugs, narcotics from his medicine bag.

A couple of days later, he joined the column of prisoners forming up on the East Road to move north, herded along by insolent Japanese with their rifles and swords swaggering to some perverted *bushido* code and reminded of brutality by the occasional rifle shot that signaled the end to another exhausted fellow prisoner.[26]

On April 10, General MacArthur issued a statement from Australia:

> The Bataan Force went out as it would have wished, fighting to the end of its flickering forlorn hope. No Army has ever done so much with so little, and nothing became it more than its last hour of trial and agony.[27]

Filipino and American troops on the Bataan Peninsula were doomed from the start. Rainbow-5 had sealed their fate all along. Relegated to defensive roles, Philippine garrisons were completely dependent on relief by a robust seaward logistical chain. The sudden Japanese attack on Pearl Harbor left a Pacific fleet crippled and unable to venture far from base in waters and airspace seething with enemy submarines and aircraft. For the time being, the Japanese owned the Pacific Ocean. The supply chain had been severed. Rescue was out of the question, never entertained as a serious option, at least not in Washington. Wise field commanders—MacArthur included—might have known also. Tactically, on Luzon, a critical flaw was MacArthur's departure from war plan Orange by dispersing troops and supplies in hopes of defeating the Japanese at the invasion beaches, an irresponsible decision considering the poorly trained soldiers at his disposal. Failure to move depots of food, medical supplies, and ammunition back to Bataan as the beach defense collapsed added to future woes of the defenders and hastened their capitulation through starvation, sickness, and lack of ammunition. Overcrowding by throngs of fleeing civilians depleted food stores even faster and, with their limited understanding of sanitation, flamed the fires of dysentery and malaria. Of course, the Bataan Peninsula was already a perfect breeding ground for *Anopheles* mosquitoes, ready to feed on infected blood and disseminate the disease in epidemic proportions—almost two-thirds were laid low.

THROUGH ALL THIS, it was remarkable that the hospitals on Bataan functioned so well for so long. It was simply a matter of the number of patients—battle and non-battle casualties combined—that completely overwhelmed the doctors, nurses, and supplies. It signaled the end of any organized, effective medical treatment. At the front, field medical care soon suffered from lack of navigable roads and continued harassment from the air by Japanese planes. By March, fallback positions hampered any expeditious evacuation and relegated life-saving surgery to doctors behind the front lines. Transport of seriously injured men was by foot, almost impossible in parts of Bataan's jungle. In the end, total exhaustion of medical supplies reduced the care of the final surge of combat wounded to the most rudimentary treatment. In the end everyone was ill and exhausted, pitiful specimens of malnutrition, dysentery, malaria, and combat wounds.

The final insult was a gruesome sixty-five-mile journey from Mariveles to San Fernando by thousands of sickly prisoners of war, far more than the Japanese anticipated. Whether the Japanese were unable to care for them all or were simply barbaric, the savagery of their treatment became legendary. But the "Battling Bastards of Bataan" succeeded in throwing off Tokyo's timeline for Pacific conquests, perhaps even forestalling invasions of the Australian mainland, New Zealand, and other islands in Polynesia so vital for American staging centers in its eventual counterthrust through the Pacific.

Part 2

Anzio

"[I]t is sad to see those dying there who have not laughed nor wept nor kissed nor cursed."—June Wandrey, 1944

7

Fickle Antium

O diva, gratum quae regis Antium
praesens vel imo tollere de gradu mortale corpus
vel superbos vertere funeribus triumphos

Oh goddess, who rules pleasing Antium
At once present to raise up mortal bodies
Or turn proud triumphs into funeral
—Horace, *Odes and Epods*, Book I-XXXV

IN THE ANCIENT SEASIDE VILLAGE OF ANTIUM, LOCATED A DAY'S JOURNEY south of Rome, the goddess of Fortune was said to reside. Worshipped in double form—*Fortunae Antiatesi* or *Sorores Antii*, the Fortunes, or Sisters, of Antium—the two rained good or bad luck with divinely perverse humor on hapless humans. They could, in a moment, turn triumph into sadness, or, in more agreeable times, sadness into joy.[1]

In the fifth century BC, Antium was home to the Volscian people, descendants of the early Latins of central Italy.[2] As the story goes, it was claimed that Antium was founded by Ascanius, son of Aeneas, whose wandering Trojan band had been welcomed by Latinus, king of the Latins. It was said that the great Roman general Caius Marcius, known as Coriolanus because of his extraordinary feats of courage in victory over Rome's archenemy the Volscians, sought refuge there. Coriolanus had been betrayed by fellow citizens at the behest of a plebian mob; the Volscian chieftain Tullus Aufidius took him in. It was here that Coriolanus won the favor of his former enemy and led the Volscian army in a series of stunning victories over Rome. It was from Antium that he surged with his legions north to Rome's very gates, its population paralyzed by fear and apprehension that a man so fearless might fall upon them in a great slaughter. It was only through the entreaties of his mother, Volumnia, who threw herself at his feet in supplication, beseeching him to withdraw his armies, that he pulled his troops back and ended the siege. The retreat from Rome fueled anger in Tullus Aufidius and other Volscians because Rome was in their grasp but Coriolanus—now viewed as a traitor—allowed the enemy respite. Conspirators surrounded and slew him. For Caius Marcius Coriolanus, his sanctuary would host his executioners. The Volscians were later conquered by the legions of Postumus Cominius Auruncus and subjugated to the rising power of the Roman Republic. The Sisters of Antium had decreed, the cycle of destiny had played out.[3]

Centuries later, Marcus Tullius Cicero sought refuge in pleasing Antium, taken by its placidity and charm. "I have fallen in love with idleness" he wrote. "[T]he mind recoils altogether from writing," and his letters and books suffered during his stay.[4] Near the mid-twentieth century, Antium, now called Anzio, birthplace of Emperors Caligula and Nero, home to Cicero and Augustus Caesar, invited the great Allied armies as the gateway to the Appian Way, the Alban Hills, and the ultimate prize, Rome. The spread of idyllic beaches would be the breach to rout another of Italy's invaders who had defiled all that was sacred and godlike. But, as with Coriolanus, Anzio and Fortune's Sisters cavorted with those warriors, first welcoming them as conquerers and then turning serene landscapes into their funeral pyres. Woe to those who wage war on the sacred lands of Romulus and Remus. As with regal Aeneas and so many of his Trojan intruders, might prevailed, but many were slain on the plains of Latium. Such were the machinations of the Sisters of Fortune. Such was the capriciousness of lovely Antium.

In kinder times, remote from antiquity, Anzio and its sister village of Nettuno, a stone's throw to the southeast, again began to attract the well heeled. Elaborate villas were built near the shore, and lovely gardens of the Villa Borghese were conceived. Just beyond the coast, though, pleasant, cooling sea breezes gave way to hot, humid flatlands. In these Pontine marshes, malaria-carrying mosquitoes bred, vectors for the misery of all. *Il Duce* Benito Mussolini changed all that. Swamps were drained, and before long, in the 1930s, the country behind Anzio was dotted with small, sturdy farmhouses and settlements to attract peasants to farm the reclaimed marshy land. Such towns as Aprilia, Carroceto Station, Littoria,

Sabaudia, and Pontinia, mostly just clusters of concrete buildings, began to populate the monotonous flatness. In the 1940s, as the Allies plotted the invasion of Italy, all were used for more-sinister purposes: to hide German troops and armor in defense. The Sisters of Fortune had not left.

At the Sextant Conference in November 1943 in Cairo, US president Franklin Roosevelt and British prime minister Winston Churchill marveled at the successes 1943 had brought the Allies. There had been stunning victories worldwide: in North Africa, in the Mediterranean, in the Pacific, and in Russia. Operation Torch, the Allied invasion of North Africa, had brought about the extermination of Axis forces in Tunisia. From half a dozen Tunisian seaside ports between Oran and Sfax and from Haifa, Alexandria, and Bengasi, the American Seventh Army under General George Patton and the British Eighth Army under General Bernard Montgomery launched Operation Husky, the invasion of Sicily, on July 10, 1943.

The towns that saw invading Americans and Brits—Vittoria, Ragusa, Campobello, Raffadali, Argagona, Pozzallo, Modica—were sleepy seaside hamlets, not inclined to showcase on the world stage, yet they were swarmed with invading troops, trucks, tanks, and heavy guns. The Allies quickly established a beachhead and thrust deep into the heart of Sicily, Patton's divisions dashing through the western half of the island, surrounding Agrigento, the "eye of Sicily"[5] and capturing Palermo by July 22. The British were more methodical but no less successful, pounding away at Axis troops on the plains of Catania, driving east toward Messina, boxing in three German divisions and the remnants of Italian troops cut to pieces by the Allies. More Germans than should have fled across the Straits of Messina to the toe of the Italian Peninsula. The long-sought-after airfields of Sicily were now in Allied possession for strikes into the "soft underbelly" of *Festung Europa* (Fortress Europe).[6]

Operation Husky had been a smashing victory. As a result, Prime Minister Mussolini was ousted by King Victor Emmanuel III, arrested by the *Carabinieri*[7] and thrown in jail on July 24, 1943. His replacement was Marshal Pietro Badoglio. Harsher treatment of the former dictator was avoided by a German *Fallschirmjager* (paratroop) unit on September 12, when he was whisked away in a clandestine operation. The former *Il Duce* was installed by German leader Adolf Hitler as the puppet head of a new Fascist state, the Italian Social Republic, in northern Italy.

The Italian boot was next. Earlier in 1943, at the Trident Conference in Washington, it was agreed that in the Mediterranean, "the great prize there was to get Italy out of the war by whatever means might be the best," according to Churchill. The occupation of Italy would afford access to friendly but neutral Turkey and its air bases to bomb the pregnant oil fields of Romania. The ousting of Italy from Axis influence would force withdrawal of Italian troops from the Balkans and would compel Germany to send precious divisions to retain control there. Of course, all was in preparation for the cross-channel invasion of continental Europe—Soviet leader Joseph Stalin was begging for it—the American pitch for the defeat of Germany. The British felt otherwise, rather focusing on soft underbellies. Roosevelt had reservations, preferring an early invasion of France. He worried that Italy might tie up valuable Allied troops in a campaign of attrition, playing into Germany's hands.[8]

Yet compromise was reached. Italy would be invaded first, giving time to beef up men and material in England for mainland Europe. On August 24, 1943, the Combined Chiefs of Staff outlined the invasion of the Italian Peninsula as a two-pronged effort, one across the Straits of Messina to the toe of Italy (Operation Baytown)—to draw off Germans from around Naples—and a second prong farther up the western coast into Salerno Bay just southeast of Naples (Operation Avalanche). The sheltered bay of Salerno would offer gentle, sandy beaches, a rolling surf fit for children—or armies and their tanks. The Fifteenth Army Group—the Fifth and Eighth Allied Armies—would carry out the task. Once ashore at Salerno, Naples was the target, then speed north, capture Rome and the airfields that circled it, and on to the Alps.

US general Dwight Eisenhower was to be supreme commander. The key feature was to be a swift defeat of Axis forces on the peninsula, quick occupation of Rome and surrounding airfields, and support to the coming Allied invasion of France, Operation Overlord, slated for May 1944. Timing and swift victories were vital.

Fearful of such an invasion and aware of the developing Allied bombing campaign of Rome, King Victor Emmanuel instituted secret negotiations in Lisbon. Eisenhower was the chief participant. Reluctant at first to accept an armistice agreement, American negotiators eventually acquiesced to Italy's surrender on September 3. The armistice was announced September 8, on the eve of the Salerno invasion. Suspecting prompt Nazi retaliation, the king and the new prime minister, Badoglio, fled to southern Italy. Not formally notified of the surrender, Italian army units mostly dissolved in despair, only a few remaining loyal to their former Axis allies. German troops moved promptly to fill the void left by deserting Italians and became sole guardians of the Italian Peninsula. Italy was now divided into two German commands: the southern commander, Field Marshal Albert Kesselring, had eight divisions at his disposal, many lucky to have made it across the Straits of Messina from Sicily. Thirteen additional divisions were north of Rome under the command of Marshal Erwin Rommel. Yet wider mobilization plans had been drawn up, reinforcing units already in Italy and transferring troops from Sardinia and Corsica to the mainland. There was no doubting the imminence or significance of an Allied invasion. Kesselring was under no illusions. Loss of Italian support seriously undermined efforts to mount a stout defense. There would be little chance of throwing the invaders back into the sea as he had hoped. It would more likely be a defense in depth, forcing the Allies to pay dearly for each mile of advance.[9]

On September 3, the day the Italian surrender was signed, Operation Baytown unfolded. Montgomery and the British Eighth Army traversed the Straits of Messina, landing between Reggio and Villa San Giovanni. A saturating preinvasion bombardment killed almost no one—the Germans had wisely withdrawn—but cratered many fallow fields. Montgomery cautiously (as was his temperament) began his march up the peninsula, hoping to tie up German troops from the main landings at Salerno. The Eighth Army was expected to link up with the Fifth Army landing at Salerno and push on to capture Naples, then Rome. General Heinrich von Vietinghoff, commander of the German Tenth Army, suspected a landing near Salerno and instructed his 16th Panzer Division to dig in on high ground bordering the beachhead. Some of the defenders were members of the Italian 222nd Coastal Division. Coercion was the carrot. Those who refused were treated as prisoners of war. Reluctant officers were shot.

Operation Avalanche began with amphibious landings in the early morning hours of September 9. The Fifth Army—the British 46th and 56th Infantry Divisions (X Corps)—landed just south of Salerno. The American 36th Infantry Division, a Texas National Guard unit, representing VI Corps, chose the town of Paestum eight miles distant on beaches named Red, Green, Yellow, and Blue. Offshore, Eisenhower kept the American 45th Infantry Division on its transports, as ready reserve. Salerno offered perfect assault beaches: a placid tide and flat, sandy dunes. The only concern was the mountainous ringing redoubts, perfect roosts for deadly howitzers and "88s."

The medical management of Avalanche was in the hands of forty-nine-year-old Colonel Joseph Martin, surgeon for the Fifth Army. Martin was a product of the Chicago Hospital College of Medicine, graduating in 1918. He was commissioned in the Army Medical Reserve that year and had spent his entire career in the military. The Mediterranean was his first overseas assignment, but he was infantry through and through, having completed the Infantry School at Fort Benning in 1927, and become a devoted advocate for field medical care.[10] Martin planned for two evacuation hospitals per division: a 400-bed, semimobile unit and a 750-bed unit. In all, four 400-bed and four 750-bed evacuation hospitals were brought in after the landings.[11] Martin wanted his hospitals ashore soon. Clearing companies were overwhelmed, and evacuation to ships was tedious and time consuming. Two evacuation hospitals had been slated for Salerno's beaches. "Evacs" (the abbreviated label) were America's signature units of combat casualty care. Mobile in design—and in terminology—they were barely so: large setups under billowing canvas with long supply trains and scores of medical personnel. Their role was surgical: care of the combat wounded, from resuscitation to reparative surgery. The chief disadvantage was their monstrous footprint. Mobility was sacrificed for capacity to handle all types of injuries, beds to recover postoperative patients, and the supporting laboratory and blood-banking services. Nevertheless, with tented housing and assigned transportation, the hospitals could be taken down, moved, and set up—but not at a moment's notice.[12]

Nine teams of veteran surgeons from the 2nd Auxiliary Surgical Group accompanied the assault phase and attached to division-clearing platoons. These surgical groups were designed to augment medical personnel of field hospitals and provided added expertise in aspects of surgical care. Most of the surgeons were fully trained, skillful, and experienced in civilian practice. They had traded their starched white lab coats for wrinkled olive-drab. Five field hospitals, used for noncombat conditions, were also added to the list. Within forty-five days of the invasion, Martin had planned an extensive hospital operation: six five-hundred-bed station hospitals added to his inventory. In all there were soon nine thousand five hundred mobile and seven thousand fixed beds available.

Troops who splashed ashore that Friday remembered Salerno—those who lived, that is. They were met by hails of gunfire and blistering artillery even before boats touched down. In the darkness, confusion reigned, with some landing craft hit and set ablaze far from shore.

Screams of burning men could be heard by those passing through. "Come on in and give up. We have you covered!" blared the German loudspeakers, dispelling any thought by Allied commanders that surprise had been achieved.[13] On the beach, bodies accumulated, "lying face inland, all in relatively the same position—with their rifles under their bodies, stomachs and faces in the sand," as one ensign from the beach party of the USS *Fredrick Funston* (APA 89) observed.[14] Medics scrambled to bring those not dead to safety. Battalion surgeons used ditches, foxholes, and sand dunes as makeshift aid stations, anything out of the line of fire. First aid was the only option, little else was possible. Colonel Edward Churchill, surgical consultant to the Fifth Army, was at Salerno. Battlefield care was stark, he observed; oftentimes the only surgical instruments were "first aid kit, extra dressings, a pocketknife and two curved clamps." "A beachhead is a hazardous place to set up a field hospital," he later commented.[15] As for any field hospital, only one clearing station was operational on D-Day, that run by the 162nd Medical Battalion attached to the 36th Infantry Division. Most wounded were run through quickly and loaded aboard departing boats for troop transports where surgeons were waiting. The USS *Joseph T. Dickman* (APA 13) received fifty-seven wounded, and the USS *Lyon* (AP 71) took in thirty-one.[16] By day's end, massive fire from big 8-inch and 14-inch guns offshore proved decisive. German strongpoints were slowly eliminated. The troops were there to stay.

Colonel Paul Sauer, a graduate of the University of Pennsylvania, landed with his 95th Evacuation Hospital on September 9, D-Day. Following him in within hours were one hundred tons of medical supplies and two hundred tons of hospital equipment—never mind the occasional artillery barrage. His hospital opened for patients three days later, near Paestum, under the shadows of Poseidon's ancient temple. Sauer's 95th Evac was set up close to a clearing station so surgical cases could be taken directly over. At first, with the usual snafu of getting equipment in, only two operating tables and two anesthesia machines were available. Nevertheless, in the first four days, the 95th saw more than one thousand patients. Sauer later reported "at times we were overfilled to such an extent that all cots were in use, other patients remained on the litters on which they had been brought to us in lieu of folding cots, and others were given 2 wool blankets to enable them to sleep on the ground."[17] Dr. Zachary Friedenberg was with the 95th. He had just completed a two-year surgical internship at Columbia University in New

York in 1939 when, as part of the Army Reserve program, he was activated and sent to Fort Benning, Georgia. From there, when war broke out, his assignment was the 95th Evac, headed for overseas duty. Paestum proved unsettling. Only the volume of work distracted him from the ominous din of combat. "It required a steady hand to repair an artery while listening to the low-pitched whistle of shells passing overhead," he recalled. "When the ward tents were filled to capacity, patients were laid on the outside along the tent walls with their heads inside and their bodies outside."[18] Nurses finally made it on September 24, after a frightening experience aboard the British hospital ship HMHS *Newfoundland* when it was bombed in the Gulf. No one was hurt, but the women were left with only the clothes on their backs. Refitted in North Africa, they made a less eventful return trip, finally wading ashore from landing craft. Nurses commented that the doctors "looked like ghosts of their former selves. They had been working night and day."[19]

Field Marshal Kesselring and General Vietinghoff were not done. Just behind the consolidated Allied beachhead, the 3rd and 15th Panzer Grenadier Divisions and elements of the Hermann Goering Panzer Division poured in as reinforcements. Kesselring stressed to Vietinghoff that victory at Salerno was imperative and "every man must know this."[20] On September 13—Black Monday it would be called—the Germans barrelled right down the Sele River corridor, almost splitting X and VI Corps.

On September 14, Lieutenant General Mark Clark, commander of the Fifth Army, came ashore to survey his battle lines and personally led a counterattack against a tank column that threatened to push them all back into the sea. Thunderbirds of the 45th Infantry Division and stupendous shelling by every gun that naval Task Force 80 could bring to bear slowly ground the Germans' advance to a standstill. The USS *Philadelphia* (CL 41) alone poured in 921 rounds of 6-inch shells; the USS *Boise* (CL 47), relieving the *Philadelphia*, added nearly six hundred rounds. Lieutenant Colonel Henry Winans, a medical officer who came ashore days later with the 56th Evacuation Hospital, saw the devastation—discarded equipment, wrecked jeeps, stained shredded clothing—and knew instantaneously, "No one who did not stand here as the shells burst among men who came ashore only with rifles and grenades or who did not make his way over a plain seeded with mines and open to attack from artillery, planes, and tanks, may complain that it took time or that once it was necessary to retreat. This was one of the most heroic deeds in all military history."[21]

Lieutenant Colonel Thomas White and his 38th Evac left Tunis on September 17. Their destination was Agropoli, a seaside town about three miles from Paestum. The 38th Evac was a large, 750-bed unit—"motorized" was the designation, not "mobile." That same night a blinding storm came through with lightning, thunder, and violent wind. Despite a scattering of equipment—mud-saturated bedding, soaked clothing, and supplies—along five miles of beach, White was able to piece together a surgical unit. In all, he somehow amassed eleven operating tables set up, staffed, and ready to take battle casualties within twelve hours. Less than two weeks later, his outfit was operating at 25 percent above capacity.

German commanders were exasperated. Kesselring and Vietinghoff had been skeptical despite the encouraging developments of September 13, and Kesselring held Hitler, who had turned a blind eye to more troops, accountable for the defeat.[22] Despite suffering heavy casualties, the Allies could not be dislodged. After a second counterattack floundered on September 16, Vietinghoff was spent, and Kesselring authorized a retreat. On September 18, the Germans pulled back. Along the way, grenadiers tore up railroad tracks, dynamited factories, scorched farmland, and slaughtered livestock. "As we push forward we leave in our wake devastation beyond anything you can imagine—whole cities battered to rubble . . . our bombing and shelling, plus German destruction, has rendered the place utterly useless," one private reported.[23] Salerno became a distant memory. Within a month, not an Allied soldier could be found; the Temple of Poseidon at Paestum was once again the sole guardian of the gulf. But the men and women of the 95th Evac were battle hardened. Exactly 2,443 patients had passed through by the end of September, and 1,223 operations had been completed.

Naples was the wealthiest and most industrialized of the Italian city-states in the nineteenth century. *Vedi Napoli e poi muori*! "See Naples and die" was the phrase, because after such a visit, there would never be anything more magnificent. In the early 1800s, French novelist Henri Beyle, writing under the pseudonym Stendhal, marveled at the panorama: "I am leaving. I shall not forget Via Toledo, nor any other of the parts of Naples; to my eyes this city has no equal and is the most beautiful city in the universe."[24]

On October 1, X Corps Commander General Richard McCreery reported to General Clark, "Today has given us one of the highlights of the campaign and Naples has fallen to 10 Corps."[25] It was a different Naples the Allies found when they entered the city. Gone were the delightful cafes, grand thoroughfares, and flirtatious *donne di palazzo*. Instead, there was total devastation. The Germans had utterly destroyed the place. A city abounding in culture was reduced to smoldering rubble, the only surviving denizens skinny rats that scurried along the waterfront. The water supply was polluted, aqueducts were brought down, and spaghetti factories, the source of sustenance for most Neapolitans, were reduced to ruins. Zachary Friedenberg remembered: "Few stores were open, many were ransacked, and food stands, mostly selling vegetables or grains, appeared on the littered streets. Meat, butter, coffee, tea, sugar, or cigarettes commanded an astronomical price on the black market . . . disease rapidly spread among the locals [with sewage lines out]. Typhus, the scourge of war for past centuries, increased in Naples."[26]

Hidden time bombs continued to detonate over the next weeks, killing and maiming many more unsuspecting citizens and soldiers. The port was clogged with every conceivable type of vessel, sunk or wrecked by the departing Germans. For a stretch, Naples's harbor was unusable until the submerged hulks could be cleared. Salerno would have to substitute, Clark's army had a voracious appetite for logistics. Yet the mood was celebratory. Gone were the Germans, fleeing in disarray many would hope. General Clark did not want to dally. "Rome by Christmas" was the scuttlebutt among his troops. Certainly Allied sympathizers and partisans trapped in Rome longed for as much.[27] Some even thought the Allies would be in Florence to celebrate the holidays. But the price had been steep. Fifth Army had suffered 7,272 casualties as of October 6, including 1,770 killed in action and 6,901 wounded, almost two-thirds American boys.

Out of Naples, the Fifth Army clanked up Route 6, the old Via Latina, toward Rome. VI Corps on the left flank and X Corps on the right, six divisions in all, swept through Cancello and Maddaloni, into the mountains above Caserta. The Greek Hoplites walked along this road, as did Hannibal's Carthaginians, Roman legions, and Vandals and Normans, and now Americans. And coming up from the toe, Montgomery's British shouldered the Adriatic coastline, a solid face of Allied might creeping beside Italy's Apennine spine. Across the swollen Volturno River twenty miles from Naples, tanks first, then infantry, Clark's Fifth Army pushed on, reinforced by additional troops and armor. Each mile traversed was punctuated by sudden explosions from German mines. Mutilated soldiers were rushed to surgeons who could do little but complete amputations, removing limbs at the knee or thigh, cleaning out mangled genitals, closing pelvises ripe with exposed bowel. The 8th and 16th Evacs were moved up to Caserta by mid-November, the 93rd Evac to Caiazzo, the 15th Evac to Alife, and the 56th Evac to Dragoni, all to shorten lengthening ambulance runs, at some points one hundred miles or longer. More beds, it was feared, would be needed. The 38th and 94th Evacs were sent to Riardo, ten to fifteen miles from the front lines. The 38th Evac had spent two weeks at Agropoli seeing more than one thousand five hundred patients with mostly nonbattle medical conditions like malaria. Its case mix soon changed to combat wounds.

The November weather turned sour to match the bloody grind: wet, cold, and gray. And ominous highlands loomed to the forefront. The Germans were determined to take a stand, with no further retreating on Hitler's insistence. Triple lines of defense formed across Italy's narrow waist south of Rome, eighty-five miles wide, with barriers named "Volturno," "Bernhardt," and "Gustav." These stretched across mountainous terrain, peaks reaching thousands of feet and flanking Route 6 through the Mignano Gap, summits with names like Monte Lungo, Monte Trocchio, Monte Sammucro, Monte La Difensa, Monte Porchia, and the massif Monte Cassino at one thousand seven hundred feet. These towering sentinels guarded passage into the Liri Valley and on to Rome. The three defensive positions were known as the Winterstellung—the Winter Line. Two corps of troops—thirteen divisions in all—now faced the combined strength of the Fifth and Eighth Armies.

By November 15, the Allies had arrived at the Winter Line. After a series of bloody mountain battles they faced the heart of the German defense, the Gustav Line, beginning at the Tyrrhenian coast, running along the Garigliano River to the Rapido River, up to Monte Cassino as the anchor.[28] With such rugged peaks, defense was simplified. Automatic weapons covered every accessible path, narrow valleys provided excellent avenues for crossfire, and strongpoints could be stubbornly held with a minimum number of troops. Fearsome German artillery and Nebelwerfer rockets backed up infantry, raining down death on slopes and passes. Allied attacks began December 1. Casualties were heavy, and evacuation down steep precipices in darkness, cold, rain, and snow was dangerous and exhausting. Of the two Corps medical battalions responsible for moving victims, the 52nd transported 25,125 sick and wounded soldiers between September 30 and December 31, and the 54th evacuated 16,186 patients in just two months, from November 15 to January 15.[29] Battles for the countless hilltops were slow and costly, and wore down combat units. High-explosive artillery shells ripped apart GIs. That meant more desperate surgery for doctors, piecing together human shreds. Snow, bitter cold, and mud made any movement laborious and wearied troops. Winter conditions imposed additional hardships on the men, and non-battle maladies skyrocketed.

From October to early December, almost four thousand patients came through the 8th Evac near Caserta. Most of these, three thousand three hundred, were "diseased, non-battle casualties," men suffering from hepatitis, malaria, respiratory infections, and psychoneuroses, all aggravated by lousy weather. Time spent on the line weakened everyone, and the constant pounding—day and night—taxed the sanity of the sanest. A dreariness settled over all, even in the comfort of tent hospitals. Little could keep out the frigid air and soaking drizzle. Surgeon Henry Winans wrote in his diary somewhere near Caserta: "The rain hammers on my helmet in good earnest and the water is flowing around the tents and in some cases, through them, where the drainage ditches have overfilled. Smoke hangs over the area and visibility is cut down to 1/4 of a mile. I slip and slide to the mess tent."[30]

Yet it was so much worse for the infantrymen. Lieutenant Avis Dagit, a newly minted nurse from Methodist Hospital in Des Moines, Iowa, was with the 56th Evac in Avellino. "Soldiers arrived at the hospital caked with mud and unshaven and they had the appearance of old men" she wrote.[31] Cartoonist Bill Mauldin captured their punishing angst in Willie and Joe's grim wisecracks jammed in freezing wet foxholes. His tribute to the GIs of the Italian campaign, *Mud, Mules, and Mountains*, seemed a fitting epitaph to the insurmountable task of rooting out an enemy holding the high ground, a ceaseless effort always up and up and up, one hill after another.[32]

At Capua, near the Volturno River, the 95th Evac wallowed in the muck and rain. Surgeons were taking twelve-hour shifts, reporting in mud-caked boots, trench coats, and helmets. Off came the helmets (put not far away) and trench coats, the mud was hosed from their boots, and on went surgical gowns, caps, and masks. There was one initial, ten-minute surgical scrub, but after that, between cases, merely a change of gloves, a hand dip in alcohol, and on with a new set of gloves. Nurses were almost indistinguishable from the men, dressed in fatigues, field jackets, and boots. Dr. Lawrence Collins, a Dallas physician with the 56th Evac, called the thick, sucking quagmire by a Southern term, *loblolly*: "We're in one big loblolly of mud . . . as though a great big egg beater had been run over the area. . . . Vehicles running through churn up a batter six inches deep everywhere, as thick as hot cake batter."[33]

All knew how miserable it was for the foot soldier up in the mountains. They saw them brought in, forced to live in the same "loblolly" but higher up, pelted by icy rain, buffeted by cold winds, not a cot or stove or tent for comfort. One wool army blanket was the only issue; it was a ghastly existence with no guarantee of survival. High German observation posts aided in raining down terribly accurate rounds on soldiers below. So-called donkey paths were so steep that not even mules bringing up food and ammunition could traverse them; the only way down for the injured was by cautious litter carry, one foot at a time. Just the dead, who could be strapped across pack animals, were afforded the luxury of quicker descent.

Early in the morning on New Year's Day, 1944, gale force winds ripped several tents of the 95th Evac to shreds, collapsing more than a few. Some described it as a blizzard. The biting cold blew among patients and staff, compounding their plight. On the east coast, the advance of the 8th Army during December essentially stopped. "We must not let this great Italian battle degenerate into a deadlock. At all costs we must win Rome," Churchill telegraphed President Roosevelt on October 26 while he was recovering from influenza.[34] Fifth Army battle casualties from November 15, the beginning of its assault on the Winter Line, until January 15, when the edge of the Gustav Line was reached, were 15,930 men, over half from VI and II Corps, American soldiers. Daily casualties sometimes exceeded fifty killed and three hundred wounded.[35] Nurse Dagit recalled: "[C]asualties were heavy. . . . Surgery once again operated around the clock. . . . Roads became quagmires. . . . Litter bearers carefully negotiated ankle deep puddles. . . . Drops of water formed on the tops of the ward tents. . . . The wounded came to the hospital after many days in water-filled foxholes on freezing, craggy mountainsides."[36]

Paul Kennedy, a surgeon with the 2nd Auxiliary Surgical Group and assigned to the 11th Field Hospital just outside Mignano, suffered through that blizzard of January 1. Some estimated the winds at ninety miles an hour. The gale, rain, and then snow scattered tents and equipment, even personal belongings. Rain-soaked doctors and nurses gave up, evacuated patients, and spent a miserable night at headquarters, at least happy to be out of the storm. But they were back at it two days later, tents braced, working through a string of wounded. On January 5, Kennedy wrote: "We've been awfully busy the past 24 hours and every case is a real emergency. One fellow came in with his brain half out—another had the entire half of his jaw shot away. We've had to remove half the bowel in some cases. . . . It's cold in the O.R.—so cold that early this morning ice formed on the sterile drapes."[37]

Between plummeting temperatures and incoming rounds—"I thought we were supposed to be out of artillery range"—it was clear to Kennedy that "the war is still far from won." Deafening booms of 240-mm "Black Dragon" howitzers and 155-mm "Long Toms" to their rear, roaring tubes sticking from camouflage netting, kept everyone's nerves on edge, always wondering if it was "outgoing" or "incoming."[38] Appalling numbers of nonbattle casualties were stacking up, reaching fifty thousand across the front. Most were victims of so-called immersion foot, that painful condition caused by booted but cold, wet feet and socks—sometimes leading to gangrene. It brought many a soldier down from the mountains and thinned Allied lines.

And still Rome was a distant, elusive prize. Churchill had emphasized at the Sextant Conference in November that "whoever holds Rome holds the title deeds of Italy," adding that "the seizure of a firm defensive base north of Rome becomes imperative. . . . [W]e cannot afford to adopt a purely defensive role [so as to not compromise Overlord, one might assume], for this would entail the surrender of the initiative to the Germans."[39] As of the first of the year 1944, those deeds were held by the Germans, the Allies lucky to retain the narrow leg they possessed. Roosevelt fretted, too. Feeling that the British were reluctant to push Overlord, the cross-channel invasion of Europe, Roosevelt saw the Italian quagmire as a hindrance. He fumed that Italy was strictly a "secondary front," a diversion. But Churchill retorted "the campaign in Italy . . . was the faithful and indispensable comrade and counterpart to the main cross-Channel operation." In mid-January, it all stagnated before Monte Cassino. Churchill had admitted to the Sextant Conference in November that the war in the Mediterranean "has taken an unsatisfactory course."[40] There was no prospect of entering Rome in 1943.

8

Codename Shingle

To snatch the Eternal City occupied all Allied thinking. Even before Salerno, commanders had flirted with an end run around German troops nearer to Rome. In fact, General Clark formed a special amphibious planning staff as part of his Fifth Army G-3 Section.[1] In Eisenhower's opinion, outflanking operations on either coast were preferable to the slow, costly batterings of a frontal assault against mountain defenses. But given the plans for Overlord, neither troops nor landing craft were readily available in fall 1943. In November, Field Marshal (General) Harold Alexander, commander of Army Group 15, proposed an amphibious landing below Rome once the Fifth Army had broken through the Gustav Line. The attack, Alexander claimed, could seize the Colli Laziali, the Alban Hills, just south of Rome. The Alban Hills commanded approach routes supplying Kesselring's XIV Panzer Corps. Possession would sever German logistics, isolating Kesselring's troops. Vital landing craft slotted for Overlord would be held in the Mediterranean until after the first of the new year. The entire business was to be codenamed Shingle.

Landing sites would be near the port town of Anzio, old Latin Antium, playground of the Roman elite. Seaside Anzio and its sister town of Nettuno sat on a low plain, open, flat terrain for maneuver and easy access to Route 6 and Alexander's Alban Hills. Suitable beaches could be found fronting Anzio and to the north and south, easily accommodating two divisions. But conservative Eisenhower worried. Such a relatively minor force would not intimidate the Germans, he felt, and probably only rouse them to fight. And unless the Allies were vigorously supplied, Eisenhower argued, it could be a catastrophe—surrounded, trapped, and choked. Churchill, pugnacious as ever, felt two divisions plus paratroopers would be fine, bursting ashore, racing toward the Alban Hills, and slashing German lines. If it was timed within days of a Fifth Army breakout at Monte Cassino, Germans in southern Italy would be finished. "[Y]ou dismiss logistics with a wave of your hand," Eisenhower responded. Indeed, Ike would have done well to remember Generalfeldmarschall Friedrich Paulus, whose supply chain had shriveled a year before, costing an entire German army at Stalingrad. But the general was on his way out, selected as overall commander for Overlord. So he did not take a firmer stand, a mistake that might have cost an Allied army.[2]

Churchill had his way. "Full steam ahead," he cabled Roosevelt on December 28.[3] Operation Shingle had been scheduled for late December, assuming the Fifth Army would be able to join within seven days. Success depended on a quick link up. But the Gustav Line held, resistance stiffened, and the timetable had to be set back. In frustration, a compromise plan developed. Shingle would no longer depend on a Fifth Army breakthrough. Landings at Anzio were now to be diversionary, disruption of enemy communication and diversion of its forces—more or less a giant commando raid. Shingle would facilitate piercing the Gustav Line. Intelligence said two divisions would be sufficient. Of course, all depended on resupply. Allied troops would be isolated. For that purpose, landing craft were critical—air drops would not be practical. General Clark cabled General Alexander on January 2, demanding enough LSTs (landing ships, tank) and other craft for a minimum of fifteen days and probably longer. Finally, on January 8, Alexander met with Churchill, who gave permission to retain twenty-four LSTs until the end of February. The prime minister then reported to Roosevelt: "A unanimous agreement for action as proposed was reached. . . . Everyone is in good heart and the resources seem sufficient. . . . Intention is to land a corps of two divisions for the assault, and to follow up with a mobile striking force based on the elements of a third division to cut enemy's communication."[4]

Roosevelt, having already been briefed on the operation, replied, "I am very glad to see that we are in complete agreement." Not all were so optimistic. Cautious Major General John Lucas, commander of VI Corps, which was slated for this assault, did not see how only two battle-weary divisions could hold a beachhead surrounded by as many as four German divisions. He wrote that "the whole affair has a strong odor of Gallipoli."[5]

Indeed, Shingle was Lucas's enigma. The mission was "to seize and secure a beachhead in the vicinity of Anzio and to advance on Colli Laziali" (the Alban Hills). Exactly how all that was to happen was a matter of conjecture and battlefield judgment and would catch Lucas squarely between the proverbial rock and a hard place. A spirit of aggressiveness could easily be offset by a thin offense, exposure of his flanks, and annihilation. On the other hand, a purely defensive presence might tie up German units bound for the Gustav Line or might simply expose Allied troops to a good, steady thrashing.

On paper, the landings called for three phases. The Star assault would be the main frontal beachings northwest and southeast of Anzio and Nettuno. For that, the 3rd Infantry Division (US), the 1st Infantry Division (British), a regiment-size Ranger unit (designated the 6615 Ranger Force—three battalions of rangers) (US), and the 509th Parachute Battalion (US) would participate. Assault beaches would be grouped into the Peter sector for the British troops and X-Ray sector for the Americans. The Sun assault involved having the 504th Parachute Infantry Regiment (part of the US 82nd Airborne Division) parachute to the rear of assault beaches, blocking enemy reinforcements one hour before the landings (General Clark canceled this airborne operation as too risky just prior to the landings; the 504th ignominiously landed by LST with the 3rd Division as regular infantry). The third phase, labeled Moon, would be strictly diversionary. A naval force would feint a bombardment and landing north of Rome at the port city of Civitavecchia. Clark had a hefty reserve force, however. For that he earmarked Combat Command A of the First Armored Division (and Company A of the 47th Medical Battalion) and the 179th Regimental Combat Team of the 45th Infantry Division (with Company B of the 120th Medical Battalion). Both would be ashore by February 1.[6] Inland of the Anzio beachhead two key towns sat astride Route 6 and Route 7 (the old *Via Appia*—Appian Way): Aprilia and Cisterna di Littoria. They would feature prominently in any attempt to disrupt these two routes of German reinforcement, resupply, and communication. It would be critical for the Allies to seize and hold what would become vital chokepoints.

Intelligence estimates put the German strength at roughly six thousand troops on D-Day, but the enemy quickly grasped the danger the Anzio assault posed to the Tenth Army on the Gustav Line and the immediate garrison was soon reinforced. By D-Day+3, thirty-one thousand three hundred troops were expected to face the Allies, and by D-Day+16, that number was expected to jump to sixty-one thousand three hundred, outnumbering Allied forces. In fact, by seven days after D-Day, the Germans had seventy-one thousand five hundred troops in place ringing the Anzio beachhead.

In the Anzio-Nettuno area, January was the coldest month of the year, averaging fifty-two degrees Fahrenheit during the day and thirty-nine degrees at night. Usually there were eleven days of rain.[7] Italian winters were hardly the images of sunny, lazy holiday stretches of summer that movies, magazines, and postcards conveyed. More characteristic adjectives would be dank, dreary, and depressing.

In charge of the medical planning for VI Corps was fifty-year-old Colonel Jarrett Huddleston. Dr. Huddleston was a graduate of George Washington School of Medicine in Washington, DC, finishing in 1916 at age 23. He served an internship at Children's Hospital in Washington and joined the army shortly afterward. During World War I, he was sent to France and the western front, a medical officer with the 1st Engineering Regiment of the 1st Division. His services earned him the Croix de Guerre. Following the war, Huddleston was a professor of military science at Georgetown and George Washington Universities. His last assignment prior to deployment overseas as corps surgeon was at Camp Beauregard, Louisiana. He was such a role model that two of his sons were army officers and a third was a cadet at West Point. In true army fashion, Huddleston did not shrink from danger. In all its chaos, the battlefield was no stranger, yet he was still amazed at the mayhem gunfire and artillery could produce. Serving as VI Corps surgeon for Operation Avalanche, D-Day at Salerno was no exception—the viciousness and carnage rattled more than a few veterans. "Great deal of confusion in landing," the colonel wrote later. "Met with a burst of 88's as we landed. . . . We got across the beach without casualties. Tough going. I see I am going to lose weight. Looked for VI Corps. Nobody knew anything about them." Where were his medical assets, he wondered. "It's a bloody bad show," was his summation.[8] And now, with the prospects of another Salerno, his pulse quickened.

Joseph Martin, Fifth Army surgeon, doled out medical units for Huddleston. His VI Corps would have the 52nd Medical Battalion, the 33rd Field Hospital, the 93rd and 95th Evac Hospitals (semimobile—four hundred beds), the 56th Evac (seven hundred beds), the 2nd Casualty Clearing Station (British), the 25th and 36th Field Surgery Units, the

3rd Field Dressing Station, and the 35th Beach Group Medical Section (all British units), and twelve teams of the 2nd Auxiliary Surgical Group.

British casualty clearing stations, staffed by surgeons from base hospitals, were a carryover from World War I and had morphed into bulky but portable surgical units. They had become the rough equivalent of the American evacuation hospital. The British also deployed field surgery units. Highly mobile, they were a combination of field dressing stations—basically similar to American clearing companies—and assigned surgical teams. Rapid intervention for the critically wounded was the purpose—the right blend of skill, technology, and mobility.[9] So impressed with their function was surgical consultant (and former Harvard professor) Edward Churchill that he copied the British system that he saw operate so efficiently in North Africa for his auxiliary surgical group. "[E]very hour added to the time-lag between injury and initial surgery increases the loss of life and limb," he wrote, attesting to the speed with which his surgical groups could respond.[10]

Auxillary Surgical Groups had been part of the Army Medical Department since the 1920s, highly specialized surgical teams that could be deployed with field hospitals to provide early surgical care of combat casualties, much like the *groupe complémentaire de chirurgie* employed by the French *Service de santé* during World War I.[11] Each Group (there would be a total of five by war's end) contained a number of surgical teams composed of a surgeon, assistant surgeon, anesthetist, operating room nurse, and two surgical technicians, along with the necessary operating room equipment and instruments. They were relatively youthful groups, the average age of the surgeons was thirty-four. Dr. Churchill had urged their broader use for Operation Torch, and now, the Italian campaign. In turn, the "Auxers," as they would affectionately be called, would be the forerunners of the Korean War-era mobile army surgical hospitals. Hand-in-hand with combat surgery was the need for blood, and with the likelihood of a bloodbath at Anzio, the British furnished the 12th Field Transfusion Service, the blood bank for the beachhead. Bottled blood brought ashore would be processed, stored, and delivered from this unit to all hospitals. Just for D-Day alone, two hundred pints were on hand. Few days would see any surpluses.

Each assault division had its own medical units, of course. For the American 3rd Infantry Division there was the 3rd Medical Battalion. The 120th Medical Battalion supported the 45th Infantry Division, and the 47th Armored Medical Battalion the 1st Armored Division. Each of these had its own collecting companies for casualty processing and evacuation, and clearing companies for early medical care. In the British sector, the 2nd Casualty Clearing Station was positioned in support of the 1st British Division. Huddleston decided to place surgeons of the 2nd Auxiliary Surgical Group with the British as well as the American 33rd Field Hospital and Ranger battalions. Offshore, three British Red Cross vessels were available on D-Day: HMHS *St. David*, HMHS *St. Andrew*, and HMHS *Leinster*.[12] In his calculations, it might barely be enough. Projected casualties were 15 percent for the first week and 8 percent for the second. After that, daily hospital admission estimates from battle and nonbattle casualties were 5 per 1,000, or 500 per 100,000 men—one half of 1 percent.[13]

From the beachhead, casualties were to be evacuated by sea. There was no land route, and air transport was never seriously considered. The G-4 (logistics) plan hinged on frequent convoys of LSTs and Liberty ships from Naples and North African ports. Supplies would be preloaded in trucks and DUKWs—massive numbers—for rapid off-loading at the beachhead. For the landings, planners felt it imperative that at least thirty-five days' worth of supplies be delivered because of those unpredictable crises—bad weather, rough seas, enemy air action—that so often plagued naval shipping. Once emptied of food, troops, ammunition, and guns. those LSTs and Liberty ships could backfill with wounded for the return trip to Naples.

Task Force 81, commanded by Rear Admiral Frank Lowry left Naples on January 21. Three hundred sixty-four vessels—242 troop carriers, mostly LSTs and LCIs (landing craft, infantry)—and 122 naval craft headed for the Cape of Anzio. The convoy split into two teams, Task Force X-Ray heading for the American sector, and Task Force Peter, for the British sector.[14] Landing craft throttled up, turned about, and were shepherded to shore by patrol boats. Overhead was a brief but thunderous rocket barrage designed to suppress any enemy reaction. Assault waves touched down on time at 2:00 AM in pitch blackness on Anzio's resort beaches north and south of town. Caught by surprise, the Germans offered little resistance. Only three engineering companies and the 2nd Battalion 71st Panzer Grenadier Regiment had been left to guard the coast from the mouth of the Tiber near Rome all the way to the Mussolini Canal south of Nettuno. Allied troops fanned out across the beaches, rousting sleeping Germans from their bunks and disposing of those who managed to fire a weapon. The American 3rd Infantry Divi-

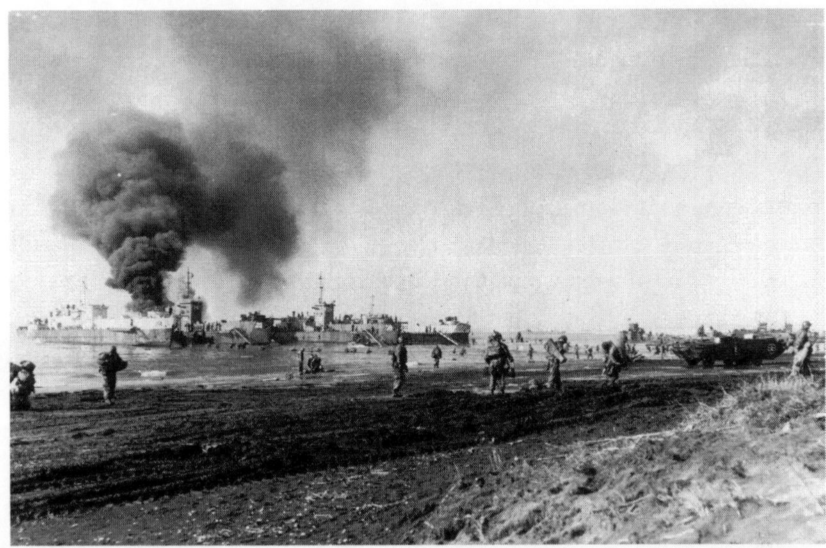

Troops and equipment come ashore on the U.S. Fifth Army beachhead near Anzio, January 22, 1944. USS *LCI-20* is burning at left, after being hit by a German bomb. At right, on the beach is a DUKW. (*National Archives*)

sion seized its D-Day objectives on the right flank and center, and set up positions along the main and west branches of the Mussolini Canal. British commandos secured the left flank to the Moletta River, and Colonel William Darby's commando-style rangers stormed through the town of Anzio, olive drab fatigues in stark contrast to pink and white vacation villas. They met few wanting to fight. To the southeast, paratroopers of the 509th Parachute Infantry swept through Nettuno. In response, the Germans managed a few paltry air attacks, most of their bombs splashing harmlessly into the sea. So far, Shingle had gone smashingly. Lucas's VI Corps was in place. By midnight of D-Day, thirty-six thousand men and three thousand two hundred vehicles were ashore. By the following day, the beachhead extended seven miles deep.[15]

Unit (Platoon) B of the 33rd Field Hospital, landed on Red beach in the X-Ray (American) sector on D-Day evening—the first medical team ashore. A temporary hospital was hurriedly set up southeast of Nettuno and saw the bulk of the casualties—mercifully few, less than one hundred. Early Sunday morning, *LST-226* carrying members of the 52nd Medical Battalion beached on Red. They were directed to the site of the nearby 33rd Field Hospital. Three collecting stations and a clearing unit were functioning by noon, and by the end of the day, 136 patients had been seen.[16] In succession Sunday, the 3rd Med Battalion came in with its three collecting teams and clearing company. Ten surgical and two "shock" teams from the 2nd Auxiliary Surgical Group joined the 33rd Field Hospital.[17] Two teams of "Auxers" were temporarily split off to support Ranger battalions. For the first forty-eight hours, the 33rd Field Hospital and its satellite teams were the main American medical complex ashore. The 33rd already had three operating tables set up, shortly working to capacity. In the Peter (British) sector, a detachment of the 35th Beach Group Medical Section, the 3rd Field Dressing Station, raced ashore and put up tents just outside of Anzio. Wounded—both GIs and Brits—were ushered off the beachhead by men of the 52nd Med Battalion, who coordinated what amounted to a well-choreographed shuttle of patients from hospital to dock to landing craft, all under the constant threat of air raids.[18]

One of the surgeons at the 33rd Field Hospital was Major Floyd Taylor. Taylor was a native Texan, educated at Baylor Medical College in Dallas. He did his surgical training—four years—at West Baltimore General Hospital in Maryland. Immediately following that, he was called to active duty in 1941 and stationed at Fort Meade in Maryland. Fort Meade had become the focal point of the army's field medicine, a major training site for casualty care. There Taylor befriended a number of surgeons, all reservists, as they rotated through—former academicians from Walter Reed and Columbia University and the University of Buffalo. After the attack on Pearl Harbor, Taylor was rushed to the Mayo Clinic for an intensive three-month course in anesthesia, then to Massachusetts General Hospital in September 1942. There he was introduced to a new concept in battlefield care: Colonel Churchill's auxiliary surgical group. Teams included a surgeon, assistant surgeon, nurse, and two enlisted surgical assistants. They were meant to provide early, life-saving forward surgical care, linking with field hospitals and clearing companies. All surgeons were young (average age thirty-four) but fully trained, many with at least a few years of experience. Taylor was part of the 2nd Surgical Group, the first to be deployed in combat. By November, his team was on a troopship to Casablanca as part of Operation Torch, the invasion of North Africa. Then Salerno, where war became up close and personal. A half-track in front of Taylor's truck was hit by a German shell and burst into flames. He watched two occupants burn alive "before our eyes." In another instant, it would have been him. Now they were at

Anzio. Taylor's team was assigned to the 33rd Field Hospital without its nurses, who arrived days later. His initial impression of Anzio: "[T]he first thing we did when we got off the beach, we'd dig foxholes."[19]

A few Luftwaffe planes buzzed the fleet on D-Day but did precious little damage. However, this was only a brief respite. Hermann Goering's air force did not sit idle. He quickly shifted fighter and bomber groups from France and Greece. Flights of Junkers 88s and Messerschmitts picked up, with hit-and-run strafing and bombing raids on the harbor every few hours. Particularly lethal were the attacks at dusk, even incorporating new radio-guided bombs. In the late afternoon of January 24, a red alert (enemy planes approaching) was called. Before long, dive and torpedo bombers were swarming the flotilla. Three British hospital ships—the *Leinster*, *St. Andrew*, and *St. David*—circled at station, well lighted and clearly marked with Red Cross identification. They were miles away from combatant ships, the closest being the light cruiser USS *Brooklyn* (CL 40). In the fading daylight, flares were dropped by enemy planes to illuminate shipping. Just after six o'clock, the *Leinster* was hit by a bomb, but the subsequent fires were quickly put out. Forty-five minutes later, more bombs fell around the hospital ships. The *St. Andrew* and *Leinster* reported near misses. After the spray and smoke cleared, officers on the *Brooklyn* could make out only the *Leinster* and *St. Andrew*. The *St. David* was "missing," and the *Brooklyn* soon received word it was sinking. Around 7:30 PM, one bomb had hit the *St. David* at the No. 3 hold near the promenade deck—perhaps a radar-guided missile. The same plane banked and dropped two more bombs, both striking amidship. The *St. David* stopped dead in the water, lights went out, and it began settling by the stern, then listing to port. Captain Evan Owens, realizing his ship was foundering, gave the order to abandon it. Just five minutes after the first bomb strike, the *St. David* could no longer be seen. Three hours later, the *St. Andrew* began picking up survivors. Captain Owens had been one of the last to leave his ship. He was seen at one point swimming in the water but was never recovered and never sighted again. Twelve crew, twenty-two patients, and twenty-two Royal Army Medical Corps staff—including Elizabeth Dixon and Winnie Harrison, two nurses of the Reserve Queen Alexandra's Imperial Nursing Service—were also lost.

On board the *St. David* had been Team No. 4 of the 2nd Auxiliary Surgical Group—an orthopedic specialty unit. Major John Adams was one of the team's medical officers. He was an orthopedic surgeon from the University of Virginia. Most knew him as friendly, upbeat "Major Johnny." Team 4 had been operating all day January 23, rested a few hours, and were up again just before midnight. Warnings had already blared that German planes were bombing harbor and beaches. Even then, the team continued on in rocking seas, many gripped with seasickness, working clear through to the early morning—seventy-eight patients passed through. By then the sea was so rough no new patients could be brought aboard. Team members thought they would have a quiet, restful day. Two surgical nurses, Lieutenants Ruth Hindman and Anna Berret, had been asleep in their cabin all afternoon when sometime after seven o'clock, explosions shook them awake. Lights had gone out. They were in total darkness. Both ran to the upper deck, where they met Major Adams, who helped them into their lifejackets. Despite a capsizing ship, Adams insisted on going back below. "I have to check on a couple of patients to make sure they got out," were his last words. There was no time for lifeboats—the ship was rolling over—and both nurses jumped. Somehow they found a raft and were picked up by the *Leinster*. Major Johnny Adams would not be rescued, however. He was the first medical officer lost at Anzio, first to be declared missing in action, then, finally, killed in action. He was not the last.[20]

Colonel Huddleston wasted no time getting his three evacuation hospitals ashore. All had been preloaded in deuce-and-a-halfs, piled full with canvas and cots and linens and bandages, stretchers, sterilizers and generators, surgical chests bursting with hemostats, needle holders, scalpels, abdominal retractors, rib spreaders, gowns and gloves—and all the innumerable T/O & E items.[21] Trucks were coaxed aboard warehouse-size LSTs at Naples and stored bumper to bumper in one big olive drab parking lot. Officers and enlisted filled in where they could, the diesel fumes almost nauseating. Some doctors and nurses boarded smaller LCIs that rocked and rolled their way to Anzio. Nurse Lieutenant Avis Dagit with the 56th Evac Hospital recalled the "choking, stale air" in the cramped bowels of their LCI, which was bouncing so violently that retching soon commenced. One bucket was the only receptacle for community *vomitus*. "Those that could not reach the bucket used their helmet for an emesis basin," she remembered.[22] Indeed, high seas and strong storms assured most of good doses of seasickness. Once at Anzio, to a person, they were ready to get ashore. Most were seasick and nervous about air raids. Anything—even enemy shelling—had to be better than upchucking over the side or being blown into the water.

Staff of the 93rd Evacuation Hospital had taken down their tents at Caivano near the Winter Line and left for Naples. The 93rd Evac first assembled at Fort Meade, Maryland, in 1942 as a four-hundred-bed, semimobile hospital commanded by Colonel Donald Currier. In April, they were shipped to Casablanca, Morocco, as part of Operation Torch and eventually were located at Oran, Algeria. Next came Operation Husky, the invasion of Sicily, and then landings at Paestum as part of Avalanche. They had moved twice since then, finally locating near Caivano. On January 19, 1944, 37 officers and 195 enlisted boarded their LST and headed for Anzio as part of Operation Shingle. On board were also members of the British 2nd Casualty Clearing Station and a number of American quartermasters and truck drivers. Belowdecks were trucks loaded with ammunition; medical officers, confined to the upper deck, were sure they were sitting on time bombs. With some relief, their LST reached Anzio intact on January 23. All departed in the middle of a red alert and took over a building in Anzio. That did not last. German artillery targeted the place and shortly reduced the quaint seaside buildings to rubble. Anzio's docks were a primary target. Explosions bracketed the 93rd, killing Sergeant Louis Bliss, who was struck in the head by flying shrapnel. That was enough for Huddleston. He ordered the hospital out, finding a wide plot of ground three miles due east of Nettuno and less than a mile from the beach. It was here that he intended to place all hospitals, brilliantly marked with Red Crosses. The Germans would even be given the coordinates to avoid shelling.

A second four-hundred-bed, semimobile evacuation hospital, the 95th, unloaded from *LST-168*—doctors only, nurses would come later. In those first days, most ships beached effortlessly—there were few air raids, no artillery—nothing like the debacle at Salerno. *LST-168* was no exception. Some speculated that it was a trap, but unloading on Green beach proceeded without a hitch, and by nightfall the hospital had set up in a bucolic expanse of grass just outside Nettuno. The 95th Evac was also a veteran unit, having seen action in North Africa and Salerno. Colonel Paul Sauer, a surgeon from New York, was the commanding officer. Chief of the Surgical Service was colorful Lieutenant Colonel Grantley Taylor, a Harvard graduate and surgeon from Massachusetts General Hospital. In civilian life, Dr. Taylor had specialized in breast diseases. He was noted for his blunt, shoot-from-the-hip comments. When asked how long it should take to examine a breast, Taylor replied, "if you take longer than five minutes it quits being scientific and becomes social." Before starting a big case, he might say, "We're not berry picking today, we're out for salmon." Being left handed, he welcomed a left-handed scrub nurse, referring to his team as the "Sinister Team."[23] But underneath the wry humor, Taylor was an intense clinician. He planned to mold a first-rate combat hospital, one that could handle any injury regardless of location and complexity. He and Sauer shared a common philosophy that every doctor should cross-train so that those patients with multiple injuries could be handled by one surgical team. Chest and general surgeons should be as adept at extremity and skeletal trauma as his orthopedic surgeons. Every surgeon was a "general" surgeon; no prima donnas would be tolerated.

On January 28, just as the nurses were arriving, Huddleston ordered the 95th Evac to tear down and set up in the same expanse as the 93rd. Disquieting features of the new compound were a battery of 155-mm howitzers to the rear, a small airstrip to the front, a radar station to one side, and a petroleum dump to the other. All were prime targets for German guns, and smack in the middle were the hospitals. Huddleston had placed his hospitals just six miles from the fighting line. The usual placement of evacuation hospitals was from twelve to twenty miles in the rear. Trajectories of incoming shells varied widely—even with detailed coordinates, errors of over 100 yards—the distance of a football field—were not uncommon. Without question, some would find their way into the compound. That plot of sacred, Red Cross ground dotted with olive-drab tents and rows of embankments would soon be called "Hell's Half Acre," not at all immune to the endless screeching, arching shells whose final destination were too often short or long—right in their midst. Nurse Mary Fisher would never forget: "[T]here was the real nuisance of the Screaming Meemies— the big Jerry guns. We could hear the report of the artillery and then the shell whistling overhead on its way to the sea. The shelling continued as long as the Allies held the beachhead."[24]

Dr. Arthur deGrandpre, a major in the Medical Corps, was a thirty-four-year-old general surgeon with the 95th. He had attended medical school at Georgetown University and completed almost eighteen months of a rotating internship at Albany General Hospital in New York. DeGrandpre then set up practice in Plattsburgh, New York, and gained more on-the-job surgical training working with an established surgeon—a not-so-uncommon apprentice arrangement. Dr. deGrandpre signed up for military service in September 1942, and, because of his experience, was designated a general surgeon. He was eventually placed in the 95th Evac and joined the unit in August 1943. By the time deGrandpre landed on Green beach at Salerno, he was already a veteran of North Africa. But even the violence of Salerno paled in comparison to Anzio, he found. His journal contained entries charged with dread as one explosion after another marked his life on the beachhead. "At Anzio life is one continuous bit of hell," he wrote at one point. "There has been no sleep in almost a week, now," an entry read on January 30.[25]

Twelve-hour shifts were the norm, sometimes longer. Trench coats and helmets were removed (until bombardments eventually persuaded them otherwise), and boots hosed off. Surgical caps and masks were donned, hands washed and dipped in alcohol. Then they were gowned and gloved by nurses in fatigues, field jackets, and boots. After each case, the gowns, gloves, syringes, and needles were re-sterilized. Nothing was disposable. Then another hand dip in alcohol, new gown and gloves, and on to the next patient.

The 56th Evacuation Hospital was known as the Baylor unit. Under the direction of Army Surgeon General James Magee, the Board of Regents of the Baylor University Medical Center in Dallas organized an army hospital, appointing Dr. Henry Winans, professor of medicine, as commander in August 1940. He was eventually replaced by Colonel Henry Blesse. The 56th Evac was a large, 750-bed unit, sacrificing mobility for size, now referred to as "motorized," not "mobile." The unit had landed at Salerno and moved to near the Winter Line at a place called Dragoni. Despite almost one thousand five hundred admissions for December, battle casualties were few—only twelve. Most soldiers suffered from some form of veneral disease, respiratory infections, hepatitis, or malaria. January was not much different, with only fourteen battle casualties. With the closing of the hospital at Dragoni midmonth, rumors ran wild that the unit was going to England, northern Italy, the Pacific, or even Brooklyn. Instead, 111 trucks and 20 trailers took personnel and equipment to the staging area at Caivano. On January 23, Colonel Blesse dispelled the rumors and announced a new assignment: Anzio. The next day, a sober medical staff boarded their boats. "We were a grim crew aboard our LCI. We believe our cohorts on the other vessels were equally grim. No one felt like talking much," the record read. And the voyage was not much help. Storms, wind, and miserable cold battered the group, rolling their LCI so drastically many thought it would capsize. Not a few lined the bulwarks, tossing army rations into the sea. The rest prayed to Saint Anthony, the patron saint of sailors.[26] Lingering off shore at Anzio was not much better. For thirty-six hours they were subjected to at least fourteen dive-bomb raids before putting ashore.

Yet their arrival on Anzio's docks was picture perfect: a sunny day, almost a postcard rendering of an Italian holiday. It was short lived, to be sure. Seeing hospital personnel lolling around taking snapshots, sentries yelled, "What the hell are you women doing here? This place is hot! Take the first vehicle you can and get out of here."[27] And with that, German aircraft screamed above, heading straight for the harbor. The first choice for the hospital had been a former tuberculosis sanitarium, but a few close blasts by German artillery changed all that. The staff spent more time huddled in the basement than taking care of casualties. Medical care was impossible with the number of incoming rounds. No one doubted that the Germans intended to pound Anzio and Nettuno into dust. It was then, of course, that Colonel Huddleston decided to move all hospitals away from town. The 56th Evac and its six teams of 2nd Auxers were the first to open in the new location on January 30. Evacuation hospitals were designed for combat, tents arranged to accommodate mass casualties. From ambulances, patients were hurried into the preoperative area, inspected, x-rayed, and sent on to one of the four operating tables in an adjacent tent. There, surgeons were waiting, assigned to eight-hour shifts, but before long, few left even after twelve hours.[28]

By February 2, all of Huddleston's hospitals were ashore. In the American sector, the new hospital site—Hell's Half Acre—was occupied by the 56th, 93rd, and 95th Evacs and two platoons of the 33rd Field Hospital. The 93rd took a site east of the 56th, and the 95th a location northwest of the 56th. In the British sector, the 2nd Casualty Clearing Station was relocated to an open area three miles due north of Anzio town just short of the Padiglione Woods, east of the Anzio-Albano-Rome highway, also referred to as the Via Anziate.[29] Huddleston now had 1,750 beds at his disposal.

In early January, comedian Joe E. Brown and tough-guy actor Humphrey Bogart had entertained troops of the 120th Medical Battalion of the 45th Infantry Division—the Thunderbirds—in the Italian village of Calvisi, a respite from their bloody work on the Volturno front. On January 24, loaded in a string of cargo trucks, the unit and its division departed for Aversa, then Naples, and onto LSTs bound for Anzio. Elements of the division had been pulled from the Winter Line and were to be reserves for Shingle. But few veterans doubted they would set foot on Anzio's streets. Not two days later, General Lucas ordered the 45th

Division's 179th Regimental Combat Team ashore. By February 1, the two remaining regiments were ashore northeast of Nettuno, filling in the center of Allied lines. The Med Battalion did not land until January 30. Few enemy planes were seen—Allied air patrols were now frequent—and only scattered artillery shells flew overhead. It was nothing like the rumors of fire and smoke and confusion that greeted other newcomers. Collecting companies deployed in support of the 179th Infantry, and clearing units set up just a mile from Nettuno. For several days, business was light. Doctors seemed more concerned about venereal disease and penile lesions than gunshot wounds. All that soon changed.[30]

HITLER WAS INFURIATED at the Allied landings, vowing to "lance the abscess south of Rome."[31] Indeed, there was a response, and a furious one. Kesselring had long suspected an Allied end run but couldn't tell where. Once he knew Anzio was the site, he activated Case Richard, a prearranged deployment of troops south of Rome. Hitler intended to hurl massive forces at Anzio, determined to defend Italy and Rome at all costs. Obsessed with the whole affair, he ordered mobilization of troops outside Italy, from France, Yugoslavia, and even Deutschland itself. Almost immediately, the 4th Parachute and Hermann Goering Panzer Divisions were on the road, and the 3rd Panzer Grenadier and 71st Infantry Divisions were brought up from the south. The 26th Panzer, the strongest German armored group in Italy, followed. By January 25, elements of fourteen divisions of Panzer and parachute troops funneled in around Anzio and ringed the beachhead. All forces were put under the command of General Eberhard von Mackensen's Fourteenth Army. Mackensen led the ruthless charge through Poland in 1939, occupied France, and battled the Soviets on the Russian front. He commanded in Italy with an iron fist and fully intended to toss the Allies into the Tyrrhenian Sea. Under his leadership, within days, the Germans had shut in the Allies, their formations a mere four or five miles from the Allied front. Distant hills bristled with artillery of all sizes, perfectly capable of hitting anywhere in the beachhead. Almost five hundred pieces were brought up and dug in: 105-mm *leichte* Feldhaubitze; 150-, 170-, and 210-mm Nebelwerfer and Kanone; and giant 240-mm Haubitze, which tossed a shell weighing 360 pounds.[32]

American and British forces were now hemmed in and targeted. Lucas had lost his narrow window for expansion. He had balked, feeling the Allies had too few troops. Determined foes now tilted and clashed in the towns and paths around Anzio, furious efforts by pompous aggressors and humbled defenders. Cisterna, Aprilia, and the roads to Rome were filled with bloodshed for months to come. The Fortunes of Antium swung from Allied to Axis as "Anzio" became synonymous with the befuddled and besieged. Mackensen was supremely confident that this would be another Dunkirk, that the Allies would be swimming before long. "Ver is der sea?" one smug German major asked his British captor in accented English, and when the direction was pointed out he replied, "Tank you very much, I vanted to know for you will soon be in it."[33]

On January 24, the bloodletting began. Irish guards of the 1st British Division ventured up the tree-lined Anzio-Albano road toward Carroceto, a waystation to Campoleone. It started out a sunny day, almost like a training exercise, Italian farmers by the side waving and clapping at their liberators. But at the outskirts of Aprilia, they ran smack into German machine-gun and self-propelled artillery fire; big 88-mm Flak cannon lowered their barrels and sent flat trajectories right into thin-walled Bren carriers. No match for that, the British beat a hasty retreat back. Next day they tried again, punching their way into Aprilia but fighting hand to hand with stubborn Germans to do so. Finally victorious, they were hit hard by counterattacks that reduced the town to rubble and reigned murderous fire on the guardsmen who were left. German gunners were uncannily accurate from their observation posts in the Alban Hills—a taste of what was to come at Anzio. Panzer grenadiers and Tiger tanks followed in and almost reclaimed the town, but the British held on. Front-line aid stations and ambulances could barely keep up with the flood of casualties, most of them victims of shelling. Desmond Fitzgerald, then a lieutenant in the Irish Guards, described the carnage at a place just outside Aprilia labeled, sardonically, the "Dung Farm" for its rotting corpses:

> The ambulance was running a non-stop shuttle service up and down the road direct to the [2nd] Casualty Clearing Station. . . . Between bandaging wounds, the medical orderlies worked to deepen the ditch and roof it with old iron fencing and earth. . . . A man denied of blood gets very cold, there is not much a man with a shattered thigh can do for himself; a man whose chest has been torn to ribbons by shell-splinters would like to be moved out of the barrage. But they did not say anything.[34]

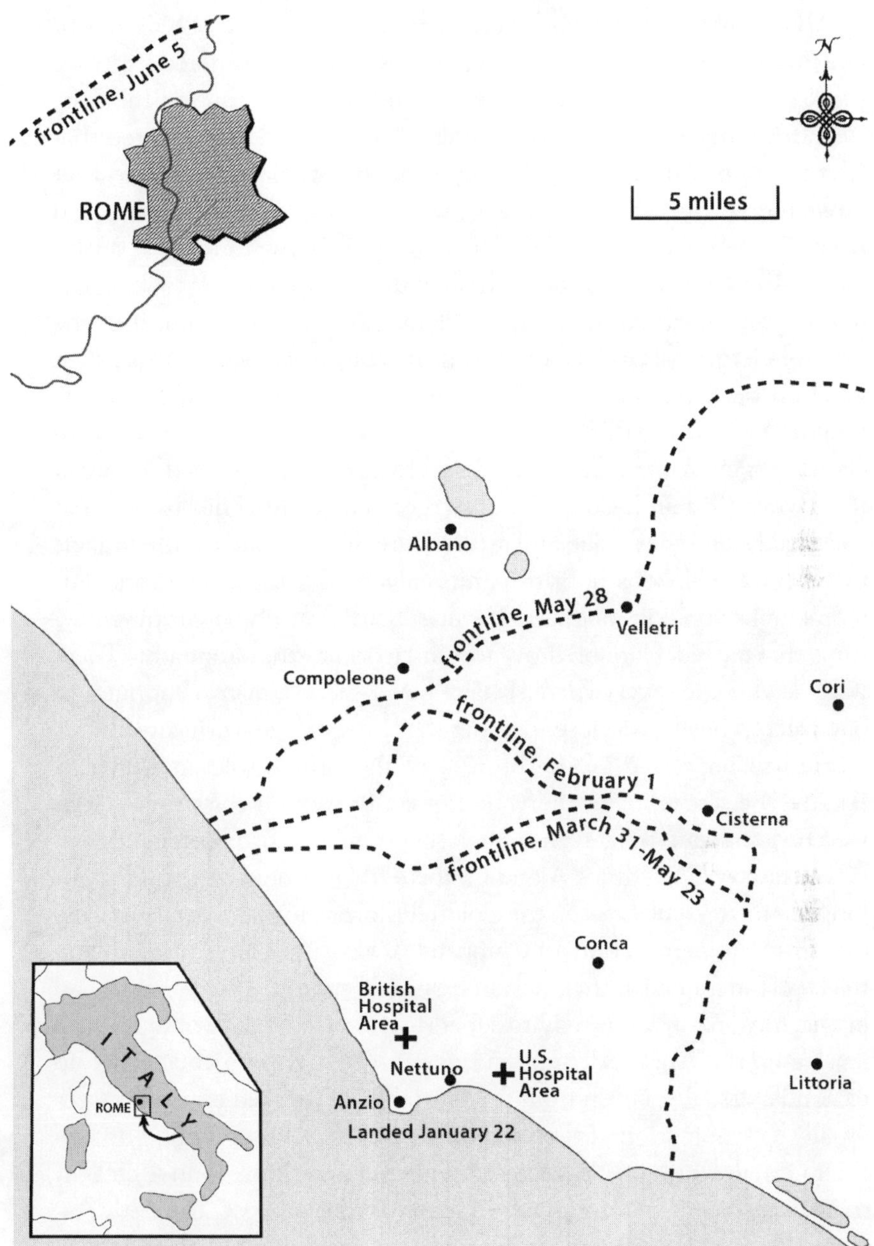

Map 2. The Anzio Beachhead, January–May 1944.

The Allies were reinforced on January 27 by the arrival of Major General Ernest Harmon's Combat Command A of the 1st Armored Division, including the 1st Armored Regiment and the 6th Armored Infantry. With his tankers on board, on January 28, General Lucas insisted that Campoleone and Cisterna were ripe for the taking—a decision that proved too little and too late. Both were access points for Route 6 and Route 7, vital objectives for VI Corps. In the western prong—the British sector—he sent his beleaguered Irish and Scots guardsmen back up the Anzio road—with Harmon's tanks flanking—straight, again, into the teeth of German defenders solidly dug in. The attack faltered in the mud and hill country, terrain not appreciated by aerial photographs and certainly not friendly to thirty-ton Sherman tanks. The behemoths soon impotently spun their treads in gullys and streams that seemed to engulf them while the bull-headed Harmon raged. The weather had turned cold and cloudy, and the smoke and artillery fire made it hard for the tankers to see. It was a bloodbath; British units pulverized in the Dung Farm, Harmon's tanks mired in mud, and German Panzers machine-gunning anything that moved. Harmon drove forward to survey the aftermath: "There were dead bodies everywhere. I have never seen so many dead men in one place. They lay so close together that I had to step with care."[35]

He was impressed by the bravery of the British soldiers that day. Amidst the screaming artillery, hail of gunfire, and incessant cold rain they had borne up well, even though half their men had been cut down.

For tanker Companies A and C, the 47th Armored Medical Battalion, commanded by Lieutenant Colonel Morris Holtsclaw, was waiting. The first treatment station for Company A was east of the Anzio-Albano road and functioned as the division treatment station. The company had moved forward on January 30 to support the western prong of Lucas's offensive up the Anzio-Albano road. A clearing station had been set up to handle casualties fresh from the battlefield. Armored casualties were usually a combination of smashed limbs, punctured torsos, and burns—the internal explosions and fires from piercing antitank rounds created murderous conditions on crews. In fact, for that purpose, the 47th Armored Medical Battalion had developed a roving surgical unit in a modified deuce-and-a-half. Tents were carried in the cab of the truck and could be pulled and deployed within fifteen minutes—and taken down just as fast. For rapid armor movement, this provided some degree of immediacy for the care of critically wounded soldiers, particularly ones in shock.[36] For most of February, with Combat Command A held in reserve,

Company A pulled back to the British hospital complex about two miles north of the town of Anzio just off the Anzio-Albano road. Company C opened a second treatment station a few miles east of the road to better service the tankers. Holtsclaw's surgical truck took care of many wounded; those more seriously stricken were stabilized and taken to evac hospitals.

To the east, American units focused on the tiny town of Cisterna, a direct route to the Appian Way. It was no better. The attack involved all regiments of the 3rd Infantry Division but was spearheaded by elite Ranger units. On the right flank, two battalions of rangers were to infiltrate and occupy Cisterna and wait for elements of General Truscott's 3rd Division. Counting on stealth and surprise, the rangers stripped down to the bare essentials: no packs, parkas, K-rations, or extra canteens. It was a monumental failure. Rangers were caught in wide-open fields by alert and well-positioned German defenders. Of 767 men who set out that night, 761 did not return, either killed or captured. The 4th Ranger Battalion attempted to rescue them but was also ambushed and ripped apart, caught between machine guns and tanks. Strings of men fell in succession, unable to evade riveting fire from crack German paratroopers. One young private witnessed the "mess": "The medic captain and the major were both crying—they knew those guys . . . the doctor was taking their dog tags. He was covered with blood, and so were the dog tags. He was crying because he knew them. We had been right behind them. I don't know how we got out."[37]

Those who remained—who did not get out—clung to the ground and were finished off by roving enemy tanks.

Mixed in with infantry were battalion medical teams. Colonel Darby, in his memoir *Darby's Rangers*, told of one battalion surgeon, "a big man with a lantern jaw and a long record of Ranger combat" from the 3rd Battalion, who was captured and apparently shot in the face and killed. Some reports indicated he refused to leave his wounded men, others, after he himself pulled a captor's sidearm and shot him.[38] There is no official record of who this doctor was or if it even happened. What is known for sure is that another battalion surgeon for the 3rd Rangers, Captain Gordon Keppel, was captured that day and spent the rest of the war as a prisoner at Stalag 7a in Bavaria. Keppel, a young medical officer from Montrose, New York, had said of the Rangers, "there was nobody like them," captivated by their resistance to fatigue and resilience after injury. So impressed had Keppel been that he wrote Colonel Darby to ask to join the Rangers. In short order Keppel was appointed battalion surgeon. His first battle was at San Pietro, on the way to Monte Cassino, near the Gustav Line. It was a frightening experience he later admitted, but he knew he had to crawl out of his hole to tend to his men. "In one hour there were twenty-five wounded, and I went to them with plasma and sulpha and bandages. It's strange, but I didn't notice the shelling at the time."[39]

The entire push on Cisterna was thrown back by a stout German defense, elements of the 3rd Division basically stalling out behind the rangers' disaster.[40] Mackensen's Panzers quickly closed any penetrations by the Americans. Even a second and a third attempt by 3rd Division troopers the next day failed, crushed by thick German defenses manned by paratroopers and Panzer grenadiers. Enormous numbers of casualties filtered back to field hospitals. The clearing station of the 3rd Medical Battalion (Company D) had arrived on January 22 and set up both hospital platoons about two miles east of Nettuno as sophisticated first aid stations. They were in position for the January offensive. Just in time, the bitter fighting before Cisterna produced a good many chopped-up infantry, bewildered by the intensity of enemy resistance. On January 30, 151 were seen, and the following day, 352.[41]

All then prepared for the German counteroffensive that was sure to come. The mission of Mackensen's Fourteenth Army was explicit: annihilate the beachhead. February became the bloodiest month of the siege by far. Over at the 95th Evac, Arthur deGrandpre found himself quite occupied those first few days of February. "Lots of hard work," he wrote. "Performing a lot of brain work . . . big German guns keep shooting at us over our heads every night—at least three of them—and scare the daylights out of us."[42]

9

Hell's Half Acre

THAT SHELLING WAS PART OF A PREPPING BARRAGE FOR THE GERMAN counteroffensive in early February. Every effort was made to destroy ammunition and fuel dumps toward the rear of the Allied beachhead—just behind Hell's Half Acre. The scream and whine of rounds coursing over the hospital compound was distinctly unsettling, and for good reason: a few fell short. On February 4, a few landed in the 33rd Field Hospital area, pulverizing several ward tents. Luckily there were no injuries. Luftwaffe bombing raids proved more lethal. The morning of February 7, twenty enemy planes strafed the port towns of Anzio and Nettuno, and bombs landed near VI Corps headquarters at the Hotel de Ville in Nettuno. These proved deadly effective. Colonel Huddleston was there, narrowly escaping injury. He pitched in filtering through casualties, indifferent to the Messerschmitts overhead, banking and turning for more strafing runs.

A few miles away at the 95th Evacuation Hospital that day, it was business as usual. Harbor raids were far enough distant that although rumbling tumbled through camp and smoke leaped from the horizon, they were mostly ignored. On that day, the hospital was at capacity with four hundred patients; the shock tent, operating tent, and x-ray tent were in full swing; and a taxi line of ambulances loaded with wounded waited in front of the receiving tent. It was then that nurse Mary Fisher heard a high-pitched whining noise. One of those ugly, tan Messerschmitts was barreling toward the hospital not more than thirty feet off the ground, chased by two British Spitfires. In a gamble to gain altitude, the pilot loosed his antipersonnel bombs and climbed steeply. The Spitfires followed, and soon the Messerschmitt was spiraling, trailing smoke, toward the ground. The pilot parachuted to safety. But his bombs found their mark in Hell's Half Acre. These were so-called Butterfly bombs: small, 2-kilogram submunitions containing 225 grams of TNT. Usually carried in packages of six to sometimes over a hundred, their kill zone reached a radius of 10 yards and could wound up to 100 yards, patterns murderous for ground troops. Six Butterfly bombs walked a pattern from one side of the 95th Evacuation Hospital to the other. Explosions and fragments tore through the headquarters tent, the evacuation tent, four feet from preoperative, midway between the receiving tent and Ward No. 1. One even hit with tragic irony on a large canvas Red Cross marker spread out fifty feet from the hospital's laboratory.

Surgeon Zachary Friedenberg ran over to the wreckage hoping not to find what he soon did: wounded and dead patients, nurses, doctors, and corpsmen. Blood ran in rivulets into the soil, he remembered. His assistant, Sergeant Watschke, lay on the floor with a jagged hole in his chest pouring blood, and a weak, thready pulse. Frantically searching for instruments, Friedenberg grabbed hemostats and was able to find and clamp bleeding intercostal arteries, which slowed the hemorrhage. Plugging the open chest wound with a battle dressing helped calm Watschke's breathing. He was taken to a neighboring hospital, his ultimate fate in doubt.[1] Bombs caught some surgeons in the middle of operations. With amazing aplomb, none even broke stride to complete their tasks. Surgeon Willard "Bob" Courter pushed his nurse anesthetist under the operating table while he finished his operation. The nurse, Adeline Simonson, managed to still keep her hand on the syringe of pentothal she was administering. He wrapped up his work as if nothing had happened. Lieutenant Colonel Howard Patterson was delicately probing a patient's skull when one of the bomblets fell close to the tent, sending hot fragments whizzing. His hands never faltered.

Others felt the full violence of the blasts. Lieutenant Virginia Barton had just kneeled to give a patient plasma. An explosion lifted and threw her against the cross bars of a cot; she was alive but temporarily stone deaf from ruptured eardrums. But two first lieutenants standing just feet from Barton were not so fortunate. Thirty-six-year-old Chief Nurse Blanche Sigman and Pennsylvanian Carrie Sheetz were both intent on starting an intravenous drip on a patient. Both were killed instantly in the blast, along with their patient. "I'm quite nervous," Sigman had writ-

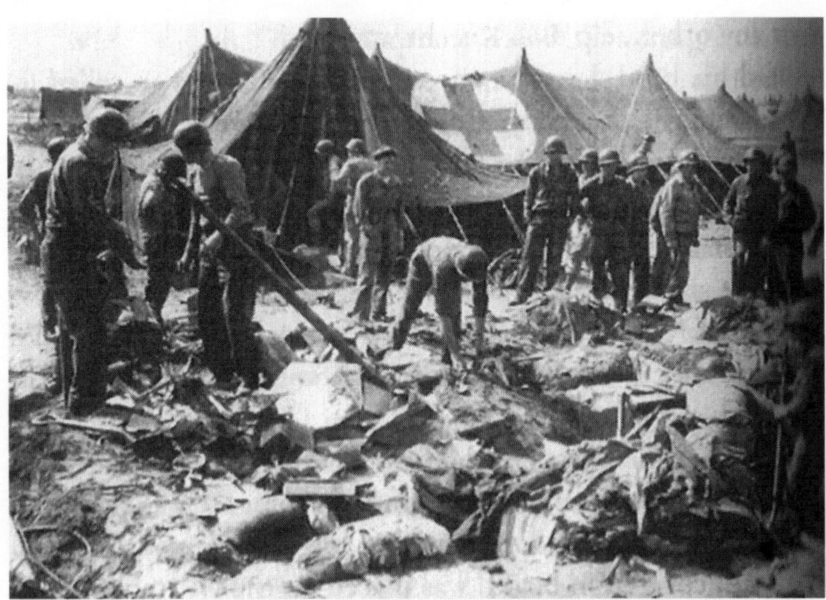

The 95th Evacuation Hospital was struck at Anzio by a German bomb on February 7, 1944, killing six patients and twenty-two hospital personnel. Fragments ripped through the administrative, receiving, and operating room tents. (*National Archives*)

ten days before, but added "we are staying in the tents so we can be near the patients" during air raids.[2] And that is exactly where she was that fateful Monday morning. Sigman and Sheetz were every bit the fiber of the 95th, always close to their patients and close to their nurses. It was what one would expect from the first officers appointed to the 95th when it was activated in August 1942 at Camp Breckinridge, Kentucky.

The carnage was indescribable. One of the nurses, Lieutenant Mary Fisher, later wrote in her diary:

> We found dead and wounded all over. Everyone got busy and first-aid was given to those who needed it. Pulses were felt of others, then [they were] covered with blankets. We had seen death many times in our hospital, but it never affected us as it did now when we faced the immediate sorrow.[3]

Twenty-six-year-old Second Lieutenant Marjorie "Gertrude" Morrow, a nurse from Fort Dodge, Iowa, had just received her first mail since arriving at Anzio. One of the blasts blew off both her legs at the hips and pulped both kidneys. Desperate efforts to save her were to no avail. She died during surgery. One of the favorites of the hospital was Red Cross worker Esther Richards. She was seen about two hours before the bombing sheepishly peering from the standard foxhole dug under her cot. She had served as an army nurse in World War I, been educated at the University of California at Berkeley and Columbia University, and had received her master's degree. The Second World War caught her too old for overseas duty in the Nursing Corps, but the idea of not serving was unthinkable. Undaunted, she signed up for the American Red Cross as a volunteer worker, ending up somehow on the Anzio beachhead. It was her last assignment. She was caught in the February 7 bombing, splattered by bomb fragments. Fellow Red Cross workers hurried her to the surgery tent, but she also died on the operating table, the first Red Cross worker killed in the war. Two officers, Captain Al Shroeder and Lieutenant Albert Heywood, both suffered fatal head injuries and died almost at once. Sixteen enlisted men, four patients, and two other military personnel were also fatalities. DeGrandpre recalled: "A boy [civilian] visiting his wounded brother, falls across him to protect him and gets killed. . . . One of my patients with a fractured skull receives another fractured skull, while being x-rayed and is killed."[4]

Hospital commander Colonel Paul Sauer was struck in the leg and shoulder. Two medical officers, Captain Henry Luce, hit in the chest, and Captain Henry Korda, hit in the chest and arm, ignored their wounds to tend the wounded and dying. Colonel Sauer was evacuated (he was soon able to return), and the command was turned over to Lieutenant Colonel Hubert Binkley. A total of four nurses, thirty-six enlisted men, and ten patients also suffered injuries. All wounded were transferred to other hospitals in the compound. The 95th Evac was rendered disabled, its operating tent and two surgical tents shredded, surgical equipment ruined.

Yet even with all the senseless tragedy, wonders still appeared. At the 33rd Field Hospital, 2nd Auxiliary surgeons repaired a ruptured popliteal artery on a wounded sergeant, a pioneering effort to save his leg. Most attempts at arterial repair failed, the usual consequence an above-knee amputation. This time, though, the operation was a success. Blood flow to his lower leg was restored and the limb salvaged.[5]

But the psychological impact on 95th Evac personnel was crushing. Dear friends and colleagues had been lost, the fabric of their unit literally torn apart. Fifth Army surgeon general Martin quickly grasped the gravity of the damage and decided to relieve the unit. They were to be replaced by the 15th Evacuation Hospital. The 95th had been a premier

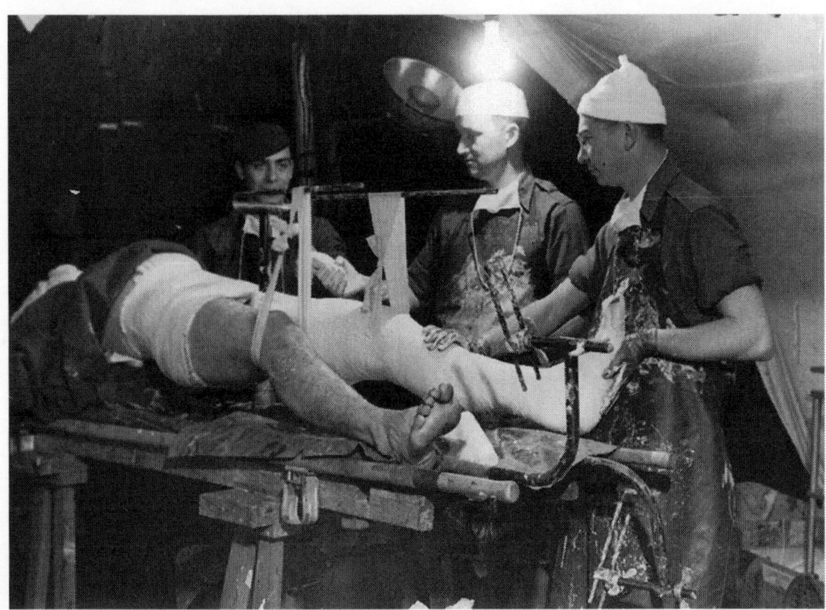

Surgeons of the Second Auxiliary Surgical Group operating at the 94th Evacuation Hospital at Anzio. (*National Archives*)

hospital. In the fifteen days of operation at Anzio, it had admitted 2,017 patients, 789 of whom were battle casualties, almost 40 percent. Four hundred fifty operations had been performed, 200 from January 24–30 and 250 the next week. Only fifteen of those patients had died of wounds, an astonishing rate of 3.3 percent.[6] And their advances in general anesthesia also were impressive, with liberal use of endotracheal intubation, providing smoother operative courses in critically injured men—and radically changing anesthetic management of those in shock. Of course, there were cases beyond salvation ("We couldn't save them all," nurse Adeline Simonson said with regret),[7] but surgical teams performed remarkable achievements, drastically reducing the number of postoperative deaths. Yet events of February 7 had made an indelible mark. Not one member of that team left Anzio unscathed by the calamity. Simonson went on to write: "I thought about Carrie Sheetz, Blanche Sigman, Esther Richards, and Gertrude Morrow as we sailed through beautiful Naples harbor. . . . I learned days after they were killed that each woman had a premonition about her death. . . . I'll never forget those four women."[8]

Up to February 8, the commanding officer of the 15th Evacuation Hospital, Colonel Frank Leaver, had been living an unobtrusive existence near Riardo, a quaint medieval town halfway between Caserta and Cassino. His unit had done well this winter, despite the lousy Italian weather. It had even celebrated its first anniversary with a party at a neighboring schoolhouse. Yes, work had been hard, shifts long, but morale was good, patient care excellent. Doctors and nurses seemed pleased with their duty station—not too close to the action—and many of the injuries challenged everyone's skill and training. But that morning, Leaver was called to Colonel Martin's office. There would be a change. Leaver was ordered to dispose of all remaining hospitalized patients. His unit was to move out, deploying to the Anzio beachhead. Without delay, the hospital was loaded into thirteen deuce-and-a-halfs and sped to the port of Naples, where they were loaded into LSTs for the thirteen-hour trip to Anzio and a nauseatingly rough sea ride. The men and thirty-nine nurses of the 15th Evac Hospital were greeted at Anzio's docks by brisk, chilling winds and a bitter cold rain. But aside from the obvious damage to buildings in the town—not one was still intact—Anzio seemed quiet and "far from the war," hardly the bedlam rumors had led them to think. "It was difficult to understand the tenseness and impatience of the port personnel and vehicle drivers to move us from the port," one observer commented.[9] But bedlam it would soon be.

The newcomers were just enjoying one of those rare interludes from Anzio's hallmark, bone-shaking barrages. In fact, the tranquillity was shattered that very night when high explosives struck the 33rd Field Hospital about fifty yards away. From that day forward, shellings were a constant accompaniment of life, happening with distinct unpredictability that amplified everyone's anxiety. Complacency was not a trait found in Hell's Half Acre. One always kept a certain tenseness for the next whine, the next whoosh that would signal a certain concussion—would it be near or far? Arthur deGrandpre knew the feeling. "Very hard to sleep," he admitted, after an incoming salvo shook him awake just before departing the beachhead. "Took Seconal for the first time."[10]

Dr. Frank Peyton was a practicing obstetrician and gynecologist in Lafayette, Indiana. After Pearl Harbor, the call went out for any physician in a nonessential role younger than fifty to be recruited. "[I]f you can see lightning or hear thunder," you would serve. Few were exempted, not in Tippecanoe County, Indiana, anyway. Peyton was to become a captain in the US Army, assigned to a gathering of medics who formed the 15th Evacuation Hospital

Now in Riardo, near Caserta, life had become routine, predictable, except for the December winds that played havoc with their tents. Christmas was spent eating turkey and trimmings, with Italian musicians and singers adding to the holiday spirit. And so entered the New Year: sometimes boring, but better than at Anzio, everyone knew. Those poor souls were being pounded daily. Then came the horror of February 7. The 95th Evac was pulling out, decimated. When its doctors arrived to take over for the 15th Evac, Peyton disapproved. "The officers as a group are a bunch of poor sissies who can't take it and no doubt are riding on the skirts of their nurses," he complained in his diary. The war had not yet come to Captain Peyton, not really. The turkey was too fresh, the wine too fine, the music too swinging. Even bouncing around in a British LSH on Valentine's Day, he joked how much fun his unit would have once they were together again. This war would finally be a great adventure. The following day, docking at Anzio, he was being hustled out of the LST by military police yelling, "Hurry up! Hurry up!" The docks were dangerous places to linger. The fun was over.[11]

That first night of his great adventure was spent in fitful sleep. "All hell broke loose for the entire night," Peyton scribbled. Four hundred seventeen remaining patients from the 95th Evac were turned over, rubble from the bombing cleaned up, fifteen damaged tents repaired, and bed capacity expanded to 570. The rumors were true. Hell's Half Acre was a perilous habitat. Only seven miles from the front, in wide-open spaces, the hospitals were clearly in enemy sights, and nearby ammo and petrol dumps—prime military targets—were little comfort. Peyton and his team felt particularly vulnerable, as if unseen eyes were constantly watching. No, this would not be fun.

Not even doctors were immune. On February 9, Colonel Jarrett "Jerry" Huddleston, VI Corps surgeon, was reviewing medical installations on the beachhead. Not one to hide behind a desk, he was constantly in motion, out on the streets, talking to his men, checking details of casualty care. It was said that Huddleston, of crisp military bearing but affectionately called "Colonel Huddle-Fuddle" by his men, carried a .45 automatic on his hip, standard sidearm for medical officers, and when Germans came over in an air raid, he boldly stood his ground and defiantly fired his weapon at the oncoming planes. That particular day he did not get the chance. In early afternoon Huddleston had just left the medical section of corps headquarters at the Hotel de Ville in Anzio. While he waited for his jeep at the corps dismount line, a high-explosive, 170-mm shell landed close by in the street—maybe a short round intended for the harbor, or maybe just for him. Fragments tore into Dr. Huddleston. He collapsed, never to get up. Colonel Huddleston, soon to be rotated to the States, would not leave Anzio alive.

His replacement was Colonel Rollin Bauchspies, who then was commanding the 16th Evacuation Hospital near Caserta. Arriving by C-47 transport and fighter escort, Colonel Bauchspies was dumped off at the small airfield near Nettuno on February 12, hopped a ride on a weapons carrier, and somehow found his command bunker in town. He was shown to his billet, the same occupied by the late Colonel Huddleston, deep in Nettuno's seven-hundred-year-old wine cellars. The new VI Corps surgeon recalled his first impression of headquarters: "About all that I can say . . . is that it was the most inhospitable place I had ever known. . . . I wondered how safe I would be. . . . These passages ended in blind alleys. . . . I calculated that a high explosive shell or bomb landing near the stairway would seal off the passage and I would be entombed."[12]

The 33rd Field Hospital, commanded by Major Sam Hanser, had been in Italy since October, coming ashore at Salerno and positioning near Bagnoli. With its attached surgical teams from the 2nd Auxiliary Surgical Group, the hospital could actually operate as three independent units, each in support of an infantry division. The army's surgical consultants envisioned these as forward surgical teams close enough for critically injured—the nontransportables. Each component unit was located with a division clearing station, providing additional personnel and beds for holding postoperative patients. While on the Cassino front, Unit A supported the 36th Division, B the 34th Division, and C the 45th. But orders came to uproot the entire hospital—all three units and their surgical teams. Something big was looming: Anzio. Unit B had landed on D-Day, the first hospital team to set up for casualties. By January 25, all three components and the headquarters section had arrived, and moved three days later to the new hospital zone east of Nettuno. And then life in a combat zone set in. "[T]he nerves of the personnel were becoming increasingly frayed. . . . A man felt strangely naked without his helmet," Captain William Hagen reported. The wail of arching artillery rounds was too familiar and too unsettling. "There was no 'going to bed.' Each night meant several dashes to the foxholes," recalled Captain Jessie Paddock, a nurse, who added, "We just kept on working. You couldn't leave your patients no matter how bad it got."[13] It might have been just as well. Barely beyond the tents shell craters crept distressingly near.

One day after Jarret Huddleston's death, the very day the 15th Evacuation Hospital arrived, artillery fire hit the 33rd Field Hospital. After one explosion, all took cover, knowing that another was sure to follow—they almost always came in twos or threes. Twenty minutes passed, and an all clear sounded. People came out of hiding and work resumed. But true to form, a second 88-mm shell came, scoring a direct hit on one of the nurses' tents. The detonation instantly killed two nurses, one attached to the 2nd Auxiliary Surgical Group, the 2nd Auxers. Chief nurse for the 33rd, thirty-year-old First Lieutenant Glenda Spelhaug from Crosby, North Dakota, and Second Lieutenant Laverne Farquar, "Tex" to her friends, from Sidney, Texas, were off duty and in the wrong place. They perished instantly. Spelhaug was decapitated, Farquar disemboweled. Spelhaug's last act was to give her helmet to a nurse who was without one. Farquar was with the 2nd Auxers attached to the 33rd Field Hospital. She had been interviewed shortly before by Rita Hume, a correspondent for the Red Cross in Italy. There was no denying that the hospital was close to the front lines, Farquar said, but, "The exciting thing is the job. To see men so badly injured you don't know how they can live and save them—that's a thrill."[14]

Major Floyd Taylor, a 2nd Auxer, took it especially hard. He had worked with Tex Farquar in North Africa and southern Italy. They were about twenty yards apart when the shell hit. Even half a century later, he remembered every detail of that day. Fragments of the shell hit the generator, plunging the entire hospital into darkness. Patients, many confined to their cots, almost panicked, but nurses refused to go to their foxholes and stayed with them. Major James Mason, a surgeon with the 2nd Auxers, continued operating, even with a spreading fire and flammable anesthetics, until firefighters from the 56th Evacuation Hospital brought it under control. Among the wounded was the hospital commander, Lieutenant Colonel Samuel Hanser, hit by shrapnel that damaged his radial nerve. He was evacuated from Anzio and replaced by Lieutenant Colonel Bennett. Also wounded was thirty-one-year-old Captain Phillip Giddings, also with the 2nd Auxiliary Surgical Group and a Harvard-trained surgeon, who was struck in the thigh. It was a gouging wound but not serious; Giddings was patched up and insisted on returning to duty. Critical patients were carried—on their mattresses, needles in their arms and plasma and blood bottles hanging—to the adjoining 56th Evacuation Hospital.[15]

Meanwhile, the generator was fixed, cots repaired, and the detritus of personal belongings scattered by the explosions swept up. The 33rd Field Hospital was back to normal operations the next day. However, many of the medical officers and nurses dug further underground, some almost five feet deep, covered with plywood and dirt—regular subterranean rooms. And for good reason: the shelling continued on the American and British hospital areas on February 12, 17, and 19 in the midst of the German counteroffensive. A Second Auxiliary nurse recorded in her diary, "air raid . . . dropped anti-personnel bombs all around us. . . . Everyone's bed is placed down in his foxhole. . . . Artillery is so heavy this morning that it sounds as if they are in the tent next to mine."[16]

On February 15, Unit A of the 33rd Field Hospital was moved even farther forward, to the so-called "Four Corners," a road junction three miles inland and "virtually in the enemy's front yard." Bitter fighting was expected. Commanders wanted surgical teams close, and, besides, the hospital compound was getting decidedly crowded. Unit A went with the 1st Platoon of the 3rd Medical Battalion's clearing company and set up in an area defended by 3rd Division troops. Sure enough, the next day, paratroopers and panzers of the Herman Goering Division launched their diversionary strike. American cannon caught them in the open, sprinkling the flatlands with dead and wounded. But not without a price. For Unit A, casualties arrived almost at once. Doctors and nurses worked around the clock for the next three days. Ninety-two critically injured were seen in just the first twenty-four hours. Sleep was a rare commodity. "[A]nother milestone in our career was passed," the official record declared. The unit was so close to the fighting that a rain of shells—almost fifty by some estimates—fell within one hundred yards. One man was killed and seven injured in the 3rd Med Battalion right next door. Medical staff deflected the danger, but it was clear all were directly in harm's way. Patients were hurriedly evacuated back to the hospital compound. Unit A and the 3rd Med Battalion followed. Crowded or not, the 33rd Field Hospital stayed put for the remainder of their stay.[17]

Yes, "Four Corners" was a good imitation of hell, but it was little safer at Hell's Half Acre. Germans had every yard of beachhead in sight. Surrounded as they were by legitimate military targets (ammo, fuel, armor parks), hospital commanders were not entirely sure of German intentions. Were the random shells meant to hit hospitals and terrorize or were they just miscalculated trajectories (those fateful "margins of error")? No need to be too visible in any case, precautions were put in place. Blackout would be strictly enforced. All light leaks were covered with salvage canvas. Outdoor activity was prohibited after sundown. Air raids, though, usually were preceded by illuminating flares dropped from aircraft. The entire compound could be lit up like a carnival—a terrifying experience. Everyone had his or her own way to deal with it. Most tried to pile as much on top of themselves as possible—and dig as deep as they could. Dr. Lawrence Collins with the 56th Evacuation Hospital barricaded his personal space, dug his cot below ground and lined it with boards. He found an antique kitchen table and perched it overhead with sandbags on top of that. His tent mate used empty ration boxes filled with sand to wall himself in, roofed with boards and more sandbags over that. Everyone—doctors, nurses, officers, enlisted—did the same. Hell's Half Acre became a subterranean community, honeycombed with foxholes and bunkers, bricked in sandbags. Some dugouts were decorated with tables and stools fashioned from ration boxes. Most people bathed using their helmets and utilized the same water to wash their clothes (hanging laundry, though, seemed to attract more artillery fire). Olive drab was the monotonous décor. At sundown, unless on duty, all retired, not to arise until dawn. "We don't have lights, but have no need for them anyway," Collins commented in a letter to his wife. Despite efforts to reassure her, he narrowly missed injury by exploding shells on more than one occasion. He never mentioned these incidents in his writings.[18] Others were not so fortunate.

There was no doubt Ellen Ainsworth was going to be a nurse. The youngest of three children, she grew up in rural Wisconsin, a free spirit some would say. She graduated from Eitel Hospital School of Nursing in Minneapolis in 1941. By March 1942, at twenty-three, she was a member of the Army Nurse Corps. Ainsworth was described as being the life of the party—dancing, drinking a little whiskey (straight from the bottle), and even smoking a rare cigar—a real beauty, that mixture of coyness and charm. Even deployment with the 56th Evacuation Hospital to North Africa and Salerno failed to dampen her spirit. And then came Anzio. Life quickly became a continuum of bloodied humans punctuated by bombing raids and random falling shells. Air raid shelters were dug for the nurses. "I'm not going to use it," was Ainsworth's response. "I'll take my chances elsewhere." The suffering, though, so much more than in southern Italy, took its toll on everyone. Ainsworth's sister, Lyda, received one tear-stained letter about the hopeless condition of many of the men: there was so much pain and so little that could be done, Ainsworth had written. It all came to an end February 12. After dark, a German air raid unloaded a number of antipersonnel bomblets on the compound—whether on purpose or prematurely no one knows. Ainsworth was in her nurses' tent. Fragments tore through, and one, the size of a quarter, ripped into her chest. She collapsed. Soldiers rushed her to the preoperative tent, awake and seemingly stable. One look at her chest, which had a large open wound, and she was taken straight to the operating tent. At surgery, it was found that the piece of shrapnel had pierced her lung, traversed the diaphragm, and lacerated her guts. Stomach contents and feces spilled into her abdomen and chest. As best they could, surgeons cleaned up the mess, washed out the slime, and sutured the holes. After surgery, Ainsworth awoke and even quipped, "Don't worry . . . I'm tougher than anything Jerry [the Germans] can throw at us." But she lost ground each day—sepsis, no doubt—organs steadily failing. Everyone loaded her dog tags with charms: a rabbit's foot, four-leaf clover, lucky-seven dice, and a Saint Christopher's medal. They were no help. Anzio's Fortunes had turned on her. On February 16, postoperative day four, she seemed to sense the end was near. The feisty brunette, so feeble now, pulled off her oxygen mask—no need for that where she was going—sighed, and quietly slipped away.[19]

The same day that bombs destroyed the 95th Evac, February 7, General Mackensen began his bid for the beachhead. Over three days, his troops succeeded in eliminating Allied gains that extended almost to Campoleone. The British lost Aprilia, now complete rubbish, in the process. By February 12, the Germans had also captured the town of Carroceto, flattening out a hard-fought salient. No Allied commander felt the Germans would be content with this. All were expecting a thrust right down the Anzio-Albano road to split Allied forces in half and take the port of Anzio itself. Ultra intercepts had said as much. General Lucas now had a full complement of the 45th Infantry Division plus all the British 56th Division; the 168th Brigade had arrived several days before. The British 1st Division, badly mauled in the fighting to take Aprilia and Carroceto, was put in reserve.

The Germans called it Operation Fischfang (Fish Trap), and it was, just as the Allies had predicted, an attack straight at Anzio. The German high command fully expected the Americans and Brits to be trapped like fish in a barrel when it was all over. Beginning February 16 and continuing until February 19, the Germans attacked in waves with enormous saturation of artillery and almost cleaved the Allied line right down the Anzio-Albano road just as they had hoped. Only heroic efforts by elements of the 45th Infantry Division and Tommies of the 56th Division saved a total disruption of the beachhead. Thunderbirds of the 179th Regiment slammed head on with German reinforcements and suffered ghastly losses. Men trickled back in small groups, crying, hysterical. Even hardened veterans broke, ashen gray, inaudible sounds escaping from their quaking lips. But those dogface Thunderbirds did not give way. Their lines somehow held. Loyals of the British 1st Division held strong as well, and a counterattack by Harmon's pugnacious tankers finally cracked German momentum. The deciding factor may have been a voracious expenditure of artillery by the Allies, delivering twenty or thirty shells for each one the Germans tossed and drenching the battleground with high explosives. By mid-February, an impressive 432 artillery pieces were in place on the VI Corps front, in addition to naval vessels offshore. And there seemed to be no limit to the supply of ammunition. Allied expenditures for February 20 totaled thirty thousand rounds. The Germans had hoped sorties by the Luftwaffe—172 on February 16 alone—would disrupt Allied shipping during their offensive, but the raids were ineffective and inflicted only modest damage. Supplies continued to pour in.[20]

In those gritty units that held the line, most of the wounded were soldiers of the 45th Division, clustered around that Anzio thoroughfare, shattered battalions that barely stopped German advances. Individual units were horribly gouged, most reduced to fractions of their allotted strength, but they held fast in the face of German tanks and waves of infantry, many times in brutal hand-to-hand combat. "These men had looked down the muzzles of cannons twenty-five yards away! Those who lived were only half alive," the 179th regimental history stated.[21] Collecting companies of the 120th Medical Battalion evacuated record numbers of casualties, braving small-arms and artillery fire on foot or by ambulance, trying to reach battalion aid stations. At the clearing station of the 120th Med Battalion, three tents were set up: one for admissions, one for treatment, and one for evacuation. Beyond simple first aid, plasma, and control of bleeding, men were sent as quickly as possible to the hospital complex east of Nettuno. In those uncertain days of mid-February, all were aware of the dangers of being overrun.[22]

Major Patrick Lawson, commanding officer of the 120th Med Battalion, wrote, "The month of February, 1944, was one that will be unforgettable in our memoirs." Those quiet days of January were gone. "[I]t was very obvious that our erroneous first impression of the Anzio beachhead and the impression of comparative peace and quiet, were to be corrected very soon." Artillery had intensified, even during the day, and frequent Luftwaffe flyovers unleashed a wealth of antipersonnel bombs on the clearing station. All were dug in, but heavy rains softened the earth, collapsing subterranean "houses" and flooding others. "It was the first time that we, as a medical installation had to be completely dug in—tentage, personnel and equipment all had their dugouts" Lawson reported. All ward tents had been recessed two feet, and a three-foot protective berm erected around them. Beginning February 7 with intensified German probing, daily casualty figures jumped from fifteen to thirty, and by February 16, at the height of Fischfang, the number reached 165 per day.[23] "The age of many of the casualties . . . proved to be young men between the ages of 18 and 21," Lawson noted. "These men came in with chest wounds, abdominal wounds, severe hemorrhage, disabling fracture, and other injuries that would give them cause for having severe shock and marked collapse."[24]

The cost in American lives was staggering. Battle casualties alone for this period amounted to 404 killed, 1,982 wounded, and 1,025 missing (presumed captured or obliterated).[25] Day crews worked on into the night and night crews into the day. "Whenever it looked like we might catch up, in would come more new cases, more than we could handle in days or weeks," Lieutenant Collins wrote from the 56th Evac.[26] Prodigious use of artillery by both sides caused most of the wounds, over 60 percent according to 3rd Med Battalion records. Some units put the figure as high as 80 percent. [27] Horrid injuries were inflicted on those found alive, fragments shattering heads, arms, and legs, and mincing lungs, bowels, and bladders. Surgeons shuddered at the wreckage presented to them, hours and hours of operating to piece anyone together—and then prayed that all held together and the wicked specter of sepsis was evaded.

German losses were not known but the battlefields were strewn with dismembered corpses, headless torsos, severed limbs, and heaps of glistening viscera. Allied bulldozers dug mass graves for an estimated one thousand five hundred bodies, eager to rid the landscape of the reek. And even the survivors suffered. For the American and British soldiers stuck in water-logged foxholes and numbing cold, there were an additional 1,637 nonbattle casualties, mostly from trench foot and exposure.[28]

The men at the front—in the gullies and caves just off the Anzio road, in the rubble of Aprilia and the pastureland known as Campo di Carne (Field of Meat), in clusters of threes and fours, maybe squads—fought off the endless tides of green-gray coated grenadiers in their coal-scuttle helmets, coming on in waves, bayonets fixed, almost suicidal in their zeal. The flatness of the grasslands around Anzio gave everyone pause. Advance and retreat were met with murderous, sweeping fire. Only the ruts and crevasses of the landscape—areas like the Cava di Pozzolana (the caves of Pozzolana) just west of the Anzio-Albano road—were any cover at all, and then Germans and Allies often mingled just feet apart, around the bend, in adjacent unsuspecting recesses and crevasses. Correspondent Ernie Pyle described it this way to the folks back home: "The land of the Anzio beachhead is flat, and our soldiers felt strange and naked with no rocks to take cover behind, no mountains to provide slopes for protection. It was a new kind of warfare for us. Distances were short, and space was confined. The whole beachhead was the front line . . . practically all farms."[29] Melons and grapes and tomatoes grew in abundance. Cattle roamed freely, now and then stepping on a buried mine or hit by a stray bullet, providing fresh meat for troops weary of C rations. But this winter season, rain and cold were everywhere, the only dry places dugouts with sturdy clapboard walls in the wadis or in what was left of Mussolini's stout individual stone dwellings built for his farming communities, those that had not already been hammered into gravel.[30] The wounded accumulated there, too dangerous to move. One British soldier, trapped with his comrades in the railway station at Carroceto, viewed the carnage around him and wrote:

> The place stinks of antiseptic and cordite and bodies. Mercifully for us, the cloud of dust and the green, yellow sickly smoke protects us from the bloodshot, questioning, burning eyes of the wounded. All we can do is stick a fag [cigarette] in their mouths and light it and when we have time, hold their hands. . . . Some of the wounded struggle so hard to tell us so much. . . . But what is there to tell? . . . Others, more hurt, either lie silent, resigned, wrapped in their bloodstained

> greatcoats, peaceful, or breathe deeply, laboriously. . . . Much of them have left us.[31]

"When a man was wounded," Pyle wrote, "he just had to lie there and suffer till dark."[32] If bad enough, he might call out to medics, who had to judge the danger, maybe make a dash for him, but mostly, one would just have to treat himself and wait for sunset. What was it like to get hit? Those artillery rounds were the most feared. Some were heard and everyone ducked, and some were silent until impact. "You never hear the one that gets you," was the common wisdom, but often not true. Many heard that eerie screech, that lonesome whine, and then all changed. Journalist Richard Tregaskis, with the troops on the Cassino front, was a victim of artillery shelling:

> I heard the scream of something coming, and I must have dived to the rocks instinctively. . . . Then a smothering explosion descended around me. It seemed to flood over me from above. In a fraction of a second of consciousness, I sensed that I had been hit. A curtain of fire rose, hesitated, hovered for an infinite second . . . an orange mist came up quickly over my horizon, like a tropical sunrise, and set again, leaving me in the dark.[33]

Tregaskis staggered, collapsed, and was left for dead until soldiers coming from the rear found him and helped him back to the rear. He had suffered a blow to the head and had a skull fracture and brain bleeding.

Private James Safrit told a tale many wounded soldiers probably could have related. A member of the 179th Infantry, he and his unit were holed in the rugged terrain in front of the wrecked town of Aprilia in late February when a monstrous Tiger tank appeared and zeroed him in. He knew what was coming but could do little to get out of the way. A scream stifled in his throat. The first shell flew by him and the second landed short. But then

> I never heard it, or if I did, the pain and shock of the shrapnel hitting my leg made me oblivious to the sound of the explosion . . . it felt as if someone had smashed my hip and thigh with a red hot spiked club. I looked down and my pants were shredded and blood began to spurt with every heartbeat. . . . I knew . . . I would bleed to death. All the while, I was yelling, "Medic! Medic!" I saw one climb over the creek bank heading for me when he caught a slug in the forehead and dropped like a pole-axed steer.

Safrit, like many wounded calling for help and watching their rescuers cut down, felt like a "sniveling yellow dog." Murder it was, he had murdered that poor fellow. At that point he took off his belt and tightened it around his thigh for a tourniquet, which quieted the bleeding. He then slowly crawled back to the platoon command post and aid station, all under his own power; Private Safrit dared not risk the life of another innocent human being.[34]

As for the truly dead, the American cemetery was so orderly; rows of wooden crosses placed with geometric precision, graves five feet deep and close together, a tidy summation after death's untidy messes. Trucks hauled the bodies in daily—from the front or unfortunate victims from the docks and tent hospitals. Graves were dug by soldiers and Italian civilians, trying to keep fifty holes ahead, the average daily butcher's bill, although on occasion that was impossible. Each corpse was buried in a mattress cover. But even the dead were not safe. Occasionally a well-placed shell uprooted a rotting body, to be buried once again. And, like everywhere on Anzio, those who dug and placed corpse after corpse sometimes dug their own grave, struck in the process by falling canisters of death.

For the GI at the front, those hunkering shadows in shallow foxholes or slit trenches, for those wretched souls who sat in knee-deep, chilled water day after day, waiting for the attack or the rumbling sound of a massive stippled German tank, there were other hardships besides bullets and bombs. Submersion of feet in that stagnant, cold water refrigerated tissues. The ordinary high-top boot issue for GIs was not waterproof and the heavy, cushion-toed, woolen sock certainly not so. Trench foot was the nemesis of Allied soldiers throughout the Anzio campaign. It was a terribly debilitating immersion injury, most often affecting dogface infantry stuck immobile in foxholes in temperatures just above freezing for prolonged periods, weather typical of Italy for January, February, and March. The first sign of trouble was a tingling or stinging of the feet caused by ischemia of the tissues. After it starts, walking causes burning pain, a serious impediment for attacking troops. With rising temperatures the feet become swollen, flushed, and agonizing. In advanced cases, blister and gangrene might develop. In milder cases, usually about one-third of those diagnosed, removal of any constricting foot gear, rest, and gradual warming of the feet is sufficient. Most could return to duty. Unfortunately, about half of victims had more severe changes with blistering, swelling, and bluish bruising. Rest, slow rewarming, and time were necessary. Even then, chronic pain developed in many, making them unfit any longer for combat. In a few, gangrene was a menace. For them, prolonged bed rest was essential, and even then tissue loss was possible—with the eventuality of amputation. The severe cases required evacuation; recuperation could be long, and there was no place near the battlefield for them. Removal of men from combat for crippling conditions like trench foot handicapped any front line unit. At Anzio it was likely as significant for the Germans as the Allies. Foot care was paramount, but for Mauldin's Willie and Joe and the other dogface boys stuck in the mud of Anzio's front, there was no easy remedy.[35]

"I have to admit I'm a bit jittery," Captain Peyton wrote on his third day on the beachhead. "I never felt this way before, but of course we've never been pinned down in such a small area hanging on tooth and toenail." He had worked all night, five "belly cases" stretched for hours. Deaths were commonplace but maddening. The reason was obvious. They were so close to the front lines that wounded were brought in who otherwise would have died in transport: irreversible shock, dismemberments, head wounds, no chance of survival. There was interminable concentration, pumping fluids, pumping blood, elbow deep in guck, then the terse report: "We lost his pulse, no heart beat. Doctor, he's dead." Several days later, the pace had not slackened. "Inherited about fifty unoperated patients this a.m. and it was 11 p.m. before they and 15 admissions were operated," he entered on February 22. He worked six hours on one mangled leg from a shell explosion, giving eight units of plasma and two liters of blood, but to no avail—off came the leg.[36]

It was the same at the British 2nd Casualty Clearing Station. With the time it took to do the difficult cases—wounds to the abdomen or chest—three or four extremity wounds could be cared for. And only half of the poor boys would survive their abdominal wounds anyway. Was that rational enough? Selection of the living over the near dead? Surgeon James Ross pondered the reluctance of some surgeons to embark on lengthy laparotomies: "It may have seemed a wasteful policy . . . for surgeons to spend valuable time on the more gravely wounded men. . . . But the 'abdomens,' if left, would certainly die. Saving of life is the doctor's aim . . . we regarded the patients in the light of the severity of their wounds and nothing else."[37]

His hospital soon became choked with wounded. Endless lines of patients meant that treating them all in a timely fashion was impossible. Surgeons' endurance, fortitude, and ethics were tested to the limit. Only at night, in the midst of sleep, could doctors sort it all out, and wonder about the poor chaps who didn't make it. Triage was imperative—picking the most critical who still had a chance of surviving. Did they pick right or did they let some die who could have been saved? "Can I forget the voice of one who cried for me to save him, save him, as he died?," soldier poet Siegfried Sassoon had written almost forty years before.[38]

Tending to the wounded seemed chaotic at times—hurried exams, blood pressure checks, hanging bottles of blood. Doctors and nurses were found in clumps huddled over individual cots and stretchers, maddeningly trying to start intravenous fluids, cutting off clothes, peeking under battle dressings. Hushed conversations in corners decided the fate of each soldier—most headed, at some point, into the operating tents. It might seem haphazard, but truly there was order in disorder. Each had a task that in the aggregate made for a methodical process. What hampered efficiency most was the Italian winter weather. Canvas invariably leaked in downpours, and while they were infinitely better than the infantryman's plight, the interiors suffered the misfortunes of wet, wind, and cold. It seemed no one could truly get dry and stay dry. In the British 2nd Casualty Clearing Station, surgeon James Ross reported:

> The preoperative ward became an unforgettable sight. . . . The . . . tents . . . let in water very freely at the junctions, and during the heavy rains it just poured in . . . till the floor became a sea of mud. On either side of the ward were placed the stretchers of men awaiting operative treatment. . . . In this ward there was a continuous movement of many men to and fro. . . . The wounded lay in two rows, mostly British but some Americans as well in their sodden filthy muddy clothes, soaked, caked, buried in mud and blood.

The clearing station clocked 1,045 operations performed by just four surgeons. Sixty-five were abdominal wounds—cases needing painstaking, time-consuming surgery. But no one was refused an operation no matter how dire their condition. "No short cuts could be taken," Ross noted.[39] In many men, who knew where to start? Rigid abdomens full of blood and stool, missing limbs, fractured skulls—all in the same patient. Combined chest and abdomen injuries taxed even the most skilled of operators: lung, diaphragm, liver, kidneys, gut all in the path. Anesthesia in these boys was critical, anesthetists learned quickly. For patients in shock too much could be lethal. Pioneering anesthesiologist Henry Beecher later observed: "It is entirely possible for an unwisely selected or incompetently given anesthetic to precipitate such profound shock in a wounded man whose status was previously not unsatisfactory that a compensated circulatory system is transformed into a state of decompensation."[40]

That was the delicate balance: too much or too little anesthetic—a task that demanded special skill and dedication. Without question, the operating team evolved in the Mediterranean theater, an interplay of talents and cooperation, with anesthetists no less vital than surgeons in an effort to salvage the unsalvageable.

Still, most troublesome were the dreadful pleas of the dying. Butchered men barely conscious clasped the hands of doctors and in a feeble voice asked, "Will I be all right, Sir?"[41] Not a few wounded fretted over the consequences of their wounds. Leg and arm injuries prompted many to worry about amputation. Blood around the genitals panicked some—would they still have a penis, testicles; would they be impotent? Nurses offered thin platitudes: "Everything will be done to save your limb." For that which could not be repaired—blindness, loss of genitalia, spinal cord transection with permanent paralysis—there were only reassurances of expert care. "Am I that bad?" some probed. "Am I going to die?" a few pressed; others, too sick to ask, lay still. Doctors moved away from the moribund; there could be no comfort in the truth. Chaplains and nurses were much better, sensing the connection so important for the frightened—even if the words were lies. While fear of dying, fear of mutilation, were real, pain was minimal. One soldier, injured by a mortar shell, suffered a meat cleaver-like slice from his fifth to his twelfth ribs near the vertebral column. Much blood had been lost—his blood pressure was steadily dropping—yet he was amazingly free of suffering. Only about one-quarter of the men admitted wanted pain medication.[42]

Tommies and Yanks laying there, patiently waiting their turn, those were a sad lot. They were brave men. There was hardly a peep from any of them—except the ones who no longer knew, the ones who were closer to the grave than to going home. For those, the agonal gurgles, groans, and incoherencies seeped out. But among the conscious, strain and terror blanketed every feature. "[D]irt and exhaustion reduce human faces to such a common denominator," Ernie Pyle observed of the wounded. "Everybody they carried in looked alike."[43] The seemingly faceless, torn bodies arranged side by side; the ghoulish chorus of moaning and labored breathing; physicians sifting through gutted and dismembered flesh—the entire spectacle was a macabre pageant. Heavy in the air, always, was the smell of congealed blood, stale perspiration, and the recently deceased. Hospitals had become Anzio's charnel houses. James Ross wearied of the sight—the bleak grime and misery; day after day he made his rounds in those sodden tents, picking out those among the throngs that he could possibly help: "I grew to hate that combination of yellow pad and bloody dirty brown bandage. Some were unconscious, these chiefly head wounds, whose loud snoring breathing distinguished them. Some were carried in dying with gross combinations of shattered limbs, protrusions of intestines and brain. Some carried in, gasping and coughing, shot through the lungs . . . all were exhausted after being under continuous fire and lying in the mud for hours or days."[44]

As for the doctors, "The rain hammers on my helmet in good earnest. . . . I am afraid I do not match up in appearance to the standards of a medical Chief," wrote Henry Winans of the 56th Evacuation Hospital. "My shoes are covered with mud as are most of my leggings. I keep my helmet on along with the raincoat because there is no place to put them."[45] "This is a good time, as is always, to be near to your Maker," Arthur deGrandpre had mused one day during his tour of the beachhead. His remedy after a particularly heavy night of flares and air raids and foxhole time: Mass and Communion.[46] "Death before Dishonor" was the tattoo on one soldier's arm. Sadly, he and his arm had become separated by a shell. Both were brought in on the same litter. The man lived. His coveted arm did not. "We made mistakes," admitted one young orthopedic surgeon with a year and a half of training under his belt. But experience was a quick teacher. "Surgeons who worked continuously in the zone of combat developed a feeling for what was a wise course of action." Mistakes became fewer and fewer.[47] But the constant danger, the imminent chance of mutilation and death, wore on many. "Poor Claire, a good surgeon from Brazil, Indiana just two nights ago was so depressed and walking about alone and insisted on getting killed here," Frank Peyton wrote in his diary. "'Frank, we'll never see our family again,'" he repeatedly said. The troubled physician was sent back for psychological assessment and rest—a so-called neuropsychiatric case.[48] It was those barrages, those damn barrages. They were endless, rounds landing on all sides of the hospital—boom! Shudder. "Keep wondering how long it will be till we catch one," Peyton finally wrote. Everyone was scared—damned fools if they weren't.[49] And Axis Sally hissed, "Go easy, boys, there's danger ahead."[50]

February was the worst month, with a bumper crop of wounded. At the 93rd Evac, the 974 operations done in January climbed to 1,187 in

February, an average of forty-two per day. The 56th Evac admitted 2,863 battle casualties and operated on 1,605 of them, including 614 major operations, an average of 22 per day. Those bloody wounds consumed 1,406 units of plasma and 603 pints of blood, mostly courtesy of the British Transfusion Service. Far too many did not escape the Grim Reaper. Twenty-two of fifty-six patients died after abdominal injuries, 17 of 131 after chest wounds.[51] They were carried in so soon after injury, picked up right from the battlefield, tossed into an ambulance, and hauled to the hospital—within an hour sometimes. Many still had a pulse but little else, some not even that—"in extremis" was the term. The bodies of victims of high explosives were riddled with holes. High-velocity shell fragments—from pea size to plate size—pierced every cavity, shredding anything in their path. At the 56th Evac, just in February, 374 patients had such injuries: abdomen, chest, extremity, and face trauma—abdominal wounding was feared. At the 33rd Field Hospital, mortality rates could be as high as one in three—and this with experienced 2nd Auxer surgeons. Chest injuries were not as lethal yet one in seven still succumbed.[52]

If that was not enough, mud, farmland, and devitalized tissue spelled gas gangrene, the nemesis of combat surgery. A gas gangrene service was started, its ward totally isolated, inmates quarantined. Lieutenant Collins was given the dubious honor of command. "I don't suppose I can be switched, at least for a while," he wrote. Once a doctor worked on that ward, he was not allowed on another ward for at least three days—there was true dread of those tiny microspores, and there would be no cross contamination. During February, Collins treated twenty-four patients in his gruesome shop. Five of seventeen Americans died, as did five of seven German prisoners. The Germans all had pitifully neglected wounds before they were captured by Allied troops.[53] Five legs came off above the knee—through the thigh. Collins had no choice. Once it started, *Clostridia* spread like wildfire. What a bloody mess, he observed. Had he been trained for this? A resounding "No" was his answer in a letter to his wife: "Have done my first few amputations. Although they are the easiest operations I've ever done, I'm plenty provoked at the shortsightedness of my superiors for not seeing to it that I was trained for such things while still under supervision."[54]

What General Mackensen could not control, and dearly wished he could, was the massive influx of men and material through the docks of Anzio—and the proficient exit of Anzio's victims. No doubt, giant Anzio

Annie and his big field guns splashed their shells in the harbor, Junkers and Messerschmitts roared overhead, and U-boats lurked underneath, but the vast majority of shipping escaped unscathed. And the Allies had made the whole venture a model of efficiency. The 36th Engineers repaired the port so that eight LSTs, eight LCTs, and five LCIs could dock simultaneously. This sped up the process of loading or unloading, and no one wanted to linger. Once emptied of their freight—foodstuffs, supplies, ammunition—landing craft were filled with human cargo, all waiting just offstage in that intricate beachhead ballet Colonel Huddleston contrived. Truck convoys seemed unbroken, flowing from postoperative wards of Hell's Half Acre—some injured only twenty-four hours before—to the rubble of seaside Anzio and onto gaping, barge-like crafts waiting at the docks. Drivers from the 549th Ambulance Company queued up their Dodge three-quarter tons, marked brightly with a Red Cross, a bit nervous at idling here, only too anxious to deposit their charges and skedaddle. It was a bucket brigade—practiced proficiency—teams at the ready, each ambulance emptied, the litters placed side by side in landing barges. Flat-bottomed LCTs were packed solid with bundled up men, quilts of brown army blankets; in others, the ambulatory wounded lined the gunwales. Within an hour, a barge could be filled. The LCTs then cast off and swung out to the harbor, ferrying men to transports or hospital ships. Transfer aboard was a seaward footwork of men and stretchers, synchronizing every step with the undulating motions of each vessel. Once boats were lashed together, wounded were passed through waterline portals directly inside and distributed to their wards. Often, LSTs beached like giant whales right on the shore and loaded men aboard. Vast tank decks were packed with cots—row after row of recumbent soldiers, their stark white bandages and casts badges of courage. A few lay motionless, others bewildered, grabbing from time to time at missing arms or legs. But there were smiles all around, the men thankful to leave that godforsaken place. A US Army Air Force B-24 crewman, ditching in the waters of Anzio, hitched a ride on one of those LSTs back to Naples. To him it was a sobering scene: "[W]e watched the medics herd them aboard. . . . [B]andaged heads and bodies with crusty red stains showing through, missing arms with flapping sleeves pinned over, chopped off legs, with blankets lying horribly flat, and stark staring shock cases."[55]

For the twenty- or thirty-hour run to Naples, each LST carried 150 or 200 litter patients and an equal count of ambulatory wounded. A doctor and numbers of enlisted from the 56th Med Battalion accompanied them. It was known as the Anzio Ferry Service. There was no dallying around port, though. Shell splashes, air raid sirens, and the ominous hum of high-level aircraft worried everyone. Not without reason. Since the hospital ship *St. David* was sunk, Anzio Harbor had claimed a number of other craft: the cruiser HMS *Spartan* and Liberty ship *Samuel Huntington* bombed and sunk, destroyers HMS *Inglefield* and HMS *Jervis* hit by guided missiles and destroyed, light cruiser HMS *Penelope* and LST-348 torpedoed by U-boats, HMS *Janus* hit and sunk by an aerial torpedo.

Lieutenant Colonel Charles D'Orsa was the executive officer for Fifth Army G-4. In one of his reports to Naples, he described a particularly active day on the docks, perhaps not different from many. It was Leap Day, Tuesday, February 29:

> The harbor and beaches were pretty hot today. It almost appeared as if they [German artillery] had observed fire. Shells landed all over the Anzio docks and Yellow Beach area with air bursts over the area. . . . Shells hit two LSTs today; one landed this morning . . . destroyed two trucks, started a fire, caused about a dozen casualties.[56]

The linchpin in the whole evacuation process was the 549th Ambulance Company, commanded by Pennsylvania native Captain Eugene Haverty. He arrived at Anzio February 1, put in charge by General Martin himself. Movement of traffic was so synchronized that wasted time was nonexistent. No casualty or ambulance team ever died during the process. But Dr. Haverty did not share that fortune. He, too, was in the wrong place at the wrong time. On that same February 29, while he was busy with the usual matters of evacuation, keeping ambulance lines moving, and watching over the handling of stretchers, one well-aimed artillery shell struck, killing him instantly. His tribute was a Requiem High Mass in his hometown of Latrobe. Later that year, his young widow, Carolyn, received the Legion of Merit and Silver Star awarded him for his gallantry. Exposed as he and his men were on those dangerous Anzio docks, it was a fitting tribute. At the ceremony, a young daughter—also named Carolyn—fondled the medals as if they were shiny new toys; the two-year-old would never know her father.

10

Stalemate

THE GREAT COUNTERATTACK ENVISIONED BY KESSELRING AND Mackensen had failed. Across the Anzio-Albano road, in Aprilia and Carroceto, in the wadis and caves and ravines of Buonriposo Ridge countless Germans lay dead, now bulldozed under. No longer would the *Reich*'s hordes be able to threaten the integrity of the beachhead—not in one massive infantry charge anyway—but neither were the Allies prepared to expand beyond it. Both forces settled down to a battle of attrition, much like trench warfare in World War I. Despite a brilliant, tough defense of his beachhead, General John Lucas was done, fired as VI Corps commander by Mark Clark on February 21. Not bold enough, he was told, unable to seize the Alban Hills straightaway, even though his orders were ambiguous, his forces were inadequate, and German strength was quickly bolstered. In all likelihood, such a daring Patton-like assault would have soon overstretched his lines and invited piecemeal annihilation of his forces. His replacement was Major General Lucian Truscott Jr., then commander of the 3rd Infantry Division, one of the pillars of Anzio.

Yet, the Americans and British were still ringed in and under siege. German siege engines—their prodigious artillery—sighted every inch of the battlefield. Steady, punishing fire was a daily occurrence. There was no let up. It was hard for a shell to fall, a bomb to drop, and not hit something—someone. Ernie Pyle had reported, "You're just as liable to get hit standing in the doorway of the villa where you sleep at night, as you are in a command post five miles out in the field."[1] And little voices in each person would say, "Will I be next?" To be sure, it was not Bataan. The Allies pumped material through Anzio at a ferocious pace. For the most part, troops were well supplied and well fed. The wounded were treated and got out. But no one was convinced it would last—not the foot soldier in the trenches, the doctors and nurses in the tents, the officers in their bunkers. And war correspondents, those barometers of disaster, fearing another Dunkirk, fled to Naples, warning of impending doom. They were not alone. British field marshal Jan Smuts cabled Prime Minister Churchill on February 23, "An isolated pocket [Anzio] has now been created, which is unconnected with the enemy's main southern front, and which is itself besieged instead of giving relief to the pressure against us in the south." To which Churchill snorted, "Naturally I am very disappointed at what has appeared to be the frittering away of a brilliant opening in which both fortune and design had played their part."[2]

Kesselring gloated at their plight. He sensed their pessimism, even as a relative calm descended over the beachhead. "Penned in as they were on the low-lying, notoriously unhealthy coast, it must have been damned unpleasant . . . with the means available we must succeed in throwing the Allies back into the sea."[3]

But disaster was not forthcoming. This would not be another Dunkirk. The month of March saw a stalemate, the flat farmlands, devoid of vegetation, began to resemble another Passchendaele, that bleak, lifeless Flanders landscape of the Great War. Troops burrowed into the ground, and existence became subterranean. Any peek above was sure to invite instant death, some sniper always at the ready. The Blitzkrieg had become a "Sitzkrieg." Each side had been bloodied and mauled to the point that neither could mount an effective attack. The Allies were stalled, encircled, and contained. The Germans resigned to surround and harass, feeling the pinch of two fronts and the consumption of men and supplies; Operation Fischfang was a distant, hollow boast. The combatants were locked in a death struggle like two exhausted boxers clinging to one another, neither willing to let go, the slender expanse of beachhead and the surrounding hills containing quarrelsome but spent foes. Skirmishes by lonesome patrols, like erratic punches and half-hearted body blows, were their maximum efforts. Knockout punches were impossible. Crack troops like the men of the 504th Parachute Infantry found themselves sealed in dugouts "living in them for weeks at a time. . . . All in all, this was not the type of combat for which the 504th was

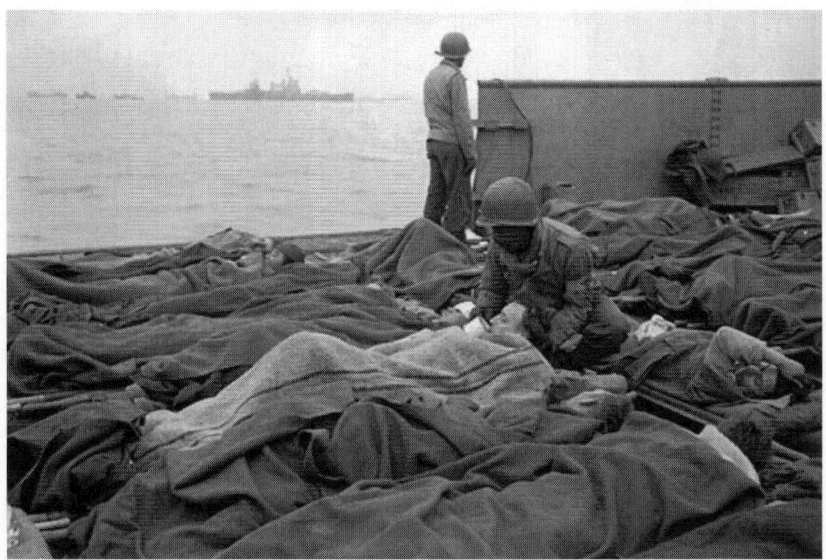

Wounded American soldiers aboard a landing craft waiting to be transfered to a hospital ship off Anzio, January 31, 1944. (*National Archives*)

psychologically suited," particularly after successfully repelling vicious German attacks down the Anzio-Albano road in early February.[4] The elite paratroopers had become mud rats, a far cry from their billowing parachutes and commando-style raids.

March was the month of artillery duels, mountains of spent cannisters piling up on both sides. German guns roared from the hills, and the Allies replied with hundreds of pieces and thousands of rounds of shells. The 701st Tank Destroyer Battalion alone fired 10,878 rounds of high explosives into German positions.[5] But for the Allies, a breakout would have to happen. Containment could not last. And so for March and April, reinforcements, artillery, ammunition, and armor poured through the docks of Anzio and Nettuno, and the battlefield swelled with men and machines. "Never had I seen a war zone so crowded," Ernie Pyle observed.[6]

Still, there was violence enough to keep doctors busy. The 56th Evac saw 1,167 wounded in March and performed 426 major operations, pouring 741 pints of blood into Allied veins. Most serious were the abdominal and chest injuries, fatal in well over 10 percent of victims.[7] Next door at the 33rd Field Hospital, 357 wounded arrived. There, too, abdominal injuries proved lethal: fourteen of nineteen patients—half of the deaths seen that month from any injury. Hemorrhage was the culprit, the number one menace for combat wounded. At the 33rd, 414 pints of blood and 313 units of plasma were emptied into those boys. With artillery now the major weapon, fragment wounds dominated; over two-thirds of casualties fell prey. Airbursts—shells detonating just above the trenches—were particularly deadly for front-line troops. Cover and concealment were imperative, but many soldiers were still caught in the open. April was little different. In groups of two or three, men were hauled in covered with slashes and gouges from shelling, with the same awful results, the same deadly outcomes. The tired litany of care—fluids, blood, surgery, and more surgery—was doled out by doctors equally tired. For health care workers, suffering soon suffocated any cheerful nature until only that part of the brain used to complete a rigid set of tasks functioned, as if doctors and nurses were simply indifferent robots manning a long and grotesque assembly line. It would only be later, perhaps much later, that the full flood of sorrow and futility and rage would engulf a mind finally awakening from the insolation it had once demanded. Mortality from belly wounds? Fifty percent still.[8]

Newcomers were struck by the utter devastation they witnessed from the docks. Anzio and Nettuno had been leveled. The violence that had caused it was unfathomable. But the first barrage they endured brought a new understanding and nerve-rattling reality. Such was the case with Captain Richard Hauver, head of General Surgery Team No. 21 of the 2nd Auxiliary Surgical Group and a graduate of Jefferson Medical College in Philadelphia. His surgical training had earned him board certification by the American Board of Surgery, and he was a fellow of the American College of Surgeons. His group had already been seasoned by duty in North Africa and Sicily. Work had been steady on the Cassino front; Team 21 linked up with the 16th Evac. Hauver had heard the horror stories of Anzio, the bombings and fatalities among medical personnel. A good place not to be, he figured. But on February 20, Team 21 was ordered into the beachhead. Onboard the *St. Andrew* there was the mandatory embarking party, "vermouth, gin, scotch, champagne, and G.I. alcohol." "[A] rousing good time is had by Americans and British." They unloaded at the Anzio docks on March 3, and, like all fresh faces, rushed "like mad" to get away before the shells began falling. Hauver's team moved in with the 93rd Evac. His first night there he made his acquaintance with "Whispering Willies," artillery projectiles that tumbled end-over-end in flight, producing a "whishing" sound. Veterans of the

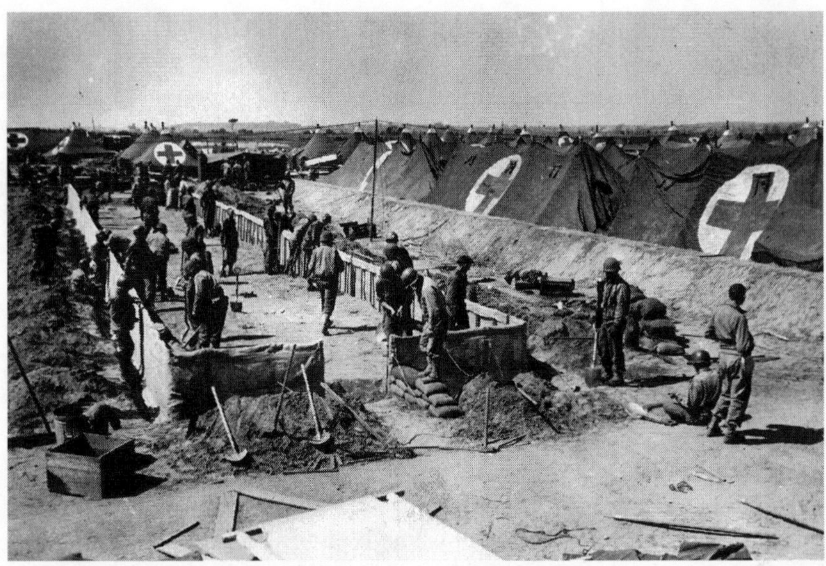

A new hospital foundation being dug in and sandbagged at Anzio in April 1944. (*National Archives*)

beachhead could distinguish them—he would soon come to understand—from "Screaming Mimis," the high-pitched whines of whirling shells sounding like the howling of the devil himself. On March 22, at three in the morning, the terrors of Anzio were upon him. He remembered "all hell broke loose," with a sweeping barrage of cannon from one side of the hospital area to the other. Hauver tried to dig as deep as he could "and believe me I was scared for the first time in this war." It was true what they said of Anzio: it was complete pandemonium. Hauver came to appreciate what any hospital denizen learned: they were all sitting ducks. Dig. Dig deeper.[9]

Invariably, rounds fell short—or reached Hell's Half Acre by grim intention. Hospitals received more than their share of hits—both British and American sectors—with an occasional sickening result. On March 17, a lone German pilot, unable to find a suitable target, dumped his load of antipersonnel bombs before heading out to sea. His package struck the 141st Field Ambulance of the British 5th Division. One full ward tent took three direct hits, killing twelve patients and two members of the Royal Army Medical Corps. Seventy-five others were wounded. Then there was the barrage that left Captain Hauver clawing at the dirt.

The 15th Evac fell victim that night. Booms of German artillery rudely shook men awake. All immediately thought of the hard-luck 95th and headed to their foxholes, awaiting the fatal blast. After a score of explosions, Captain Peyton ran out to survey the damage. Ward 18 had been hit, the smell of cordite still thick, the smoke blinding. He grabbed a body, a young man gasping and bleeding from a throat wound, fragments right through the larynx and carotid arteries. The lad didn't last fifteen minutes. Another with massive chest and abdomen injuries died just before dawn. In all, five patients were killed and eleven wounded from just one blast. Peyton recalled "this mess or shambles of blood, groans, smoke, odor, upset [disheveled] ward was the worst I ever expected to witness." One officer's tent, not too far away had recently been sandbagged. An 88-mm warhead struck, detonated the sandbags, energy spent on thick sand. It failed to penetrate but still macerated everything inside. The three inhabitants were all nurses. Chief Nurse Maurietta Shoemaker had been asleep in her cot, dug down below ground, a barracks bag suspended overhead. That bag, her clothing, and the tent were shredded. "It looked as though a nest of rats had spent the winter in that bag," the new 6th Corps surgeon, Colonel Bauchspies, commented.[10] If she had been at ground level, there would have been little of her left. Dozens of fragments pierced Colonel Peyton's tent too. His overcoat, trench coat, raincoat, jacket, and suitcase were all holed. Those barrages frayed everyone's nerves. "Are we developing '88itis?" Peyton wondered. "This sort of thing is unpleasant and everybody seems to notice them more." The remedy: a few slugs of cognac helped.[11]

General Truscott inspected the damage the following day. The bombardment was intentional, he felt. Moving the compound was out of the question. There was no place any safer on the beachhead. The only solution was to dig deeper yet. Sixth Corps Engineers set to work. Layers of earth were scooped away, three or four feet worth. Fortunately, winter rains had let up and the water table receded. Everything was sunk in: ward tents, operating tents, and personnel tents—dug in and sandbagged, not only in the American sector but the British too. A thousand combat engineers from the 36th and 39th Engineer Regiments jumped at the chance, anything to get them away from inglorious duty along the Moletta River. Ward tents were then placed end to end in each excavation and earth revetments were built over three feet thick and five feet tall around the tent walls, veritable Red Cross fortresses. Sandbags were added as a final reinforcement. Two-inch-thick planks of plywood covered the operating tents as some protection from falling flak fragments. Hell's Half Acre was reduced to a fortified underworld—"artillery proofed"—shielded from everything but a direct hit, a proposition that many feared was still a distinct possibility.[12]

But all Truscott's work added zero immunity from aerial bombings. To bear that out, a neurosurgical ward of the 93rd Evacuation Hospital, shielded by berms and sandbags, took a direct hit from a German flyover, starting fires and killing three patients as well as their two enlisted attendants. Fifteen others were injured, including four officers. Dr. Floyd Taylor with the 33rd Field Hospital told of hearing planes coming in while they were operating, knowing full well bombs were soon to fall. Ack-ack fire from antiaircraft batteries confirmed their suspicions. All put helmets on and stooped low to the ground. Surgeons covered operative fields—open abdomens and chests—with towels. Anesthetists ducked under the tables still squeezing their ventilator bags. Then, after the drone of engines receded, all stood, removed towels—some containing bomb or ack-ack fragments—and resumed operating as if nothing had happened. "This was nearly a daily occurrence," Taylor insisted.[13] On the wards, patients held on for dear life, confined to cots, strung up in traction, unable to move. They clung to their nurses, who refused to leave. Of course, there was the usual nervous chatter. During one nighttime air raid, a young soldier chirped, "Nurse it's a beautiful day, isn't it?" The unfortunate chap had lost both eyes. When told it was the middle of the night, he only apologized, "hope I didn't awaken any of the boys."[14]

Amid the bombings and shellings and parade of wounded, life on the beachhead assumed a perverse normalcy. Nurse Avis Dagit marveled at the trappings of civilization she observed strolling through the compound: "The ditch beside the hospital took on the appearance of an underground city. Foxholes and bunkers honeycombed the bank. Many were elaborate, with tables and stools made from ration boxes. Others found furnishings in surrounding homes."[15]

From above, Goering's Luftwaffe tangled with Allied fighter-interceptors. During the day, spectacular dogfights could be seen high in the sky, with zigzag contrails more reminiscent of peacetime air shows. Doctors and nurses peeked from their sandbags and gawked in amazement.[16] Baseball games were held on the beach in the afternoons, all within sight of German field glasses miles away. The British had a band of bagpipers who marched and practiced every afternoon, to the irritation of their German counterparts in the hills. They were the Scotch Highlander's

Bagpipe Corps and even put on shows for hospital personnel—Brits and Yanks. Stop or we'll shell you, the Germans demanded—and the Americans too, for that matter. The parade fields were only a few hundred yards from the hospitals. The Scots refused to stop, and the Germans shelled. More close calls. Distressed Americans drank homemade gin and dutifully crawled into their holes.[17]

On March 27, a wedding ceremony was held in the movie tent of the 93rd Evac. Lieutenant Genevieve Clarke married Lieutenant Thomas Ross of the 3rd Infantry Division Signal Corps. Even photographers and correspondents were there. Following the ceremony, the twenty-six-year-old bride cut her wedding cake with a trench knife. At the reception, revelers carried on as if at a posh country club, with wine and GI alcohol in grape juice.[18] Captain Hauver was there. "Everyone is good and drunk" he wrote. Shortly afterward, the area was bombed. Apparently Germans, eyeing the whole scene from miles away, felt the empty ammunition crates used as seating for the three hundred wedding guests were full and being stored under the protection of the Red Cross. Dr. Quinby Gurnee, an orthopedic surgeon with the 93rd, received a Bronze Star that day for refusing to stop operating in the midst of explosions. Not far away, Private John Ramsey, a litter bearer, was killed when Ward 14 received a direct hit.[19]

No amount of ingenuity could resurrect Anzio, though. General Mark Clark called it a "barren little strip of hell."[20] Hell's Half Acre was a microcosm of the subterranean civilization Anzio had become. Sinners here clawed the earth to escape damnation, not to enter it. Random shellings and air raids were a fact of life, safety found only below ground. What bothered the most was their illogical nature. Why now, why here? Why him and not me? Sure enough, sooner or later, some other innocent would fall, one more Purple Heart. "Well, another bomb hit our area just now, and one of our nurses got a chest wound, and a doctor . . . got a leg wound. . . . It was a phosphorus bomb," wrote Lawrence Collins to his wife on March 29. Clark had just visited the hospital when an enemy flight passed overhead, dropping bombs that ranged from the 93rd Evac across to the 56th. One of the bombs hit directly into the fifty-foot Red Cross sign painted near Ward 26, as if these were bullseyes for bombardiers. Four patients were killed, nineteen wounded (again). Lieutenant Helen McCullough, one of the nurses, was hit in the chest by a fragment that caused a jagged, sucking wound and lacerated right lung. She survived. Private Nick Gergulas with the 56th died of injuries he suffered that day. The randomness and suddenness psychologically knocked people silly. After a while there was a look about some, a blank, faraway look. "Anziating" it was called—the "thousand-yard stare": the mind numb, the nerves frayed. "The bur-r-rUMP came so close on my right that I knew the next one would be on my left or on top of my head. . . . I died once again, waiting for the next bomb to put me out of my misery," Lieutenant Collins remembered weeks later.[21] Inexorably, the roster of casualties among medical workers expanded. Including collecting and clearing companies 82 were killed, 387 wounded, 19 captured, and 60 reported missing in action.[22] According to records from the 15th Evac "casualties were admitted almost as frequently from service troops as from troops on the line."[23] Would anyone even leave this place? Would one giant German attack round them all up, wipe them out? Would they end up as prisoners of war? Would there be executions? No one felt secure.

Kesselring, Goering, and Mackensen were not so sure. There was no stopping the Allies from replenishing their troops. LCTs and LSTs plied the Naples-to-Anzio route daily, Liberty ships from North Africa weekly. Anzio became the seventh busiest port worldwide. An immense load crossed the docks: 60 percent ammunition, 20 percent fuel, and 20 percent rations was the usual distribution. Sometimes special convoys brought even more. For January and February, daily averages approached three thousand five hundred tons, and in March an all-time high of five thousand one hundred tons were delivered each day. On the way out, casualties filled the boats—33,063 American and British wounded and sick in total—with not a single loss of life in the process.[24] It was a quartermaster's nightmare, though, orchestrating flow of material in and wounded out, timing motorized caravans between Luftwaffe sorties or Whistling Willies or Screaming Mimis. To be sure, the waterfront streets of Anzio were no safer than trenches astride the Anziate.[25] Lieutenant Colonel Cornelius Holcomb, commander of the Quartermaster Corps, told a gruesome tale from those docks. He was supervising unloading one day, standing in a doorway of a waterfront building when he heard the whining sound of a bomb. The colonel jumped downstairs to the basement and yelled for his young lieutenant to do the same. The bomb hit at the front door, sparing the colonel, but the lieutenant's head was found lying in the corner of the room.[26]

On March 22, new medical units arrived. The 94th Evacuation Hospital, with elements of the 402nd Collecting Company and the 161st Medical Battalion, came ashore, dodging the usual artillery fanfare in the harbor. They arrived the same day shellfire clobbered the neighboring 15th Evac. For the next four days, men of the 94th frantically dug in and piled solid berms and sandbags all around, trying to figure out rhyme or reason to their new assignment. Nurses joined them March 27, their appearance baptized by a flyover of three dozen enemy planes and a good deal of falling flak. Several men caught in the open narrowly escaped injury. By March 29, four hundred beds were ready and the first patients appeared. Anzio was different than anything the 94th had seen so far. "Artillery fire was almost constant. . . . It was a tragic sight to see ward tents and equipment go up in a puff of smoke," the official record read.[27] "On April 2nd, at night, there was a continuous shelling with several landing near. Two went in our motor pool," nurse Ramona McCormick wrote.[28] Journeys outside tents were made frugally and hastily, furtive scurries, even to the latrines. Whistling shells were unnerving; the fact that many were headed for the harbor reassured few. Who really knew where they would land? Almost every day in April, diary entries divulged: "Air raid at 2300 hours," "Air raid at 2130 hours," "Air raid at 0330 hours," "enemy shells coming in about 1730." On April 4, thirty shells landed nearby. Fortunately, most were duds, an observation that comforted no one. Some were chillingly close. It wasn't until April 9 that there was a day free of raids and artillery. But that was the only respite. Every other day in April was laced with bombings and artillery fire, some coming "very close." Patients were invariably rattled by the whole affair, feeling so helpless that they pined for those awful days in front-line foxholes rather than lying in cots under flimsy canvas tenting.[29]

Even religious services were put on hold. "Common sense instead of relying upon prayers is the most dependable protection here," said the Catholic chaplain for the 15th Evac. For "padres," praying in April played second string to dodging "Jerry's" shells. Everyone, it seemed, shared that philosophy. "We could hear their muzzle blasts, sounding like kettledrums," surgeon George Tipton remembered.[30] Anyone out in the open was at risk. Rounds fell during a baseball game near the 56th Evac April 3, killing one man. "Such a silly thing to be doing up in this area," surgeon Frank Peyton thought.[31] Axis Sally had just blared "Hi, fellas of the 56th Evac. I hope you're enjoying the ball game and your camp."[32]

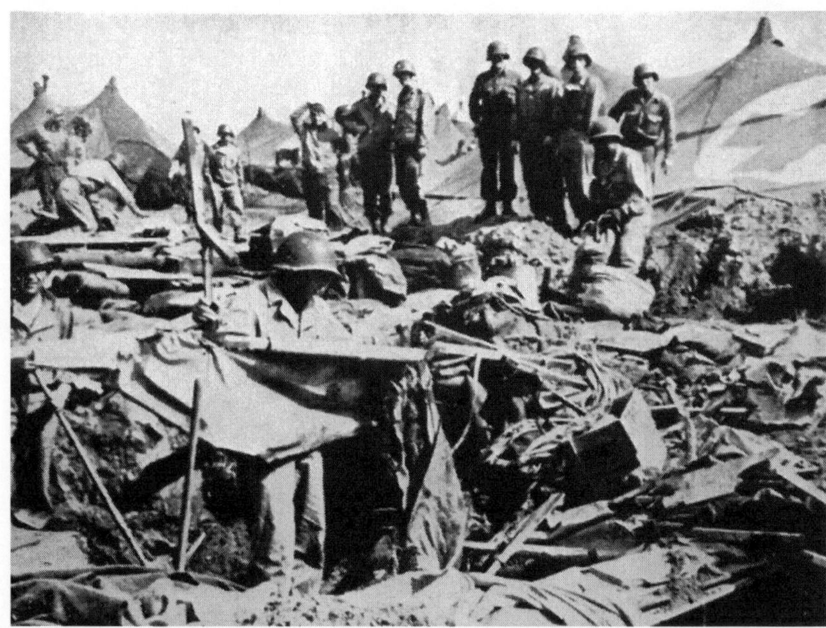

56th Evacuation Hospital following the shelling on April 6, 1944, that destroyed one surgical ward. Fortunately, this time, no medical personnel were killed. (*Army Medical Department*)

Three days later, shells landed in the 56th Evac, destroying the post exchange, one of the surgical wards, and enlisted men's tents. Pete Betley, one of the laboratory technicians, had jumped into his foxhole, safe he thought, and began shining his shoes. But a shell followed him in—one of those rare direct hits—and blew off both his legs at the hip. In one of those despicable ironies of war, those shined shoes would not be needed. "Please God protect us because I want to go home again," nurse Dagit prayed. Captain Hauver over at the 93rd spent too much time building and rebuilding shelters, almost to the point of exhaustion. The bombardments consumed what little spare time he had. "Everyone jumpy," he scribbled.[33] Wrote one surgical nurse, Lieutenant June Wandrey of the 56th Evac, "We live down under the ground in sand-bagged damp, smelly foxholes, like moles in a blackout."[34] And the violence gave birth to its victims with sickening regularity. Captain Peyton worked straight through the night of April 16, one soldier with a traumatic amputation of his left leg and right foot and another a belly case with a ruptured kidney and transverse colon. Two days later, his hospital was swamped with twenty-two cases all at once, eighteen the result of one shell landing in the midst of 45th Division soldiers in formation standing down for a briefing.[35]

Officers, nurses, and enlisted were not allowed to leave the compound and had to remain on duty 24 hours every day—all within the barriers of their restricted confines. Rest, when it did occur, was spent in cramped tents, foxholes, or dugouts. Even ventures out in the open were hazardous. The "Anzio walk", a jerky, crouching "dance" from one point to another, all the while listening for the scream or whish of an incoming round, characterized sojourns outside of tents. Most latrine visits were done at night, in darkness. More often nurses simply used empty plasma cans in their tents and then dumped them in the morning. Hair washings occurred only when it rained, showers once weekly at best; helmet baths were the norm. Laundry was rarely done.[36] Colonel Bauchspies could tell the effect on hospital personnel. Shellings, bombings, the loss of friends and colleagues, the continuous presence of wounded and dying, long hours of work, lack of recreation, and little rest wore down the morale and resistance of even the most resilient doctor, nurse, or enlisted man: "I noticed an increased loss of efficiency, a lack of interest in the daily activities, and that the usual cheerful spirit and feeling of physical well-being of the personnel were diminishing. The personnel had haggard and weary appearances . . . or had no expressions at all; they had become listless—there was no laughter—no kidding—no griping about their plight."[37]

On April 6, Axis Sally dedicated "Happy Days Are Here Again" to the 56th Evac, announcing they would soon be leaving the beachhead. How uncannily accurate she was. The next day Colonel Blesse, the commanding officer, told the medical staff they were being relieved by the 38th Evac and would be departing. Two days later, on Easter, the unit was in trucks heading down "Purple Heart Highway"[38] past the rubble of Nettuno and Anzio and boarding LSTs for the ride to Pozzouli and its next duty station at Nocelleto. No one objected. "We're in tents . . . in a valley so quiet and peaceful our ears ring," Dr. Lawrence Collins wrote on April 10. Rats were no longer a problem. Their new mess hall was "infested, literally infested, with Italian waiters," Collins mused.[39] It was night and day.

Replacing the 56th Evac was the 38th Evac, another 750-bed motorized hospital, a veteran unit of North Africa and landings at Salerno. Activated in early 1942 at Fort Bragg, North Carolina, the nidus were doctors and nurses from Charlotte, but eventually the 41st Evac was folded in to provide fully authorized strength. Second Auxers were also part of the unit: two general surgery teams, a chest team, and a maxillofacial team. Some members had already arrived at Anzio and been assigned to other medical units. Since November, the 38th had been stationed at Tavernanova, a small town north and east of Naples. But beds stood empty. Activity on the Cassino front had drawn down, mostly a stalemate. By March the hospital held only 150 patients. Enjoying the slack, many officers and enlisted spent free time in Caserta, Naples, and Capri. Life was not too bad, with opera, fresh eggs, oranges, clean bedding, Italian servants, and marmalade. There were rumors of Anzio, mostly ignored. Rumors were just rumors. One of the physicians, Captain Stanton Pickens, even wrote of an impromptu dance party: "With the club room and the orchestra . . . and with plenty of food, Coca-Cola and coffee, all we needed was some girls . . . we needed more females."[40]

All too brief, most would say. On March 24 orders were received to pack up and move to Nocelletto, closer to the front, but almost as soon as staff arrived there new orders came to prepare for Anzio. So it *would* be Anzio. With some understandable apprehension hospital personnel dutifully loaded their belongings. It would be one of those typical arrivals for Anzio's rookies. On April 9, military police greeted them at the docks with shouts of, "Step lively! Step lively! Shells landed right here yesterday morning and killed four men." One doctor, Hunter Jones, recalled his first impression of the beachhead: "As soon as we arrived in the harbor these shells started coming over. I got into a two-and-a-half-ton truck with some fellows and we started out, and the shells were coming over. . . .Then we saw tremendous holes on the ground right beside our tent. . . . That's what the Anzio Express did [he was told]."[41]

Homes were well-worn dug-in tents and dug-in cots left by the 56th Evac. The men and women of the 38th Evac were alerted to the bombardments and the killings—by then the beachhead had acquired quite a reputation—but, like most, could not fathom the danger. That is, until the first barrage, the first air raid. Then the howl and whine and ear-splitting blasts shook everyone from their wits. Sandbags were their new best friends and reinforcing shelters was their new pastime. So shell shocked were they that any idleness fueled fears, but fortunately there was little of that. Once tent flaps opened, patients rolled through. Ward work and operating were healthy distractions from falling flak and random rounds. In the first twenty-four hours, 193 patients arrived. By the end of April, the census had risen to almost seven hundred. The pace was so frenetic that some almost became complacent to the danger, the dread of errant ordnance dulled. But commanders insisted on protective measures. Helmets were to be worn—there were checks, to be sure—and blackout conditions at night were to be strictly enforced: "All personnel are reminded that helmets will be worn at all times. . . . Every individual will be held responsible for his quarters [blackout precautions]. Flashlights will not be used outdoors by any member of this command. . . . Smoking outdoors is prohibited during blackout hours."[42]

Captain Pickens, forbidden to identify his location ("'Anzio Beachhead' will not be mentioned in any correspondence," the official dictum read), wrote home about life in "the camp"—air raids ("Here it is entirely too close for any comfort"), and artillery ("There must be a million guns and they all fire at once"). Helmets were a necessary accouterment, everyone agreed—no argument there—falling flak the major hazard: "You wear your helmet all of the time except in bed and sometimes there, if a system is worked out where it is comfortable. It gets heavy and burdensome and hot, but it has saved people so we keep it on. No one wastes time in open spaces. . . . We are reasonably busy with patients."[43]

For the combat soldier, Mauldin's Willies and Joes, April was no different than March. Life was grindingly familiar: trench routine, patrols, short, violent firefights. Then nothing, just the perpetual awareness of sudden death from the skies. Like March, it was a month of back-and-forth cannon duels. Canoneers were prime targets; so were tankers—anyone next to a big gun. Even individual GIs were sometimes bracketed. Any movement on the battlefield was picked up by high-powered German binoculars, coordinates sent back, elevation and fuses fixed, powder adjusted, and lanyards pulled. Exploding shells invariably caught someone, sometimes whole groups. "Sometimes it was worse at the front; sometimes worse at the harbor," Mauldin observed.[44] Victims were picked up and hauled back—some able to walk—holed with fragment wounds. Collecting and clearing companies, such as the 3rd Medical Battalion, reported a majority of their wounds were caused by high explosives. So much so that across British and American sectors, for all the boredom and backyard brawling, there was a steady butcher's bill:

on average, over a hundred a day—maybe twenty killed outright, a few missing, the rest injured.[45]

Tar Heels at the 38th Evac saw it, a grisly assortment of dismemberments and disfigurements. For the next couple of months, almost three thousand five hundred battle casualties, including several hundred German prisoners of war, passed through their subterranean hospital. Surgeons busied themselves with the onerous task of repairing 136 abdominal wounds, 322 chest wounds, and 83 traumatic amputations, their registry enumerated. Curious wounding patterns were observed: a large number of Yanks—almost three hundred—were peppered by shell fragments up and down their backs and rumps. The reason: instinctive hunching over—fetal position—in a foxhole, or hugging the ground as a round came in, backs and buttocks exposed. Despite airbursts and ground bursts and tearing shrapnel, the staff did marvelous deeds. Only 104 died—97 percent survived their injuries.[46]

But artillery was not the only threat. There had long been worry about the bordering Pontine Marshes and nefarious German efforts to dismantle Benito Mussolini's benevolent canals. Mussolini had boasted of his program called *bonifica integrale*—reclaiming the land—a sweeping policy of agricultural reform. It was part of his efforts at national independence and sovereignty. Italian marshlands were notorious habitats for malaria—*mal aria*—carrying *Anopheles* mosquitoes, the bane of Italy from the time of Rome. By 1933, Mussolini declared that almost 19,000 square miles had been recovered. Marshy Littoria was transformed. But then two mad Nazi scientists, Eric Martini and Ernst Rodenwaldt, ruined it all. Littorian grasslands once again flooded, *Anopheles* flourished, and malaria reigned. Italian soldiers quartered there were felled at a ferocious pace. Almost 60 percent became infected. And in 1944, there would be a fiftyfold increase in the number of malaria cases involving Italian civilians.[47] By spring it was feared the area would revert to the pestilence of ancient days.

Sixth Corps surgeon Rollin Bauchspies knew well the ravages of malaria. Troops involved in Operation Torch, the invasion of North Africa, had shown a high infection rate. *Plasmodium* parasites were found in blood smears taken on hospital admissions for other reasons. Thousands harbored the microbe. Would that the hell of Anzio be spared this additional insult. The Allies had been fortunate so far. Chilly January and February brought a reprieve. At the 95th Evac, only about thirty cases had been diagnosed. But warmer spring temperatures and rainy days would provide optimum breeding conditions. Unchecked malarial outbreaks might affect thousands more troops. Truscott had already accosted his corps surgeon. "Bauchspies, what are you doing about the malaria situation here on the beachhead?" This was his counter. Beginning in March, every unit down to company size implemented an antimalaria program, distributing early suppressive therapy (Atabrine) and forming details for local control of mosquito breeding. Every soldier would be monitored for measures to reduce infectivity: proper clothing, mosquito netting, and the hated Atabrine.[48] Heavy equipment from the Corps of Engineers also set to work ditching and draining any remaining swampy areas. What could not be filled in or diverted was liberally sprayed with DDT or Paris green. The 42nd Malaria Control Unit dusted 107 miles of streams and static pools, even ranging into no-man's land. So effective were these measures that the 3rd Division surgeon reported no cases of malaria in replacement troops coming to the beachhead from malaria-free areas. By April and May, according to Bauchspies's report, daily surveys "failed to discover the presence of either adult or larvae of the Anopheles mosquitoes on the beachhead." Victory over *Anopheles*.[49]

11

Breakout

Breakout of the beachhead was inevitable. A two-prong thrust, up through the Winter Line, past Cassino, and into the Liri Valley linking up with VI Corps busting out of Anzio was the plan. Still, on both fronts, the winter and early spring saw a costly stalemate. Allied gains were almost imperceptible. Yet it was a meat grinder. From the middle of January to the end of March, the entire Fifth Army, including VI Corps, suffered over fifty-two thousand casualties in seventy-six days. And by the middle of March, the Germans had amassed almost sixty-six thousand troops surrounding the Anzio beachhead. For a time, a renewed offensive was contemplated, driving again down the cratered Anzio-Albano road or out of Cisterna, but Kesselring scrapped the plan, unwilling to commit vital reserves to General Mackensen around Anzio. By April 10, enemy strength had increased even more, to roughly seventy thousand troops—but there was still no green light for an attack. On the Allied side, American forces had been boosted by Combat Command B of the 1st Armored Division, the 34th Infantry Division, and, later in May, the 36th Infantry Division. The British had two infantry divisions in the line, the 5th and the 1st. Generals Alexander and Clark had finally devised a breakout plan called Operation Buffalo. American divisions would strike toward Cisterna, cutting off Highway 7, and continue northeast to the town of Valmontone. Eventually, forces would cross Highway 6 and trap German troops filtering out of the Liri Valley. British forces would hold the left side of the beachhead perimeter, paralyzing facing German units. The Allied counterpart to Buffalo on the

Cassino front, code named Diadem, would be an all-out offensive involving the Fifth (II Corps) and Eighth Armies. Major General Geoffrey Keyes's II Corps along with General Alphonse Juin's Free French Corps would shift to the Garigliano sector west of Cassino, and the entire Eighth Army would then focus on Cassino itself. The Allied right flank extending to the Adriatic was thus only lightly defended. Because of this weakness, the realignment required extraordinary stealth and cleverness—piecemeal—in April and May, leading Kesselring, perplexed by Allied strategy, to think that the real effort would be another amphibious operation north of Rome at Civitavecchia. If all went well, the Eighth Army, driving up from the south would join in, smash the Gustav Line, and fling German troops back through the Liri Valley toward Rome.

On April 16, the 11th Evacuation Hospital arrived to replace the battle-weary 93rd, now on the beachhead for four months. During its tenure, the 93rd Evac, under the command of Colonel Donald Currier, had admitted 5,596 patients and performed over three thousand operations, almost one thousand two hundred in February alone. Only forty-seven patients were lost—for them, too, a remarkable 98 percent survival rate. Feared epidemics of malaria cases were almost nonexistent. Only 143 patients were treated, virtually all because of disdain by soldiers for Atabrine therapy.[1] Its replacement, the 11th Evac under the command of Colonel Raymond Scott, was a four-hundred-bed, semimobile unit. Scott's hospital had seen action in North Africa and Sicily and had been in Italy since January. Its first location was Vairano, near the Gustav Line, but it switched in March to Casanova, closer to the Garigliano River. Little more than a month later, on April 12, orders were received to proceed to the Anzio beachhead. Scott arranged the standard surgical configuration: two connected operating tents for two surgical teams working at once. Each team that landed on April 16 had seven physicians, one nurse anesthetist, and one enlisted anesthetist, enough for alternate twenty-four-hour shifts.[2] First impressions were deceiving. Anzio was quiet that April day. "11th can't see why anyone would get jittery up here. WAIT AND SEE," 2nd Auxer Captain Hauver wrote in his diary.[3]

As a general surgeon with the 2nd Auxiliary Surgical Group, Major Luther Wolff landed via LST at the Anzio docks on May 7. He was a product of the University of Pennsylvania School of Medicine and had done surgical training at the Mayo Clinic before entering the service. "Will I ever see this beautiful country again? Will I ever feel the love of my wife and children?" he remembered thinking on February 20, 1942, as he boarded the train for Camp Kilmer, New Jersey, the likely debarkation station for overseas. Although the landings at Salerno had been something of an adventure, he and his team had stayed safe the past few months—as of late with the 10th Field Hospital at Carano—watching the Allies bang their heads against Monte Cassino and taking care of a steady trickle of casualties. Then, on May 6, "Colonel Forsee called and told me to get packed up, Anzio-bound, it seemed." Word was Anzio had become a mark of manhood. Wolff gossiped, "There have developed two cliques back at headquarters, the Anziites and non-Anziites. The former look down their noses at the latter."[4]

He would now be among the former. At Anzio, his team was assigned to the 11th Evac. "They are apparently going to give us mostly chests and bellies to do," he learned. "I don't think we will work too hard." On a tour of the beachhead, Wolff had visited the British 14th Casualty Clearing Station and met one of his fellow 2nd Auxers, a Kentuckian named Robert "Red" Robertson. Robertson had been attached to the British hospital from the start, his sense of humor and storytelling earning him an honorary place among the British. He had befriended a number of resident surgeons, including a Mr. Rodney Smith, later to become Lord Rodney, one of the pioneers in liver and bile duct surgery. "Red Robby," as he was called, welcomed Wolff with British-style tea and crumpets—and a double rye.[5] "All in all, this Anzio deal is not nearly as rough as . . . back at the Minturno Gap [on the Winter Line]," Wolff wrote, while preparations were underway for the big breakout.

On May 11, Prime Minister Churchill cabled General Alexander, "All our thoughts and hopes are with you in what I trust and believe will be a decisive battle, fought to the finish."[6] Diadem began that very day with a stupendous artillery barrage. Over the succeeding days, elements of the Eighth Army and Fifth Army II Corps breached the Gustav Line, pushing the German Tenth Army back to new defensive positions called the Hitler Line. These, too, were attacked and breached, forcing Germans up the Liri Valley toward Rome. Then on cue, with Germans in full retreat, the beachhead breakout occurred. It was early in the morning of May 23. Colonel Bauchspies, corps surgeon, watched the show from the roof of the Hotel de Ville in Nettuno—or what was left of it. "[E]very piece of artillery at the Corps command let loose and pounded the enemy lines for three-quarters of an hour."[7] Stocky Major General John "Iron Mike" O'Daniel's 3rd Infantry Division spearheaded the effort in an attack toward Cisterna supported by Harmon's armor and General William Eagles's Thunderbirds. A bloody affair it was, the Wehrmacht weakened but not finished, giving ground grudgingly. All along the battlefield, especially around Cisterna, losses were alarmingly high. Field units were suddenly swamped. Clearing Company, 3rd Med Battalion, admitted 572 wounded on May 23 and 444 the following day. Harmon's 47th Armored Medical Battalion saw 336 wounded in the first seventy-two hours of combat; in the 120th Med Battalion supporting the 45th Division, admissions from battle wounds on May 23 jumped tenfold.[8]

At the 11th Evac, Luther Wolff had it all wrong. "We are all practically dead with fatigue. Started at midnight, worked until 11:00 A.M., got three hours' sleep, and started in again," he reported on May 24.[9] Hell's Half Acre was jumping. To keep pace with the breakout, the 33rd Field Hospital disassembled into component units. On May 23, Unit A followed combat infantry, setting up south of the small town of Cori on the way to Valmontone. In the first thirty-six hours, the unit received sixty critically wounded men. Then it was directed to the Aprilia sector, a former no-man's land still cluttered with unburied American and German corpses. Unit C relocated just to the northeast of Cisterna just as the beachhead emptied in the dash for Rome. "So accustomed were the nurses to their dug-down tents that sleeping above ground for the first time in four months seemed strange and made them apprehensive," the nursing report read.[10] Unit "B" stayed put. Numbers of critical wounded tripled from April. "We were 72 hours behind in surgery, and the patients still arrived. The overtaxed personnel of our hospital, working day and night, handled this situation in a manner worthy of the highest commendation," the record read.[11] Over at the 94th Evac, the scene was similar. "At 0600 hours on the 23d of May we started receiving our first rush of casualties. . . . All that day, that night and into the next day casualties came in fast and heavy." And yet the shelling continued, some falling very close to the hospital tents.[12]

Richard Hauver had been on leave in Naples: sunshine, vineyards, and welcoming Italians. Diadem cut that short. Back at Carano with Wolff's former 10th Field Hospital, he found himself deep in "two bellies," sorting out shredded bowel. On May 22, he was ordered back to Anzio with the 94th Evac—and the graveyard shift at that. The first night he did eight cases, including one laparotomy and three amputations. The following day he was back at work at 2:00 PM and did not leave until 4:00 AM the next day—twenty more cases logged. "[A]wfully tired," he wrote. By the next day, after another fourteen hours, thirty-eight cases were still waiting. The 94th was now doing about 125 operations a day. "Never have been so tired even after a day's sleep. . . . [It] has been a hard grind," he wrote.[13] Across the compound at the 15th Evac, an "all time record" of 378 patients were admitted on May 31, including 167 battle casualties, almost all needing major surgery.[14] Captain Peyton wrote in his diary on May 23, "Casualties high—probably 1,000 today or 1,500. We have around 300 alone, several very sick. I worked until 7 AM."[15] By May 26, Captain Wolff had about had enough. "We are still working eighteen to twenty hours a day, sleeping very badly in the afternoon, and we are getting punch-drunk, and tempers are getting pretty short." Cases consumed hours of surgery—wounds of chest and abdomen. Spleens, kidneys, parts of liver all ended up in buckets.[16] Colonel Bauchspies estimated that during the first five days of the offensive, the casualties exceeded four thousand, almost twice as many as losses in the German raids of February.[17]

Nurse Wandrey, now with the 94th Evacuation Hospital, could not reconcile the daily destruction that passed before her eyes. Unlike some who tried to impersonalize it, to her each case was a separate catastrophe, the ruination of lives yet to be lived. Her sterile clinical expressions belied a deeper hurt and incomprehension:

> We're working now from 12-15 hours a day, never sit down, except to eat, all day long. . . . [W]e see war at its worst. . . . Such young soldiers. . . . Nineteen-year-olds and they can't even vote. . . . Bed 6, penetrating wound of the left flank, penetrating wound face, fractured mandible, penetrating wound left forearm. . . . Bed 5, amputation right leg, penetrating wound left leg, lacerating wound of chest, lacerating wound right hand. . . . Bed 4, massive penetrating wound of abdomen. Expired. . . . This field-nurse business is not for the faint of heart.[18]

On the backs of these young boys, the siege of Anzio officially ended, after 123 days, on May 25, as elements of the 36th Engineers (VI Corps) linked up with the 91st Cavalry Reconnaissance Squadron of II Corps at the small town of Borgo Grappa near the Pontine Marshes. With remarkable speed, after the capture of Cisterna, American troops swept through the countryside. The stream of wounded slackened. As the Germans' resistance was broken, they managed a steady retreat and paltry resistance to Allied forces. Elements of the 1st Armored Division entered the Eternal City on June 4. Julius Caesar could not have had a more jubilant reception by Roman citizens.

One hundred twenty-three days of conflict had produced 33,128 patients, 10,809 of whom were battle casualties funneled into Hell's Half Acre. [19] Success was realized not by brilliant strategy—of that there was very little—but by human tenacity and the agonies of true heroes. From front-line Willies and Joes to quartermasters, enlisted, and officers, the list of honorables is endless. As for the medical personnel and their efforts, Colonel Bauchspies summed it up in his gallant tribute: "No impressive array of figures can accurately express the total character of medical accomplishments. . . . As long as memory exists, these men and women of the Medical Department, the Courageous Medics of Anzio, will not be forgotten by the grateful host of men they served."[20]

In his memoirs, Churchill said of those months on Anzio's beachhead, "Such is the story of the struggle of Anzio; a story of high opportunity and shattered hopes, of skilful inception on our part and swift recovery by the enemy, of valor shared by both."[21]

For Luther Wolff and all the doctors and nurses who had endured at Anzio, the return to America at war's end was almost a dream, and matters of the heart, fueled by survival, took over: "As soon as we were allowed off post, I called my wife. Everything else . . . was completely and thoroughly dismissed from my mind as being inconsequential. I was home again!"[22]

And the thousands of young soldiers they worked on? Fifth Army surgeon Joseph Martin, now a brigadier general, made it clear to the public their wounds would endure a lifetime. For many, the battle would not be over when they returned home; families should be prepared: "It is an unfortunate psychological shock that awaits many families in the United States who after the war must give sympathy and consideration to their invalids. Medical men are not miracle workers. We can only do our utmost to save lives and prevent permanent disability to those under our care."[23]

"The tumult and the shouting dies . . . Still stands Thine ancient sacrifice . . . Lord God of Hosts, be with us yet, lest we forget—lest we forget!"[24]

Part 3

Bastogne

"Bastogne was a German job of death and destruction and it was beautifully thorough."—Martha Gellhorn

12

Arduennam silvam

FOLLOWING THE NORMANDY LANDINGS IN JUNE 1944, VICIOUS fighting continued on the Cherbourg Peninsula until July 25, when the Allies finally broke out of their coastal enclave. Paris was officially liberated a month later, and Allied forces sped across northeastern France. On August 15, French and Americans under Lieutenant General Alexander Patch's Seventh Army landed in southern France, linking up with George Patton's Third Army on September 10. Many thought the war in Europe would be over by Christmas. By then Allied forces were poised to enter Germany. The First Army had seized crossings over the Rhine, and the Third Army was at Mannheim. December witnessed a tremendous force of three Allied army groups spanning the frontier before Germany: Lieutenant General Jacob Devers's Sixth Army Group in the south, Major General Omar Bradley's 12th Army Group in the center, and Field Marshal Montgomery's 21st Army Group to the north. But failure of the Allied Operation Market-Garden in the fall to effect a pincer movement through Holland to trap German forces located in the Ruhr industrial districts ended all hopes of a quick surrender.[1]

With the steady German retreat across France, Hitler gave orders in September to raise twenty-five new divisions to be combat ready by December 1. These were Volksgrenadier divisions, largely recruited from second-rate inductees who would populate the Siegfried Line, basically cannon fodder for elite Panzer units. Racked by jaundice and fever in his redoubt at Wolfsschanze (Wolf's Lair) in East Prussia, Hitler was unwilling to settle for a defensive battle of attrition on the eastern and western fronts. Instead, a bold stroke would split the capitalist and communist alliance. A sudden, surprise thrust in the west—such a move in the east against the Soviets would be suicidal—was his plan. Disrupt Americans, British, and Canadians, weaken their resolve, and fracture the fragile link with Stalin. Drive a wedge between Allied commands and seize Antwerp, the port now so vital for supply. Hitler's entry point would be the thinly held Ardennes sector of Belgium, the same location where his Panzer units had flooded into France in 1940. Surprise would be essential, and the thick woods of the Eifel would hide troops and tanks.

By late October, troops began shuffling to the Aachen region, under the code name *Wacht am Rhein* (Watch on Rhine). Wacht am Rhein was largely delusional; most staff officers nodded in agreement but doubted that anything close existed in the true reality of the war, only in Hitler's deranged mind. Hitler called for three entire Panzer armies; the sixth, under Waffen-SS general Josef "Sepp" Dietrich just south of the Hurtgen Forest, would carry the main thrust, protected on its left flank by General Hasso von Manteuffel's Fifth Panzer, and turning left to block Patton's Third Army to the south, was the Seventh Panzer under command of General Erich Brandenberger. Hitler's generals were skeptical, especially the head of *Oberbefehlshaber West* (Command West), the aging General Gerd von Rundstedt, who knew "all, absolutely all conditions for the possible success of such an offensive were lacking" but sensed the desperation of his armies. In the end he echoed his Fuhrer's mandate: "We stake our last card . . . we cannot fail"—the very survival of the Reich was in jeopardy.[2] Key points in the Ardennes were the crossroads towns of Malmedy, Saint Vith, and the thriving community of Bastogne. Wacht am Rhein was inexplicably changed to the equally deceptive name Operation *Herbstnebel* (Autumn Mist) in early December.[3] Mechanized units would burst out of the forest, catch Americans napping, take over petrol dumps for their thirsty tanks, and drive on across the Meuse River to Antwerp.[4]

The Ardennes. "Arden" was the Celtic name for forest. In his commentaries on the Gallic Wars, Julius Caesar described the Ardennes of present-day Belgium and Luxembourg: "Arduennam silvam, quae est totius Galliae maxima atque ab ripis Rheni finibusque Treveroroum ad Nervios pertinent milibusque amplius quingentis in longitudinem patet." (The Ardennes forest, the largest of all of Gaul, reaches from the banks of the Rhine to the frontiers of the Treveri and Nervii, clearly more than five hundred miles in length.)[5] In this heavily wooded, sparsely populated area of Belgium, Luxembourg, and western Germany were the Gallic Treveri and the warlike tribe of the Nervii living among beech, alder, oak, and silver fir indigenous to the region, thriving on its abundant wildlife. Their forest was their fortress; even seasoned warriors like Roman legionnaires could not penetrate it. Roads were infrequent and unknown to all but the natives. So formidable was the place that Romans declared Diana a goddess there, hoping to curry her favor. She was sometimes called Arduenna—the huntress of the Ardennes. It would make little difference—they would never penetrate it.

The Meuse River divides the geography of Belgium. To the north the country is flat, gently sloping to the north and northwest. To the south the horizon quickly rises, forming the uplands known as the Ardennes. On maps, the forested areas appeared as a dark smudge, almost incapable of habitation. Some of the Ardennes is often described as mountainous but is not really so. It is deeply cut, though, by steep-sided valleys, carpeted by extensive areas of forest, at times almost impenetrable, in antiquity a wooden barrier between Celtic tribes to the west and Frankish tribes to the east. Yet the eastern regions known as the "haute-Ardenne" (High Ardennes) display mountains reaching more than two-thousand feet in the Hohe Venn, gradually blending into the Schnee Eifel near the Rhine River.[6] Travel was arduous; there were few trails to traverse the many hills and valleys of the seemingly endless expanse of greenery.

East of the Meuse, at a crossroads deep in the Ardennes, perched on a rise, is the city of Bastogne. "A rich, handsome town" of two thousand inhabitants, some would describe it in 1833, known for the excellence of its hams, a vast corn market, woolen manufacturing, and leather dressing.[7] In fact, the grain and cattle fairs of Bastogne were so well known that Italian diplomat Francesco Guichardini labeled it the "Paris of the Ardennes." Others were not so kind. Bastogne was described in one travelogue of the nineteenth century as evoking few romantic memories, the area around "the dreariest part of the Ardennes, the grim capital of which is Bastogne." So wrote British journalist Dudley Costello during his sojourn down the Meuse in 1846. In Costello's mind, the Paris of the Ardennes bore "a better resemblance to a new settlement in North America." All this amid the "most picturesque scenery in Belgium." He entered Bastogne after sunset, finding little comfort or food. And, upon leaving early the next morning, bereft of its famous hams, he once again entered the "last woody outpost of the Ardennes" at dawn. "[N]ever had

I witnessed a more glorious effect" than seeing the rising sun through the trees "like a vast red ball of fire"—apparently a welcome relief from the bleary disappointments of Bastogne.[8]

Astride trade routes, Bastogne probably always enjoyed prominence in the Ardennes as a city of commerce. It is likely some community existed there as early as the second century AD. The ancient Treveri probably inhabited the area, perhaps carving out livable quarters atop the gentle plateau. A village called Balsoniacum, corresponding to the present-day Bastogne, was mentioned in the Antonine Itinerary of the second or third century AD.[9] Bastogne, or its urban predecessor, lay in the path of the Roman road constructed from Rheims to Cologne and may have been a way station in the journey, perhaps following older tribal trails. A developing commercial hub in the first millennium, tiny Bastogne soon linked England, Flanders, Champagne, and Italy. Merovingian king Childebert II probably held a judicial assembly at Bastogne in the sixth century when he ruled over Austrasia, that Frankish kingdom incorporating present-day Belgium and Luxembourg. The name "Bastogne" can be traced to at least 634 AD, when records showed the city was bestowed as a gift to the Abbey of Trier. By the tenth century, Siegfried, "Count of the Ardennes" and the First Earl of Luxembourg, had built a fortress there, attesting to its strategic location even then. The castle was destroyed by the feudal armies of Liege in 1236, rebuilt, and finally dismantled by order of French king Louis XIV during the Nine Years' War in 1688. John the Blind, Count of Luxembourg, granted the city a charter in 1332 (before he was killed in the Battle of Crécy). A wonderful church, Eglise Sainte Pierre, began sometime before the tenth century was restructured in the sixteenth century in a more contemporaneous Gothic style. The square bell tower, reflective of older Romanesque architecture, still commands a dominant position in the town. In 1944, Bastogne became the hub of the Ardennes—most serviceable roads to the Meuse passed through it—a tactical linchpin for any counteroffensive on Allied maps, right in the center of the weakest sector of the American line.

Seven roads intersected at Bastogne, and along those roads were dotted towns and villages like beads on a rosary. From the north, along the Houffalize road, lay Noville and Foy, little more than a string of scattered stone huts, the small, spired Church of Foy a distinct landmark. From the east, the towns of Longvilly, Magaret, and Marvie. To the south off the Neufchateau road were Assenois and Sibret. Toward the west lay

Mande-Sainte-Etienne and Senonchamps, with Longchamps to the northwest.

Winters in the Ardennes—the wettest and coldest region of Belgium—were typically cold, icy, and barren, the forests appearing from a distance as blankets of pine and fir strewn over hills and valleys. Hitler and his high command well knew this. Frosts there are long and severe, snowfall abundant. Days were brief, and what daylight there was dampened by overcast skies. It was a time for hibernation, for winter quarters, for inactivity. All were concerned with keeping warm. Certainly it was not a time for war. In front of the Schnee Eifel, those rolling mountainous ridges, all was quiet. They were impassable. Uninhabited frontiers. Such was the terrain in 9 AD when Teutonic warriors, expertly concealed in thick timberlands encircled, ambushed, and massacred three Roman legions under Publius Quinctilius Varus. Now, much like the Romans of antiquity facing warlike Germanic tribes, the Americans were spread thin along the Ardennes, peering at the enigmatic Eifel. They settled in for an uneasy wintry peace. With sound muffled by snow, it was a quiet place to rest tired divisions.

In December 1944, the task of defending the Ardennes sector fell to Major General Troy Middleton's VIII Corps of the American First Army. Most Allied forces were clustered to the north and south. Middleton placed three US divisions along his eighty-five-mile front. The rookie 106th Infantry Division, fresh from training camps in America and loaded with replacement troops, held the left, abutting the 99th Infantry Division in V Corps. Some felt they were deplorable. Author Kurt Vonnegut, a member of the 423rd Infantry, saw his fellow soldiers as "poor physical specimens" who should never have been accepted in the army, much less the infantry.[10] He himself had no prior infantry training, his advanced instruction had been as an artilleryman. The "Golden Lions," as they called themselves, actually were stationed eight miles across the Our River into Germany. Frontage for the 106th Division alone covered twenty-six miles, over five times the width recommended by The US Army Service Manual. The veteran 28th Infantry Division was the anchor, smack in the center, and the war-weary, but seasoned, troops of the 4th Infantry Division guarded the far left (south), along with elements of Patton's Third Army on the division's right flank. A Combat Command of the untested 9th Armored Division (Combat Command B) occupied a narrow sector to the left of the 4th Division. And facing the Losheim Gap, that five-mile-wide valley at the western foot of the Schnee Eifel, rested some nine hundred cavalrymen of the 14th Cavalry Group, pinched between the V Corps sector to the north, held by the 99th Infantry Division, and the 106th Division to which it was now attached—a thin trip wire for any enemy advance into Belgium. It was through the Losheim Gap in 1940 that Rommel's Blitzkrieg roared to reach the Meuse River and across France, the only reasonable route for mechanized forces out of Germany. Occupying the northern shoulder of the Ardennes, in Major General Leonard Gerow's V Corps, was the green 99th "Checkerboard" Infantry Division.[11] Like the 106th Division, the 99th was untried in battle, having arrived in France just two months before. On their left, though, was the 2nd Infantry Division, veterans of Cherbourg, Saint-Lo, and, recently, attacks on the Roer River dams. Both divisions were arrayed in the Elsenborn-Krinkelt-Wirtzfeld area to block the northern network of roads funneling through the town of Saint Vith. In the opinion of Allied commanders, a thinly held VIII Corps front was a "calculated risk." Winter in the Ardennes rendered continuous logistical support unlikely, limiting any far-ranging objectives of a German counteroffensive. And the only reserves in the entire Allied Expeditionary Force were two divisions of the XVIII Airborne Corps, the 82nd and 101st Airborne Divisions, both resting and refitting near Rheims, France, following their grueling campaign in the Netherlands called Market-Garden.

In fact, most combat units were so overstretched that commanders placed company-size units with an eclectic mix of artillery and armor at strategic hamlets and crossings. In between, patrols roamed the countryside, mostly confined to roads, as passage through woodlands was laborious and almost impossible for mechanized infantry. Foot patrols were conducted simply to keep in touch with neighboring friendly units. In reality, during tranquil days of November and December, neither Americans nor Germans expressed much desire for hostilities. Often, troops of both sides were in clear sight, out of their foxholes, enjoying rare days of sunshine. Bedford Davis, an Emory-trained battalion surgeon for the 109th Infantry, watched as Major General Norman Cota, head of the 28th Division, asked a young private why he was not shooting at the enemy, quite visible to both. The private responded that the enemy soldier might shoot back. Laughter. All, including the general, seemed satisfied with the status quo.[12] On the German side, appearances were deceptive. Just behind those lazy, lolling troops was an inexorable buildup of men and material for the coming offensive.

Colonel Richard Eckhardt was the surgeon for VIII Corps. He had set up his command in Bastogne alongside Middleton's VIII Corps headquarters. His corps medical support centered on the 64th Medical Group, furnishing people and ambulances to divisions and corps medical teams, including field and evacuation hospitals. Eckhardt had four hospitals at his disposal—one field (42nd) and three evacuation (102nd, 107th, and 110th).

The 42nd Field Hospital had landed at Normandy on June 9. It had endured Normandy's grinding campaign, treating over one thousand one hundred patients in a week. After the breakout, the hospital split into three platoons, each supporting an infantry division racing across France. Now, in December, commanded by Lieutenant Colonel Fred Lahourcade, unit No. 1 of the 42nd was stationed at Wiltz, almost due east of Bastogne, supporting the 28th Division's clearing sections (Company D, 103rd Medical Battalion). Unit No. 2 was at Walferdange, just north of Luxembourg City, next to Company D, 4th Medical Battalion of the 4th Division. At the crossroads town of Saint Vith to the north was Unit No. 3, supporting the clearing sections (Company D) of the 331st Medical Battalion of the 106th Division. Each of the three units had been augmented by surgical teams from the 3rd Auxiliary Surgical Group.

The 102nd Evacuation Hospital had moved in late November from lavish quarters in Libin, Belgium—the elegant Chateau de Roumont—over one hundred rooms. The operating room had been put in a former ballroom, with elaborate drapes, mirrors, and rose-satin brocaded walls. Crystal chandeliers still hung undisturbed from the ceiling, and there were waxed, hardwood floors underfoot.[13] Yet the chopped up chambers made patient care following surgery less than desirable. Now the billets were more plebian: the agricultural college in Ettelbruck, less than six miles from the front lines. The 107th Evacuation Hospital was set up in German prefabricated buildings in fields just west of Clervaux, Luxembourg, affectionately known to their people as "the mud hole," and the 110th Evacuation Hospital was located on the French border at Esch-sur-Alzette, to the south of Luxembourg City in an abandoned, three-story school building, much better than the wet, muddy tents across France.[14] In V Corps sector, Unit No. 1 of the 47th Field Hospital and its attached surgeons from the 3rd Auxiliary Surgical Group were located at Waimes, east of Malmedy, and Unit No. 3 was at Butgenbach even farther east, almost within a stone's throw of the front. Both supported clearing sections of the 324th Medical Battalion of the 99th Division. On the southeast edge of Malmedy were set up the 44th and 67th Evacuation Hospitals in school buildings. Empty beds and idling surgeons backed up V Corps troops of the 99th and 2nd Divisions.

As Christmas 1944 approached, "Im Westen nichts Neus"—Nothing new in the West—as Erich Maria Remarque would have written. On Saturday, December 16, Omar Bradley, commander of 12th Army Group, had picked his way on icy roads through Luxembourg to meet with General Eisenhower at Versailles to help him celebrate his fifth star. Champagne was poured, oysters and scrambled eggs served. And in the nearby Ritz Hotel, Ernest Hemingway and his cronies were drinking and littering the floor with liquor bottles as bare-breasted girls did the hootchie cootchie.[15] Eisenhower later said "the responsibility for maintaining only four divisions on the Ardennes front . . . was mine."[16] His strategy was attack, attack, attack on both flanks of the Ardennes—but not the center. For now, it was a place of rest, recovery, and replenishment. Caesar's *Arduenna silva* would be a peaceful, frosty respite.

Troubling reports of increased vehicular activity behind German lines, refugee accounts of massed German equipment in the woods near Bitburg, and information from captured German prisoners of fresh troops pouring into the camps were largely ignored and not even reported to VIII Corps Headquarters.[17] On the eve of his great offensive, Rundstedt issued a proclamation (in leaflet form) entitled, "A Last Attempt." In this he stressed that all must go well: *Es geht ums Ganze*, "Everything is at stake." His last phrase was ominous, admonishing his troops that if all else fails "save what still can be saved —your life (*dien Leben*)." Intelligence officers of the 99th Division picked up the intercept.[18] What did it mean, some wondered? Most did not.

The holidays became raucous affairs. Leggy Marlene Dietrich sang and danced for the boys. Screaming Eagles of the 101st Airborne ogled after her at Mourmelon. One paratrooper remembered, "She had that sexy gown on and on stage she looked like a million bucks." Yes, and even at the front Dietrich pranced and slinked—and not a better time. Sentimental times for many, who were long removed from loved ones at home. For most, it was the first experience away from families. Her performance was good for morale and let the men know what they were fighting for. Always mindful of the lowly GI, she went where they went—mud, cold, tents and all—insisting on the same chow—and chow lines—as them. "She was witty, she was brilliant and kind, and she possessed a voice that raised glandular hackles," Lieutenant Brendan Phibbs, battalion surgeon for the 12th Armored Division, remembered.[19] By December 15, Dietrich was near the front lines on the border of Germany in the hamlet of Diekirch, teasing men of the 28th Division's 109th Infantry in her skintight dress and no underwear. Few foot soldiers were privy to the likes of Bob Hope or Bing Crosby in balmy rear areas where quartermasters pampered the privileged far from the grit and grime of battle. But here she was in windy, damp woodlands playing for unshaven men, crowding around in web gear with slung rifles. The next day at Verciers, she tossed off her baggy fatigues and steel helmet, slinking around the stage singing "Lili Marlene" to a howling audience. There had been thunder now and then, an occasional artillery round. Little did she know the Germans were tuning up. "If your men can be there, I will be there," she had said, not at all put off by a little danger. "There was an emotion close to furious tears when she sang goodbye and drove off in her truck through snow and ruins to the next division," Phibbs observed. "Take care, Marlene! Never die!"[20] Would that all could. It was the last time many saw the radiance of a woman.

"Guess we'll be stuck in this mud-hole till the spring," they were saying at the 107th Evac.[21] And it was only December 16. The night before, many had been out celebrating, enjoying the Christmas holidays. The morning of December 16, all still blissfully quiet in his area, Major Henry Swan, fresh from a surgical residency at the Peter Bent Brigham in Boston and now with the 4th Auxiliary Surgical Group, wrote his wife "Fletchie": "Yesterday was fun. I took a little trip up front to see how things were. . . . The front is rugged these cold days, and men are living in hovels. . . . Can you tell me why human beings constantly subject themselves to the indignity of warfare?"[22]

Yet with the winter snows, the landscape took on the look of a picture postcard, Martha Gellhorn thought, with "smooth white snow hills and bands of dark forests and villages that actually nestled."[23] But for the men settled in this picture-postcard setting, mud and snow and cold brought another set of tragedies. Swan's "fun" would not be an adjective used to describe the next few weeks. All the while, on that fateful Saturday morning, as Dr. Swan penned his letter, thousands of German troops were silently crossing the Our River in boats and building bridges for Tiger tanks and StuG cannon. Six divisions would be poised to attack the 28th Division alone, guarding what would be known as the Bastogne corridor. In total, VIII Corps (and the lonely 99th Division) stood directly in the path of three German armies in their rush to Antwerp and the North Sea.

13

Blitzkrieg in the Ardennes

At half past five in the morning on December 16, Americans sleeping in countless farmhouses, huts, and barns to escape the icy cold were awakened to a furious barrage of German artillery, their retreats specifically targeted as likely places troops would inhabit. Rolling thunder from the discharge of hundreds of cannon rattled windows, shook the ground, and turned heads to the east. Houses disintegrated in balls of fire, and plumes of smoke and earth filled the horizon. It was enough to stampede any living thing, including lonely GIs who jumped from their foxholes and headed west. Citizens of these scattered townships panicked, seeing their barns and haystacks set ablaze. A number of innocent victims—men, women, and children—were caught unawares in the apocalypse and blown apart. Those alive loaded their belongings and scooted down farmpaths and country roads toward sounds of silence. Directly in the path of Kampfgruppe Joachim Peiper and the rest of the 1st SS Panzer Division barreling through the Losheim Gap[1] was the 14th Cavalry Group, which put up a valiant fight in platoon-size clusters in remote outposts like Weckerath, Roth, Kobscheid, and Manderfeld Ridge against overwhelming odds. Neighboring elements of the 106th Division to the south were frustratingly out of contact—as it turned out, wires had been cut by infiltrating Germans—so a coordinated defense was impossible. But it was a losing proposition anyway. They were seriously outgunned and outmaneuvered. Gradually, and under pressure, cavalrymen of the 14th withdrew, thinking the neighboring troopers of the 106th were doing the same. This opened a wide avenue for Germans to spill through and around their comrades to the south.

In the panic that quickly developed, medical care was delivered on the run. For the first few days of the offensive, combat units were in disarray, many quickly surrounded, and evacuation routes cut off. Collecting points became meaningless, ambulances scarce, and litter teams needed more for defense than transportation. Even field hospitals were in danger of being overrun—some actually were—and spent a considerable amount of time on the move, usually westward and to safety.

Company A of the 331st Medical Battalion, 106th Infantry Division, headed by Captain Bob Mitterling, was assigned to the 14th Cavalry and was to furnish ambulances for evacuation to its clearing section located back at Saint Vith. They enjoyed a pleasant duty station on the east bank of the Our River near the town of Andler. That is, until Saturday morning. Instead of the usual admissions for trench foot, a flood of battle casualties arrived with shrapnel wounds from high explosives. Reports soon poured in that Germans were in the battalion rear and had even stopped one ambulance en route from a battalion aid station. Soon all communication with forward aid stations stopped. Cavalry group headquarters informed the 331st that its position was tenuous and advised the company to withdraw to Heuem, Belgium, along a route that led by the tiny village of Schonberg. Dropping German shells forced a quick trip through—Schonberg had been targeted by enemy artillery—men diving for cover with each incoming *whoosh.* Yet their stay in Heuem was short lived. German penetration west of Schonberg, just up the road, forced a further withdrawal to Saint Vith the following day. There the town hall served as a new collecting station, catching the wounded straggling in from units farther east. But few were cavalrymen. By that time, contact with the 14th Cavalry Group had been lost. Many troopers had been encircled and surrendered as they ran out of ammunition and hope.[2]

Company D of the 331st Med Battalion—the clearing company—had, just a few days before, taken over buildings occupied by the clearing station of the 2nd Division in Saint Vith. During the two-day transition, the ten medical officers and two dental officers of the 331st absorbed valuable information from a unit that had extensive battle experience. Once the 2nd Division vacated, Company D organized in much the same fashion. For the next few days, most admissions, maybe six per day, were trench foot or upper respiratory infections; few were battle wounded. Early Saturday morning, shelling was heard. Two hours later, a throng of wounded arrived with myriad fragment injuries clearly from artillery. Doctors counted over 270 men, many from the 424th Infantry (106th Division). Twenty-five were critically wounded with chest, face, and limb injuries. Those were given emergency care, packaged, and sent to the 42nd Field Hospital, where surgeons with the 3rd Auxers were stationed. Rumors soon circulated that Saint Vith was directly in the path of German attack, maybe even already surrounded. Tanks were headed their way. "The day passed in utter gloom," records read. Casualties stacked up despite efforts by auxers to move patients along, a number suffering deep internal damage and scrupulous repair.[3]

Sunday found an even worse situation. Artillery blasts were almost continuous, some disturbingly close. Ground shook and plaster fell from the walls, meddlesome distractions for painstaking surgery. Team leader Major Phil Partington was trying to control bleeding from an axillary artery injury when there was an explosion in the courtyard, blowing out lights and windows, felling assistant Captain Al West, and leaving Partington alone, one hand on the bleeding artery and the other "groping for a ligature." The normally meticulous Partington, feeling that Germans were just around the corner, quickly ligated the artery and closed the wound, the only illumination the beam of a flashlight.[4] Reconnaissance patrols had already been sent out to find fallback positions, the town now soon to be overrun. Twelve miles west was the town of Vielsalm, so far out of danger. Word soon passed to evacuate. Patients and personnel hurried to get on the road, all equipment left behind. Traffic was paralyzing. Tanks, troops, and vehicles were moving east, trying to get to Saint Vith, while civilians and panicking GIs headed west. "It was a case of 'every dog for himself.'" "It was a retreat, a rout," according to one armored officer.[5] Local citizens suffered the most, especially peasants displaced from their humble huts, now torched and smoldering embers. One surgeon observed "the risk and mortalities of war are unequal and the poor carry the biggest part of the risk." He later felt guilty of his relatively safe environment, even during those harrowing few days of the Ardennes offensive.[6]

At one point, the surgeons' truck was pushed completely off the road, with priority given to long lines of armored units snaking their way to the front. Yet Vielsalm was equally chaotic. Disorder and confusion ruled, spreading like a human plague.

The hospital platoon and surgeons arrived after sunset. A pathetic scene greeted them, one that spoke bewilderment, disorder, and terror. Numbers of wounded lay unattended, brought in by any convenience, set down, and abandoned. By flashlight, many were found pale and almost lifeless, dying of shock or peritonitis. Some had barely received first aid. By midnight, a Catholic boarding school had been found to use as an operating room. With the little surgical equipment salvaged from Saint Vith—and with little anesthetic—surgeons set about the painful task of salvaging whom they could. Company D of the 331st Med Battalion arrived just before dawn the next morning. It had been traveling fourteen hours, caught in the same roadbound human misery. None too soon, the men of the 331st brought much-needed surgical supplies: suture, clean instruments (hemostats, knives, saws, retractors), sterilizers, plasma, intravenous needles. That day alone, sixty-four battle casualties were treated. The count soon reached 170, but amazingly, with all the bedlam of those days, only two patients died.[7]

In the German Blitzkrieg, regiments of the 106th Division had been caught in the open, directly in the path of Panzers and hordes of foot soldiers. Eighteen- and nineteen-year-olds—many draftees hardly prepared for combat—faced battle-hardened Grenadiers emerging from fog-cloaked Schnee Eifel, camouflaged in white snow garb and their distinctive Stahlhelme. It was either fight or run. Most stayed put in their foxholes and fought, a few at the point of their bayonet. Some ran, throwing down their weapons—even screaming in fright—and "bugging out."[8] Many heard relief was on the way—the 7th Armored. But there was no such luck. The boys of the 106th were surrounded—the 14th Cavalry had already pulled back and left them. Help was never even contemplated. German troops were fanning out around and behind them. Collecting Company B of the 331st, supporting the 423rd Regiment, found itself cut off near Buchet. The last message received was from a Sergeant Murphy, surprisingly unruffled: "Casualties being received from anti-tank and service companies. Enemy using 88s, mortars, and small arms. Casualties show a slight increase. . . . Situation remaining the same as reported on previous messages."[9]

Within two days, the 422nd and 423rd Regiments had been pinched—ensnared—by German forces, with no escape. Ammunition was gone, artillery support nonexistent. Further resistance was suicidal. At the 422nd aid station, food, medicine, blankets, and water dwindled and were soon gone. Lieutenant Colonel Thomas Kelly of the 589th Ar-

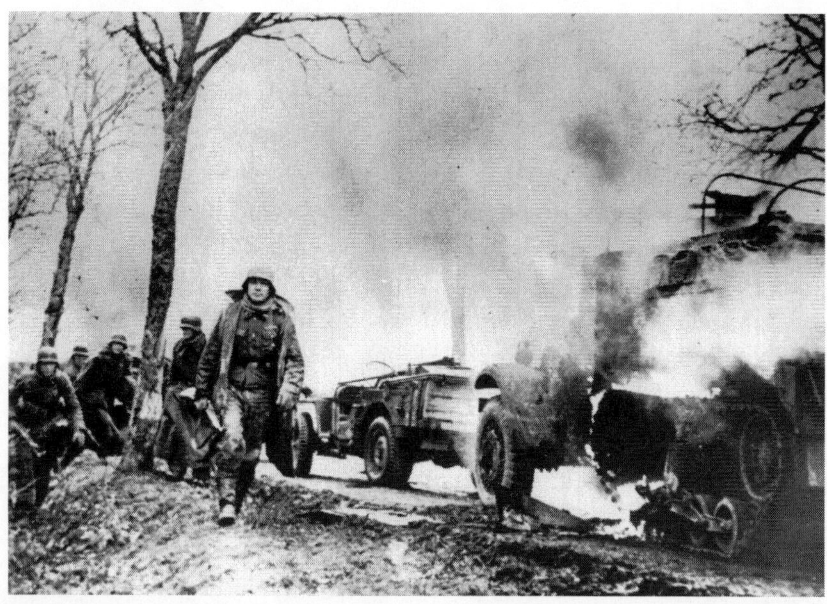

German infantrymen pass burning American vehicles during the Ardennes offensive in December 1944. This photogaph is part of a reel of film captured from a German soldier. (*National Archives*)

tillery later remarked "there was a steady stream of wounded . . . and without dressings or blankets there was nothing we could do except let them lie in their gore and shiver—with the most goddam pitiful look in their eyes."[10] The commander of the 422nd, Colonel George Descheneaux, having been given orders to fight his way through, knew his men would be "cut to pieces." Next to his command post he could hear the moans and cries of the wounded and dying. As a casualty passed him on a stretcher, one leg missing, blood dripping in a steady stream, he exclaimed, "My God, we're being slaughtered." His decision was obvious—to save as many men as possible. He implored the commander of the 423rd Infantry, Lieutenant Colonel Joe Pruett, to do likewise.[11] On December 19, around seven thousand American soldiers—the exact figure will never be known—capitulated, the largest surrender of American forces since Bataan. Some escaped, but medics, battalion surgeons, and patients of Collecting Companies B and C were rounded up, unable and unwilling to leave. What was an embarrassment to higher command was looked on by their officers as an act of humanity. Just to the south, the 3rd Regiment, 424th Infantry, managed to stabilize its front, thanks to the intrepid actions of one Lieutenant Jarrett Huddleston Jr., who led a group of soldiers to fight off encircling German efforts. "Jerry" Huddleston was the son of Anzio's late VI Corps surgeon, Colonel Jarrett Huddleston.

North of the 14th Cavalry Group, in V Corps sector, SS Oberstgruppenfuher Josef Dietrich's Sixth Panzer Army collided with elements of the 99th Infantry Division. Dietrich dearly wanted the road network leading northwest to Bullingen, Butgenbach, and on to Malmedy and west to Buchholz, Schoppne, and Faymonville. He unleashed all the artillery his Panzers could muster. The barrage was thunderous. GIs thought all hell was breaking loose. Never had veterans of the Checkerboard Division seen anything like it. Towns were crumbling, buildings smashed by a rain of shells. All that is but Monschau, a favorite town of German honeymooners and, so it was said, of Adolf Hitler himself. Volksgrenadiers pressed forward, emerging from the mist as ghostlike figures. The Americans held, felling Germans in gigantic numbers.

Aid stations were never far from the action. Hunnigen, site of first aid for the 394th Infantry, caught repeated shelling. The wounded, fresh from shelled foxholes, wondered if they would be blasted again. In Bucholz, a battalion aid station was repeatedly hit, ruining bottles of plasma and packets of morphine and forcing an evacuation. Litter bearers were scarce, and buddy carry was the only alternative. Ambulances were no safer, running a gauntlet of enemy fire on any serviceable road—all had been ranged in beforehand by German artillery. Medics and doctors were advised to pack and leave, back to Butgenbach, where the 47th Field Hospital was. But many injured were stranded, unable to move. Heartbreaking stories abounded. Soldiers of the 393rd Infantry helped a wounded comrade whose right arm was attached only by shreds. He was in shock, his body trembling—the cold almost unbearable. "Get me out of here! For God's sake get me out of here," he kept saying. His medic, trying to comfort him and administer plasma, was shot clean through the head. There would be no getting out of there, not for a long, long time. One infantryman remembered being in a foxhole with his buddy: "Gordon got ripped by a machine gun from roughly the left thigh through the right waist. . . . We were cut off . . . by ourselves . . . we both knew he was going to die. . . . We had no morphine. We couldn't ease [the pain] so I tried to knock him out. I took off his helmet, held his jaw up, and just whacked it hard as I could . . . that didn't work. . . . Nothing worked. . . . He slowly froze to death, he bled to death."[12]

Captain Fred McIntyre, battalion surgeon for the 393rd Infantry, stayed with 15 victims, many too critical to move, when his battalion withdrew from enemy pressure. He and his patients were later taken prisoner.[13]

Merciless German behavior added to worries. There was never certainty that surrender would mean survival. The division surgeon, Lieutenant Colonel K. T. Miller, reported:

> Medical Department soldiers were deliberately killed in spite of Red Cross brassards on both arms and four red crosses on white, circular backgrounds 4 inches in diameter on the helmets. It is further known that vehicles transporting wounded and plainly marked with Geneva Red Cross were deliberately riddled by enemy small arms fire . . . in one instance, a tank at close range fired an armor-piercing shell through an ambulance operating in an adjacent Division.[14]

To the north of the 99th Division, troops of the 2nd Infantry Division wisely began a choreographed withdrawal to the twin villages of Rocherath and Krinkelt and along high ground of the Elsenborn ridge. Evacuation routes from clearing companies to clearing station were quickly cut. Only one small field hospital near Nidrum remained, and that unit cared for over one thousand three hundred wounded, including several hundred battle casualties. In Rocherath, leading toward the Elsenborn ridge, the 2nd Med Battalion—Company C—found a building near the center of town. Everything possible was done to mark the place as a hospital. Ambulances were parked out front, Geneva markers were placed on the roof; windows were sandbagged. Still, doctors in Company C were bewildered. The arrival and sorting of wounded had deteriorated into a jumbled collection of frightened, bleeding youngsters dumbfounded at the explosive onslaught of mechanized warfare. Doom was thick in the air. Rumors of onrushing Germans were everywhere. Who knew? The next minute might bring a flash of rifle fire or the deafening blast of a grenade.

Casualties tumbled in day and night, but total care was impossible. No one could tackle serious injuries. Bandaging, splinting, plasma was all that could be done. Evacuation was high priority, getting them in ambulances and on to surgeons, evading onrushing Germans. Inexplicable scenes unfolded. One aid station was located less than one hundred yards from a road junction occupied by enemy tanks. A single ambulance made ten trips to this station in less than twenty-four hours, all in full view, tracer rounds crisscrossing the village streets. Men dashed out, stretchers in hand, and filled any vehicle available. Once loaded, the jeeps, trucks, and ambulances took off, dodging German troops and tanks, and ran the gauntlet from Rocherath to the twin village of Krinkelt, a short distance away. Most made it. A few did not. Three jeeps and one Dodge ambulance were destroyed, killing one patient and wounding another (again).

Over the next few days, fighting spilled into Krinkelt, becoming as chaotic as the scene in Rocherath. Seventy-ton German Tiger tanks roamed the streets, crushing ambulances, blasting structures point blank with 88-mm cannon fire. Artillery rounds fell, shattering windows and partially destroying one wall of the building the regimental aid station occupied, just arrived from Rocherath. Men inside could see a Tiger only twenty-five yards away, the tank commander shouting commands in English for Americans in trucks and jeeps in the area to "dismount and be recognized." Those who did were shot in cold blood "where they stood." Two such victims were dragged to the aid station, where they died of their wounds despite efforts to save them.[15] Delayed, yes, but not repulsed, Germans kept coming. Finally, there was no option but to abandon Rocherath and Krinkelt for the safety of the Elsenborn Ridge. Unbelievably, all medical personnel and their wounded withdrew without harm. The Germans left them alone.

On the morning of December 17, the second day of the offensive, men of the 3rd Platoon (Unit No. 3) of the 47th Field Hospital at Butgenbach, a town not far from the German border, heard distant rumblings but as yet were unaware of any danger. They had stumbled onto a battered schoolhouse without light or heat just a few days before, but it at least provided shelter from the snow, wind, and cold. There they set up cots, tables, and equipment. Now, outside, the clanking of tanks, jeeps, and half-tracks picked up in tempo, passing in both directions—to the front and away from it. Pedestrian traffic also increased; many were disheveled American soldiers shuffling hurriedly west. Some kind of German probing, many surmised. "[O]ur troops would chase them back in short order," doctors boasted. Others thought that gun and artillery fire was from a 2nd Division offensive toward the Roer dams. But the snarl of overloaded jeeps and personnel carriers moving west and packed half-tracks and antitank guns moving east finally convinced the 47th commander, Major John Henderson, that something momentous was happening. What was concerning were the worn-down soldiers tramping west, with little order or purpose and without rifles, packs, even helmets. Captain Claude Warren, a 3rd Auxer, had just finished operating on a double amputee—both legs blown off by mortar fire—when he heard rifle shots down the road. Jeeps were speeding by, heaped with armed soldiers. The air was electric, as if a crisis was approaching. Warren and his fellow surgeons were excited, glad that they would be operating on battle-wounded men instead of the rare appendicitis or rotten toes from trench foot. He stopped one infantry officer to get a report on the front. The officer, quite nonplussed, asked what he was doing there. "We are running a hospital," Warren replied. "You better get yourselves some guns or you will be operating on Heinies [Germans]," the officer shouted. Germans were already in Bullingen, perhaps a mile away, and, by all reports, rolling onward. Evacuation orders were quickly given. Nurses left first, to Elsenborn and on to the 2nd Division Clearing Station—no baggage, just what they could carry. Then, later, doctors, patients—including the double amputee, his guillotined stumps soaked in blood—medics, and technicians, all grabbing whatever vehicle they could, sure that Germans were just around the corner, the popping of small-arms fire now distinct.

Henderson's unit was soon on the road to Waimes. Its destination was the 1st Platoon of the 47th located there. It was slow travel, weaving in and out of refugees and oncoming traffic. Once at Waimes, he found out that the 1st Platoon had already evacuated to Malmedy, its place deserted. Nurses, doctors, and patients had been hustled out only hours before. Henderson hurried his group to Malmedy, afraid he was already too late. They passed a checkpoint on the way, a hamlet called Baugnez. Not two hours later, dozens of captured American troops were senselessly murdered by men of Colonel Peiper's Panzer column—even medics and wounded. It was a close call for Henderson. At Malmedy, doctors, nurses, and medics of the 47th moved into an old school building with other medical refugees, men and women of the 44th and 67th Evacs. But not for long. More rat-tat-tat of automatic rifle fire and shouts of, "The Germans are coming." Colonel John Blatt, commander of the 44th, shouted, "Hurry up! They're coming down the road!" "There was no longer any desire to be a hero," surgeon Warren remembered. "We were in a tight spot." Thoughts of excitement quickly faded.[16]

Malmedy derived its name from the Latin *a malo mundarum*—cleanse from evil. And there would be plenty of cleansing to do that December.

Shells began falling near the 67th Evac in Malmedy early Saturday morning, the 16th. Germans had targeted the area as another vital crossroads town, hoping to catch any American troops marshaling there. Before long, rounds were landing at a regular pace, rattling dishes, knocking out plaster, and cratering streets. Services at the twin-towered Catholic cathedral were just ending, people filing out its doors, when explosions tore into the brick pavement—and the parishioners milling outside. Two American soldiers walking out of Mass had gone to the aid of wounded civilians. More explosions. Fragments tore into both, killing them instantly. One of them was a medical officer, commander of the 464th Medical Collecting Company, Captain Alfred Duschatko of Scarsdale, New York. He was twenty-six. Duschatko had been a star scholar and all-around big man on campus at Columbia University. Later, in medical school there, he married a fellow student, Elizabeth Lambert. A son was born to them, now nine months old, hours after he shipped overseas.[17]

Malmedy, too, was soon evacuated. Germans had broken through, it was said. Shellfire bracketed buildings housing the 44th and 67th Evacs, endangering everyone inside. Nurses and doctors were hurried out to the 4th Convalescent Hospital, in Spa, Belgium, safe for the moment but, as it turned out, still uncomfortably close to the German advance.[18] Several men and women from both hospitals volunteered to stay behind; critical patients yet needed surgery. During a night filled with peril, ten operations were done on those casualties. Miraculously, all made it out the next day.[19]

The 28th Infantry Division, the "Keystone Boys," held the center of VIII Corps, blocking the Bastogne corridor.[20] General Cota was in command. His "Keystone Boys" were right in the path of two Panzer divisions, three infantry (Volksgrenadier) divisions and one Fallschirmjager (parachute) division under Prussian general Hasso von Manteuffel. Manteuffel wanted Wiltz, which lay on the route to Bastogne, and he wanted Bastogne. The 28th Infantry would catch hell in the process. That morning, GIs in the town of Grindhausen heard what they thought was "incoming mail,"[21] probably miles away. Artillery bombardments had begun. Shells were headed for Marnach and soon into Clervaux, Heinerscheid, and Munshausen not far from the German border, in Luxembourg. In these towns were stationed company-size units of two battalions of the 110th Infantry, spread across a ten-mile front west of the Our River, including the north-south thoroughfare from Saint Vith to Diekirch called by the Americans "Skyline Drive."

Before long Wiltz itself, headquarters of the 28th Division and about eleven miles from Bastogne, was being shelled. Along the Bastogne corridor, explosions wrecked buildings and flamed farm fields. Soon, from the woods emerged thousands of Germans. Easy targets, these were Manteuffel's Volksgrenadiers, massed formations of foot soldiers who were to open the way for his 2nd Panzer Division. They were cannon fodder. GIs dropped Germans every step of the way. Mortar fire tore limb from limb, decapitating, eviscerating. The dying screamed "Kamerad," but there would be no mercy, not now, not without a white flag. All along Skyline Drive, Americans and Germans collided; even some artillery units engaged in hand-to-hand fighting. Yet despite fierce resistance, vast numbers of enemy troops slowly pushed through, exploiting wide gaps in the thinly held American line. By the afternoon of December 17, Colonel William Fuller, commander of the 110th, who was holed up with his headquarters staff in the Claravallis Hotel, was surrounded. Germans were firing directly into the windows. Regimental surgeon major Lester Frogner had set up his aid station in the basement. In the pitch dark, what emergency care was possible was given—but little comfort. As Germans encircled the town, it was unlikely anyone could be evacuated. There was no way to make it to the 103rd Medical Battalion, now at Kautenbach, just south of Clervaux. Roads there had already been severed by German forces. Fuller eventually gave orders to get out any way possible. Amazingly, many were able to evade enemy troops and somehow make their way to Esselborn.[22] Major Frogner and his wounded soldiers were not so lucky, and were taken prisoner.

Maunteuffel's men bowled forward. Clervaux fell that Sunday, then Marnach, Munshausen, Holzthum, Weiler, Hoscheid, and a number of small villages west of the Our River. Defenders of Hosingen finally waved a white flag after tying up two regiments of enemy troops sorely needed elsewhere. Any delay was invaluable to Americans. It gave precious time to regroup to the west. Casualties were mostly cared for at aid stations, battalion surgeons battling hemorrhage, shock, and cold. Dr. Brendan Phibbs was one of those, desperately trying to stem bleeding, bide time, somehow get his patients to surgeons. He wrote:

> [W]e've learned to concentrate our skills . . . where they do the most good. . . . Wounds in bellies, heads, and chests are beyond definite help here: we can only support life with plasma, adrenaline, caffeine, and morphine, and ship them off for surgery. . . . We pray for speed.

. . . We concentrate on bleeding from the extremities, the neck, and the face; by stopping this bleeding we can stop dying.[23]

The 103rd Medical Battalion's collecting companies did what they could, setting up straggler points for wandering soldiers, checking them over. Those fit enough were directed back to combat units. Serious wounds were a problem. Roads had become deadly passages, and ambulances were few and far between. As it was, twenty-one medical personnel were captured. Still, over one thousand five hundred wounded were seen and treated. For the clearing platoons—now there were three, one per regiment—doctors busied themselves in the most remote locations, under fire and in danger. Nowhere was safe. Somehow they were able to treat almost two thousand wounded, even some German casualties.[24]

The Keystone Boys were hit hard. By December 18, what was left of the 110th Infantry withdrew west. Some survivors headed north, joining other units; some made it back to Wiltz, the division command post. Estimates put losses in the range of 2,750 men killed, wounded, or captured. To the north, the 109th Infantry had been pressed hard by mobs of German troops, cut off from the 110th Infantry, and began falling back on Diekirch and then Ettelbruck. To the south, the 112th Infantry put up stubborn resistance, but the German tide forced it back to Wiltz. Panzers were soon on the outskirts of Wiltz, the last stop to Bastogne. In Wiltz itself, combat engineers, bandsmen, paymasters, and telephone linesmen were thrown into the defense. On December 19, General Cota had moved his command to Sibret, and by nightfall the defensive perimeter was pierced, defenders falling back to the center of town. By the next day all was lost. Small groups of soldiers fought their way out to the west, already encountering enemy roadblocks toward Bastogne.

Unit No. 1 of the 42nd Field Hospital in Wiltz was located in an almost fairytale setting, the Castle of Wiltz, completed by Count John VI in 1720. The castle, partially used as a convent, was placed high on a rocky promontory, looking out on acres of manicured lawns and gardens, and beyond, mile after mile of Ardennes countryside. The town of Wiltz was spread out below, with rows of French provincial whitewashed homes and businesses. Teams of the 3rd Auxiliary Surgical Group were based with the 42nd Field Hospital, headed by Majors Charles Serbst (Team No. 11) and Duncan Cameron (Team No. 15). Events happened quickly after December 16. In two days, the Germans punched salients to the north and south of town, soon enveloping it.

Communication with the 64th Medical Group in Bastogne had been lost. Not knowing whether to evacuate, Major Serbst made his way to Bastogne, dodging shells but discovering nothing—the medical group was just as confused as those in Wiltz. By the evening of December 18, Wiltz was surrounded. Orders from division headquarters were given to move out. What to do with nontransportable patients?[25] Should they stay and risk being captured by the Germans or leave, even though some patients might die on the road? Serbst and Cameron decided to split the hospital into two sections, one to leave and the other to stay with the twenty-six most critical patients. The truck convoy moved out after dark carrying all transportables, most platoon personnel, nurses, and surgeons. Arriving in Bastogne with the Germans only three miles away, they found an empty monastery and a thin defensive perimeter of 10th Armored Division troops. Realizing they would likely soon be captured here, too, they moved on to the 107th Evacuation Hospital at Libin, and the nurses on to the 42nd Field Hospital unit across the border in Sedan, France.

For those remaining in Wiltz, German shelling soon blew out windows of their sanctuary, forcing them to move all patients to the basement. There was total darkness, casualties and wounds inspected only by the beam of a flashlight. The following day, December 19, machine-gun and rifle fire drew closer. Major Henry Huber tied a bedsheet to a pole, went outside, and flagged down German paratroopers. The Germans approached and lined up American staff in the courtyard, scrutinizing each one. Papers on Captain Harry Fisher were examined, and he was called out. "Jude" (Jew) was heard as he was gruffly taken away. Hearts sank; all feared he would be shot. The rest were informed they were now prisoners of war and would be allowed to remain to care for their wounded. Soon a German Hauptverbandplatz, or dressing station, the rough equivalent of an American clearing station, was brought in and set up, but it was woefully short of supplies. Only the amputation knife wielded by a German surgeon was impressive and used liberally. Amputees, German doctors declared, could be discharged in a few weeks; a man in traction with a plaster cast would tie up a hospital bed for months. Over the next few days, dozens of wounded Americans were brought in. Without blood, heating, or supplies, many died either of shock, peritonitis, or gangrene. Although American surgeons collegially shared a Christmas dinner with their captors, by December 27 they were hustled out onto the road and took a long journey into Germany and Stalag 12. To their amazement—and joy—they met up with Harry

Fisher, who recounted unbelievable tales of the battle for Bastogne—from the Germans' side. He had been pressed into service in their medical units. Better than a round to the back of the head, he knew.[26]

Resistance in the Bastogne corridor was buckling. Middleton had insisted these checkpoints be held at all costs, but it was not to be. Brigades—called combat commands—of the 9th Armored Division in outposts like Allerborn and Trois Vierges in Luxembourg withered under superior German firepower and sheer numbers. Retreat forced all back through Longvilly—soon a scene of confusion and ripe with rumor—and farther west to Margeret. Soldiers were exhausted, cold, hungry, and thoroughly whipped. Second Med Battalion medics and doctors practiced medicine on the run, hurriedly setting up field stations and just as quickly tearing them down as the Germans drove on. Company C, supporting one of the 9th's brigades, had run from Allerborn down through Longvilly and finally was lucky to make it into Bastogne on December 19. It dragged along as many wounded as it could but left not a few poor souls dead along the way.[27]

Clervaux, Luxembourg, is another of those charming Ardennes towns of whitewashed villas, an abbey, and churches. The focal point is the majestic Castle of Clervaux, first begun in the twelfth century. On December 16, some at the 107th Evac "mud hole" near Clervaux heard distant thumps of shelling—like the stompings of some colossal giant—almost, it seemed, getting louder by the hour. "Sheer imagination" the denial went. The next morning doctors, nurses, and technicians were awakened to the shouts, "Get the hell out of bed, throw your cots on the trucks, grab some chow, and be ready to move at a moment's notice." The sky was vibrant with flashes of artillery, searchlights, and antiaircraft fire. Rumors of street fighting in Clervaux spread. Stragglers reported horror stories. "The Kraut is taking no prisoners," bedraggled, drained soldiers were saying. They would gladly leave, but not for an anguishing five hours, a lone tank finally leading the way. "The Jerries are right on my tail," the tanker said.[28] Everything was left but the patients. Long underwear, fatigues, and quilted combat pants were the standard garb, for work and sleep. The weather was bitterly cold. Their destination was Libin and the grand Chateau de Roumont, recently occupied by the 102nd Evac. Wounded were carried up four flights of a magnificent marble staircase until the rooms were packed with over four hundred patients. Within days, the bone-weary men of the 42nd Field Hospital arrived—and in good time. Help was needed for a backlog of wounded.

In an eighty-hour period, almost four hundred operations were performed, many on serious chest, abdomen, and brain trauma, most fresh from battalion aid stations. It was backbreaking work, hours of resuscitation and operating. Surgeons worked straight through, rarely taking breaks. Others—officers and enlisted alike—would put in a twelve-hour shift then fill in as litter bearers. No one slept.[29]

December found the 102nd Evac in Ettelbruck, along with a clearing station of the 28th Infantry Division (2nd Platoon, Company D, 103rd Medical Battalion). Ettelbruck, like Clervaux, was yet another picturesque Luxembourg village. The quarters in the agricultural college were spacious and comfortable, with hot and cold running water, cots, and warm food. There was over seventy-three thousand square feet for the hospital proper. Trench foot was the most serious challenge—until December 16. Wounded Keystone troops flooded in, hammered by advancing Germans. Diekirch, just three miles away, was under attack, the injured taken directly to Ettelbruck, not even stopping at aid stations. Serious injuries—nontrasportables—likely died on the spot. Few made it back. With Diekirch in danger of falling, the 102nd was ordered on the road. The medieval town of Huy was its destination. It was lucky to reach it. The convoy became split. Trucks, doctors, and nurses "wandered around for two days on Belgium roads," according to its chaplain, Ren Kennedy.[30] It was a miracle they all were not captured. In Ettelbruck, thirty-five seriously injured patients were left behind—head, chest, and belly injuries, some fresh from surgery. Three doctors and a score of enlisted stayed with them. Not until December 22 did they make it safely out.[31]

All eyes were now on Bastogne, the intersection of vital roads leading to the Meuse. Advancing German troops had been slowed but not stopped. Bastogne was next, gateway to the Meuse. Two crack German divisions, the 2nd Panzer and the elite Panzer Lehr, took aim. Late Saturday afternoon, December 16, aware that the Germans had broken through at a number of points in the Allied line, Eisenhower consulted with his pal General Bradley and dispatched the 10th Armored Division, the "Tiger Division," from Patton's Third Army to the Ardennes area. It was placed under General Middleton's VIII Corps command. He had already called the 7th Armored Division down from the north to aid in defense of the northern shoulder. Aware that Patton would not be pleased losing one of his armored divisions, Eisenhower added, "Tell him . . . that Ike is running this damn war."[32]

Combat Command B of the 10th Armored Division, four battalions of tank, armored infantry, and armored artillery, had been resting, a period called "rehabilitation," in France near the Luxembourg border. Within twenty-four hours of Eisenhower's call, troops and tanks were on the road, through Arlon and on to Bastogne. Commander Colonel William Roberts had gone ahead to meet with General Middleton in Bastogne. Roberts decided to split his forces into three teams. "Team Desobry," headed by Major William Desobry, would be placed five miles north of Bastogne at the small village of Noville. "Team Cherry," commanded by Lieutenant Colonel Henry Cherry, would travel east to Longvilly, already defended by units of the 9th Armored Division, and "Team O'Hara," led by Lieutenant Colonel James O'Hara, would be placed southeast near the town of Wardin. "Hold these positions at all costs," was Middleton's directive. He knew there were now only skeleton forces between Bastogne and Longvilly. And he suspected the Germans dearly wanted Bastogne. From the west, Middleton's Screaming Eagles were on the way.

14

Screaming Eagles

On June 25, 1940, the War Department directed the formation of a parachute test platoon, located at Fort Benning, Georgia. The troops would be a rapid-reaction force intended to seize and hold tactical objectives lightly defended—usually in the enemy's rear areas—until ground troops could arrive to reinforce them. It was a novel idea, a force of air commandos. The nucleus would be the 82nd Division, the "All American" Division of World War I fame. In July 1942, the 82nd would actually split into two divisions, the 82nd and the 101st. The 101st Division was called the "Screaming Eagles," presumably after its mascot, the bald eagle Old Abe from Civil War days, when it was the 8th Wisconsin Volunteer Infantry. Each division contained parachute regiments, at least one glider regiment, and batteries of artillery. Men would be carefully selected, intensely motivated, and rigorously trained. All would be equipped to survive for periods of time behind enemy lines. Even among hardened combat veterans, paratroopers were supremely testosterone driven. Hard-charging and often hard-partying misfits, they dwelt on the fringe of sane behavior. With blackened faces and Mohawk haircuts, it was as if a band of renegades had jumped into the fray. There was a propensity, even, for hand-to-hand combat, razor-sharp knives preferred to eight-clip Garands. Paratroopers for the 101st were more likely to identify with their individual regiments—the 502nd and, eventually, the 501st and 506th ("Parachute Infantry")—and for "glider" infantry the 327th and 401st.

Glider troops rode in on plywood gliders, cut loose from tow planes, totally then at the mercy of winds and air currents. Landings were white-knuckle affairs—basically controlled crashes. Hoping to better concentrate troops and heavy equipment, gliders were the stealth technology of the day. In theory outwardly noiseless, they could approach and touch down without raising a great deal of suspicion. But theory was not practice. Glider infantry faced even more danger than paratroopers, entombed in "silent wings" as they descended to the ground. Some called them towed targets, easy prey for German gunners, who were too often not fooled, drawing beads on the flimsy planes. General James Gavin, commander of the 82nd Airborne, commented, "It is a chastening experience. It gives a man religion."[1] The most commonly used glider, the Waco CG-4A combat glider, was forty-eight feet long and built of steel tubing with plywood flooring and covered in fabric. It could be loaded with over a dozen troops or a combination of heavy equipment—jeeps, howitzers, and trailers—and troops totaling almost two tons. Once released from the tow plane, usually a C-47, two pilots guided their plane in at seventy miles per hour hoping to hit the ground in some type of aerodynamic fashion (or maybe not). Of course, anything in the way—tree stumps, telephone poles, ravines, even heavy brush—would aid in dramatic deceleration. So any number of configurations resulted: pancake landings, full-speed crashes, jackknife buckling, and somersaults. Few landings were perfect, maybe less than one in four. Pilot and passenger casualty rates reached 40 percent: wrenched backs, fractures, sprains, and cracked ribs. Some landings proved fatal.[2]

The 101st saw action during the Normandy invasion in June 1944, parachuting at night behind the beaches. Later in 1944, another large airborne drop, Operation Market-Garden, tried to outflank the Siegfried Line in Holland. After weeks of brutal combat, the Screaming Eagles were now enjoying a period of rest and refitting at Camp Mourmelon, a former French artillery base just outside the village of Mourmelon-le-Grand, twenty miles from Rheims. The 101st Airborne and the 82nd Airborne, as part of XVIII Airborne Corps, were designated the reserve component for the entire Allied Expeditionary Force. There were lazy days at Mourmelon for men of the 101st, it being reminiscent of their home post of Fort Bragg, North Carolina. Soldiers had hot meals, regular showers, haircuts at French parlors, football leagues, and even thirty-day furloughs back to the United States.

Major General Matthew Ridgeway, commander of XVIII Corps, was at the rear headquarters in England, and Major General Maxwell Taylor, present commander of the 101st, was all the way back in the United States when word reached Eisenhower and Bradley that the Germans were driving out of the Ardennes. The assistant division commander, Brigadier General Anthony McAuliffe, a former artillery officer, was the acting division commander. On Sunday, December 17, McAuliffe called his staff together and announced, "All I know of the situation is that there has been a breakthrough and we have got to get up there." By the afternoon of December 18, over 380 trucks were rounded up to transport eleven thousand men of the 101st Airborne. "The 101st . . . has no history, but it has a rendezvous with destiny," men were told.[3]

The medical backbone for the 101st were self-contained collecting units and field hospitals, the 326th Medical Company. Like all division medical support, the 326th had a headquarters section and platoons servicing each of the regiments with litter bearers, ambulances, and field hospitals. Major William Barfield, a thirty-two-year-old Georgian, had commanded the 326th from the outset and went with his men into Normandy and Holland. All members of the medical teams were volunteers, and, like all paratroopers, energized and superbly conditioned. All had gone through paratrooper jump training. Ordinarily, on airborne missions, one officer and fifteen enlisted men would jump with each regiment—or land by glider—bringing in eighty-five containers of medical equipment: ampules, plasma, dressings, sterilization equipment. There would be five bundles full of surgical gear, one of which was entirely orthopedic. While major surgery would be unlikely, a number of debridements, wound explorations, and splinting could be performed. The enlisted men each carried two units of plasma, debridement sets, two sterile hemostats, a sphygmomanometer, a pair of scissors, scalpel, dressings, a can of alcohol, twenty morphine ampules, wire splints, tetanus toxoid, Novocain, gas gangrene antitoxin, aspirin, sodium amytl, and Vaseline gauze. An entire medical team was loaded on the same plane to jump together. They would be expected to function for forty-eight hours without relief or resupply. The plan was to swiftly locate some structure, usually a farmhouse or barn, and set up an aid station. All life-and-limb-saving efforts would be in their hands.

Team No. 20 of the 3rd Auxiliary Surgical Group, headed by Major Albert Crandall, was attached to the 326th Medical Company. Crandall was a big man, described by team members as "fearless." "Just to be near him gave you a feeling of security," his surgical technician remembered.[4] The 3rd Auxiliary Surgical Group had outfitted two airborne surgical teams, an all-volunteer—and all male—unit. Crandall and his team were designated the 1st Airborne Surgical Team. Not jump qualified, they had landed in Normandy by glider packed in with a quarter-ton trailer containing all their equipment. Just in case, each man also carried a canvas field kit with the same medical gear carried by paratrooper battalion surgeons. There was a second glider insertion during Market Garden. This time sympathetic Dutch nuns directed them to a tuberculosis sanitarium as a haven where they treated over three thousand wounded during the three-week operation.

Their present assignment would not be a parachute or glider mission. Cloud cover and fog put any type of air drop out of the question. Trucks and trailers carried the men this time. They were loaded in such a hurry that many left without rifles, helmets, and ammunition, and were packed in like sardines. Their convoys snaked along traffic-clogged roads, headlights blazing to make time, knowing the danger of enemy nighttime air raids. Talk was of a village named Bastogne. They would be posted in reserve, so the rumors went. Some kind of irritating German probing, it seemed. But one never knew for sure in this war. First Lieutenant Charles Phalen, a medical officer, recalled that "shadowy figures of men and women lined the streets of Mourmelon, waved and shouted '*Bon Chance*,'" not sure either about the fate of their beloved Yanks.[5]

So on December 17, three units converged on Bastogne: Combat Command B of the 10th Armored Division, the 101st Airborne Division, and the 705th Tank Destroyer Battalion, then stationed about sixty miles north of Bastogne in Kohlscheid, Germany, released from the 9th Army to Middleton's VIII Corps. The Screaming Eagles' sister unit, the 82nd Airborne, had initially been slated for Bastogne but at the last minute was redirected to the northern border of the German offensive. As convoys neared Bastogne, men of the 101st were appalled at the stampede of civilians and soldiers west. One paratrooper recalled: "I'm telling you I never seen men with a look like that in my life, running, scared to death. No helmets, no weapons. They threw everything down, they threw their bandoleers down, they threw everything down. The kids were out of breath, yelling, 'Don't go up there, there are so many Germans, they're gonna kill everybody!'"[6]

Paratroopers insisted on scavenging as much as they could from the troops passing by. Boots, coats, rifles, field packs, anything of standard

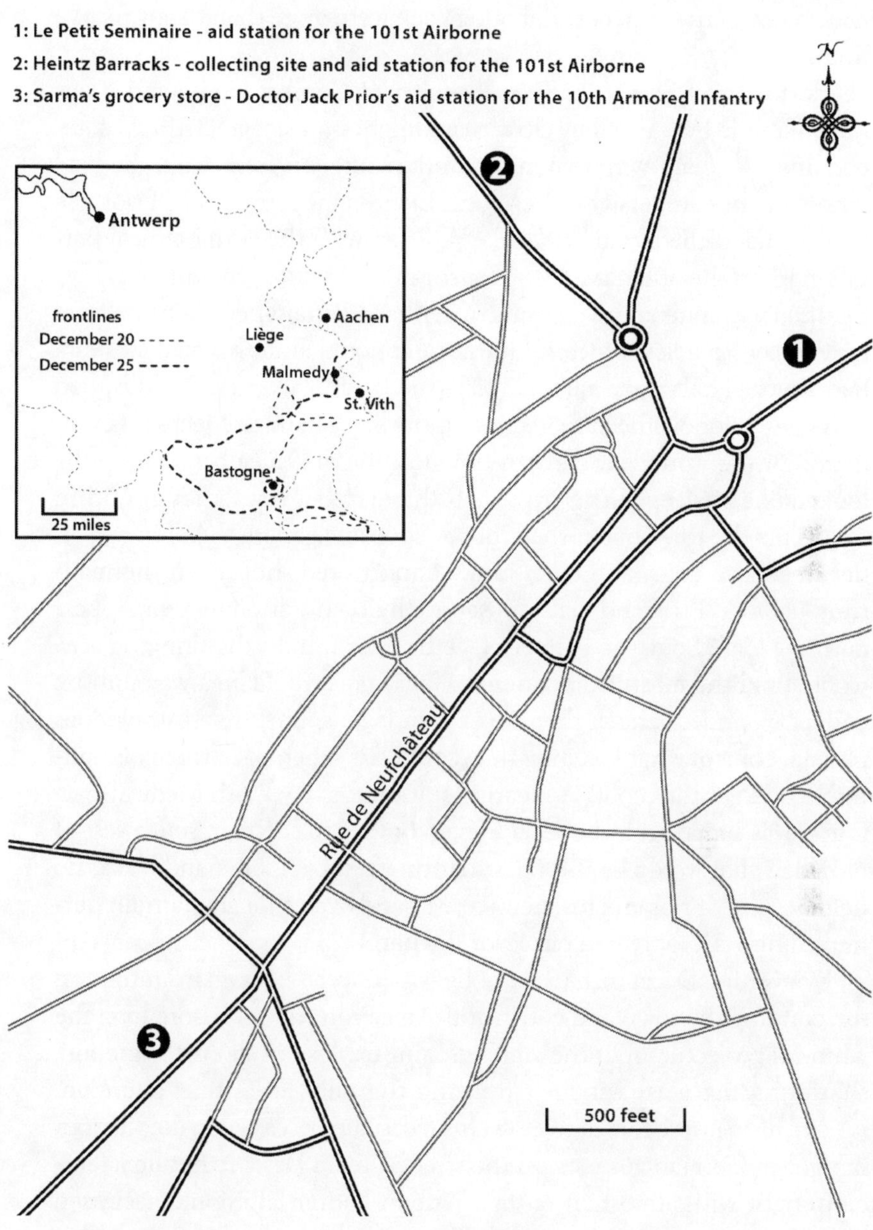

Map 3. Bastogne, Belgium, December 1944.

issue was taken—and most hobbling back were more than happy to give it up.

Northeast of Bastogne, Team Desobry of Combat Command B entered Noville by way of Foy close to midnight on December 18. Accompanying the team was a young battalion surgeon fresh from medical school at the University of Vermont, Lieutenant John "Jack" Prior. He had been detached from his regular position with the 80th Medical Battalion when the original surgeon for the 20th Armored Infantry was hospitalized with pneumonia. He and a dentist, Captain Lee Naftulin, were now the two medical officers. Like most armored units, his medical team had armored half-track ambulances—the Purple Heart Boxes (they had only canvas for overhead protection in the bed)—and two jeeps for evacuation of the wounded. Early in the morning of December 19, Noville looked like a "sleepy little crossroads" hamlet, but not for long. Within two hours the town had turned into a "shooting gallery."[7] Automatic rifles, machine guns, and even tank cannon fired shot down the main thoroughfare. Prior and Naftulin set up their aid station in a small local pub, the Café Louis—a perfect place in their minds: the drinking area would hold the most litter patients. Café Louis would be a way station: collect wounded, check them over, bandage, splint, start intravenous plasma, control what bleeding they could see. Then pack them on half-tracks and get them out. A clearing station for the 326th Medical Battalion was supposed to be set up several miles to the rear, southwest of Noville. That would be their destination. Combat Command B had no field hospital. Prior and his crew were it, and even though Naftulin outranked him, Desobry had put Prior in charge.

By evening December 19, Noville was a hotbed, Germans intent on surrounding the town and cutting off American troops. Before long the whine of projectiles split the air. Deafening explosions shook the ground, shattering the glass windows fronting the pub. From that point on, medics inside were forced to crawl from casualty to casualty, keeping out of sight of German gunners. In the streets, Team Desobry put up a ferocious fight with almost an entire German Panzer Division, exacting a horrible cost in tanks and troops. The main thoroughfare was soon littered with burning vehicles and clumps of lifeless forms. Yet despite the efforts of the Screaming Eagles from the 506th Parachute Infantry, German armor pressed on, clanking down side roads into town and zeroing in on Desobry's command post. Late that afternoon, point-blank cannon fire blew through one wall, killing Lieutenant Colonel James LaPrade, commander of the 1st Battalion, 506th Parachute Infantry. Fragments of that same shell struck Major Desobry in the head, almost enucleating one of his eyes and knocking him unconscious. He was rushed by medics to the 506th aid station and then to the 326th Medical Battalion hospital near Herbaimont. Auxers of Team 20 were able to save his eye.

No one was immune from danger. Captain Joseph Warren, surgeon for the 1st Battalion, 506th Parachute Infantry, was felled by a blast while pulling injured men to safety. One of his medics, Owen Miller, bandaged both of Warren's wrists and moved him to the 506th aid station. Major Louis Kent, the regimental surgeon, stepped in to take over. Shortly he reported that he was caring for "about fifty 1st Battalion casualties."[8] His aid station was packed. Some were gruesome sights indeed. One young private stumbled onto a soldier sitting on a block of wood. "His skull on the upper right side has been totally torn off by a huge chunk of shrapnel. His brains are showing." A medic knelt and dabbed at his skull. Another paratrooper was screaming for a medic, "his guts trailing in the dirt behind him." Buddies washed his entrails with canteen water and pushed them back inside, bound him up, and dragged him into a ditch hoping he would soon be located by medics.[9] Finally, two deuce-and-a-halfs were found, casualties lifted in, including Captain Warren, and set off for Bastogne with the regimental dentist, Captain Sam "Shifty" Feiler, in charge.

By the next day, German troops and armor had encircled Noville. The Americans fought valiantly but were pushed into smaller and smaller pockets. Orders came to pull out toward Bastogne. The corridor back, all knew, would be lined with Germans. The only salvation was a dense morning fog that brought visibility almost to zero. Even then, everyone prepared for a bloody shellacking. By that time, Lieutenant Prior had a macabre collection of gravely wounded men, hardly ready for evacuation. Among them, one had a shaggy wound of the abdomen caused by a one-inch fragment and was unconscious, "pale and waxy-looking as a corpse." Another was sitting up, fidgety, one eyeball "hanging halfway down his cheek in a bloody, viscous mix of goo."[10] The only humane decision was for him to remain behind at the café. So there he stayed, expecting to be captured while the tavern owner and his wife fervently prayed their rosaries. But rescue was at hand in the form of departing tankers who ripped doors off their frames, strapped the patients down, and loaded them on their tanks. At one point, after Prior and Naftulin had hoisted four stretcher cases on the back of a half-track marked with a big Red Cross, a German tank came around the corner and put a round squarely in the center of the cross. Unbelievably, the round went straight between litter patients, through the cab, and out the engine. Prior and Naftulin quickly unloaded the wounded, uninjured by the blast, under the gaze of the German tank commander, who muzzled his gunner.[11]

Schutzen skirmishers and Panzergrenadiers made the trip down the Houffalize road a gauntlet of destruction, stalking the column and sweeping it with automatic fire whenever the fog cleared. The five miles took three hours. German volleys peppered the column, forcing all to scramble into roadside ditches, rounds chipping away only inches from their heads. Some wounded were so critical that they could not be left alone and certainly could not be moved. Bullets pinged on armored siding as damaged men strapped inside screamed to be taken off. Common soldiers without hesitation popped up and rushed to their aid, trying to get them out. On the shoulders of the paved road, mud became a problem. Vehicles with injured aboard that were forced off stuck in the soft ground and had to be extricated with winches, paratroopers and armored infantrymen all dismounting to give a hand. Medics treated the injured right in the midst of crisscrossing rounds and exploding ordnance. Their gallantry did not provide immunity however. One medic, caring for an armless soldier, caught the blast of an artillery shell just above him. "Hey Charlie! I'm hit," he cried and then went down, a hole in his chest pumping blood onto the pavement. He lived only seconds.[12] Up and down, the convoy scenes were the same. Ordinary men in extraordinary times, as Prior later recalled: "Many of our enlisted men demonstrated great bravery on the road, pulling tankers from their blazing tanks, driving jeeps with the injured on the hood to our Aid Station. . . . This observation was to be pounded home again, time after time, in the months ahead. I have never learned who to predict will be a hero."[13]

The column inched past the settlement of Foy and reached Bastogne after dark, some tanks now driven by paratroopers, unfamiliar with armor but insistent that they would learn to drive "the son of a bitch."[14] Of fifteen tanks Team Desobry took to Noville, only four returned. Half of the almost four hundred soldiers were also killed, wounded, or captured. An additional 212 paratroopers of the 506th were lost. Prior himself had loaded and returned 112 casualties to Company B of the 80th Armored Medical Battalion, a collecting company. All but sixteen were battle casualties, most, fortunately, "lightly wounded" from shrapnel injuries.

Seven, though, were much worse: chest injuries, head wounds, dozens of fragment holes. From the 80th Med they went to the 107th Evac outside Libin. Some had already been taken to the 326th Medical Battalion at Herbaimont. Exact numbers will never be known. No records were kept. Reports from the 80th Armored Med Battalion failed to break out individual units, mentioning only that evacuation from December 17 to 26 "was neither adequate nor systematic."[15] But "Tiger" Division tankers and Screaming Eagles had exacted a horrific price from the Germans, killing hundreds and delaying the advance on Bastogne.

The town of Noville was wrecked. Hardly a building stood intact; homes lay in ruins. Families were forced out with only the clothes on their backs. Beasts of burden—cows, horses—and farm animals lay dead. More tragically, on the heels of the 10th Armored departure, the Gestapo moved in. Behind Dr. Prior's aid station, behind the quaint little Café Louis, seven citizens—including the schoolmaster and village priest—were shot in the head, the penalty for American collaboration.[16]

Prior found Bastogne almost deserted. Many civilians had fled, and those who stayed were holed up in their homes. Now officially attached to the 101st Airborne, he first set up his aid station, the only one for his tankers, in a garage on one of the main streets along with Lieutenant Talbot of the 80th Armored Medical Battalion, but two days later moved it to a larger, private, three-story building, called Sarma, a local grocery store on the main thoroughfare, the Rue de Neufchateau. The first floor was the store with a kitchen at the rear, and the upper two floors were living quarters. There was also a spacious basement. But Prior had salvaged almost nothing from Noville. Even scalpel blades were in short supply. For infections, he had only hydrogen peroxide, no other antiseptic. Even supplies of morphine were soon exhausted. His men fanned out scavenging anything, even private doctors' offices. There would be little hope for the critical wounded, he feared. "The patients who had head, chest, and abdominal wounds could only face certain slow death," Prior wrote later. It was that next day, December 21, while his team foraged, that he met Renée Lemaire and Augusta Chiwy, two nurses who volunteered their services at the aid station.[17]

As units of the Screaming Eagles moved into Bastogne, the 101st Division surgeon, Lieutenant Colonel David Gold, and the division supply officer, Lieutenant Colonel Carl Kohls, picked a location for the 326th Medical Company's division hospital about eight miles west of Bastogne in what they considered the rear area. Unbeknownst to them, there was no rear area. Germans were drifting to the north and south of Bastogne in a deliberate attempt to avoid a frontal assault, flooding porous American defenses. Their directive was to get to the Meuse, so further combat with American units around Bastogne was shunned—time was wasting. Yet even then, some 326th officers were nervous. Why so far from Bastogne? Why so removed from the protective paratroopers? Gold was reassuring. It was a linear battlefield. Keep hospitals in the rear, away from artillery and combat. Few were unaware of the fast pace of the German offensive, of roving Panzer units and wide gaps between American forces. Still, surgeon Crandall felt commanders were too casual about the situation; too little was known of the German presence. "[W]e should have been more familiar with the current military situation," he reported in 1945. "[W]e should definitely have posted sentries and have established some type of reconnaissance."[18]

But to most it was business as usual. Soon after arrival mid-morning on December 19, men of the 326th Medical Company erected their tents in a broad meadow, close to the crossroads town of Herbaimont. In the distance was the Bois de Herbaimont (Herbaimont Woods). All appreciated the meadow's wide-open spaces. There was almost no cover or concealment and plenty of warning that this was a medical outfit. Red crosses blared "Geneva Convention"—or so they hoped. Enlisted surgical technician Emil Natalle remembered well: "When we arrived at Herbaimont, we could hear gun-fire in the distance. And it wasn't very far away either."[19] Yet commanders felt the location crucial, next to a road network that would allow ambulance transport from all directions. Auxiliary surgical teams would be poised to tackle seriously wounded, the nontransportables—head, chest, and abdominal trauma—then hustle them off to the 107th Evac in Libin. It all seemed perfect.

Yet right away there were ominous signs. Captain Ed Yeary, acting commander, was bothered by the steady stream of civilian refugees heading west, loaded with possessions, typical of populations pushed ahead by advancing enemy. They were a grim lot, he saw, none of the smiling and shouting he had witnessed back in Mourmelon. "They walked without looking at the Americans," Lieutenant Charles Phalen, evacuation officer for the 506th Parachute Infantry, was told.[20] By noon, though, business had picked up; casualties were arriving, and the operating tent filled. Everyone focused on the work at hand, plenty of damaged men from Noville. That same afternoon, Captain Yeary, still worried about the exposed position of his unit, traveled to the division headquarters in Bastogne and expressed his concern. The hospital could be overrun, he told General McAuliffe. McAuliffe replied, "Go on back, Captain—you'll be all right."[21] By late afternoon of December 19, all ambulances had been sent on into Bastogne to battalion aid stations for more wounded. In the meantime, three cross-country ambulances loaded with fifteen litter and walking wounded departed the clearing station headed for the 107th Evacuation Hospital in Libin. They were the last wounded out.[22]

Sometime around 9:30 PM, two vehicles were sent with casualties from the 501st Parachute Regimental Aid Station in Bastogne to the 326th hospital. Two hours later, they had not returned. At midnight, Lieutenant Phalen tried to transport wounded from the 327th Glider Infantry to the hospital. Not far from Bastogne, he was met by paratrooper sentries and told to turn around. Something had happened at the field hospital. In fact, something was very wrong there. Two hours earlier, Sergeant Natalle, asleep in his foxhole, was awakened by what sounded like a machine-gun barrage. Peeking over the rim, he saw tracers racing just over his head. In moments, American vehicles were on fire, hit by cannon, and the screams of those trapped inside could be heard. Natalle crawled from his foxhole over to the surgical tent and peered in. "It looked like a morgue," he recalled. Everyone had hit the ground and lay motionless, afraid to move. "Some men were quaking with fear. Some sobbed quietly. Some moaned." "I was practically lying on my stomach operating on patients," Captain Charles Van Gorder, one of the 3rd Auxiliary surgeons, remembered, "because of the shooting coming right into the tent."[23] Major Crandall was also on the floor. Suspecting they had been overrun, he quipped, "It looks like Germany for us."[24] Captain Gordon Block remembered being woken by German "burp" guns. He bolted for the evacuation tent: "Machine guns opened up . . . tracers tore through the canvas. The wounded lying on stretchers groaned as some were hit a second time with fragments. I remember thinking 'Son, you've had it now.'"[25]

In fact, an enemy force estimated at six armored half-tracks and tanks and one hundred infantry had motored down the Houffalize road from the northeast and stumbled onto the tented compound. Not immediately identifying Red Cross emblems, they opened fire. Even after vehicles were aflame, illuminating the crosses, firing continued, at least for a few moments. Finally an enemy officer in a pressed uniform with shined black jackboots and a monocle approached Lieutenant Colonel Gold, who had ventured outside the tent, and demanded a surrender. The German commander allowed the unit thirty minutes to gather patients and equipment and load them up. Before long a convoy, loaded with eighteen officers, including four Auxer surgeons from Team 20, and 125 enlisted men were snaking their way back up the Houffalize road and on into Germany.[26] One of the patients rounded up in the attack was Major Desobry, who narrowly escaped capture in Noville. They all would be prisoners of the Third Reich.

Around midnight, Company B of the 401st Glider Infantry was sent to the crossroads to check out some reported gunfire. As they positioned themselves on a ridge overlying the hospital compound, they could hear Germans talking and see trucks burning. After a brief firefight, the Germans fled, but the paratroopers still did not know the hospital had been captured. At dawn, Private Carmen Gisi and other members of the 401st approached the now-deserted compound, tents ghostly in the dense morning fog. As they entered, the place was eerily quiet. No signs of life. Equipment and personnel were simply gone. "It was even worse when we got into the operating tents," Gisi recounted. "We saw two paratroopers on gurneys ready for surgery. Apparently they were too severely wounded for the Germans to take them prisoner so they'd cut their throats."[27] Word reached headquarters of the 101st Airborne Division in Bastogne that morning. Casualties were quickly rerouted southwest to the 429th Collecting Company at Molinfaing, directly down the Neufchateau road. But by late that evening that route, too, was cut by Germans. It was the last road out of Bastogne. McAuliffe had returned from a meeting with Middleton on that same road not thirty minutes before. No doubt, Middleton's parting advice was ringing in his head: "Now, don't get yourself surrounded." Bastogne and its garrison of eighteen thousand soldiers were surrounded.[28] The vice had shut. Up to forty-five thousand Germans waited to do the tightening. Nothing would get in or out by ground. And a long trial awaited the wounded, in confinements primitive and cold, with doctors short on talent and shorter on supplies.

Within Bastogne's perimeter, any shelter served as a collecting point for casualties. Better locations were brick-and-mortar buildings in the town itself. The 501st Parachute Infantry set up its aid station in the chapel of Le Petit Seminaire on the eastern edge. Wooden pews were ripped out to make room for wounded, the sacristy cleared out as an operating area—it was quiet and out of sight of injured men. With no evac-

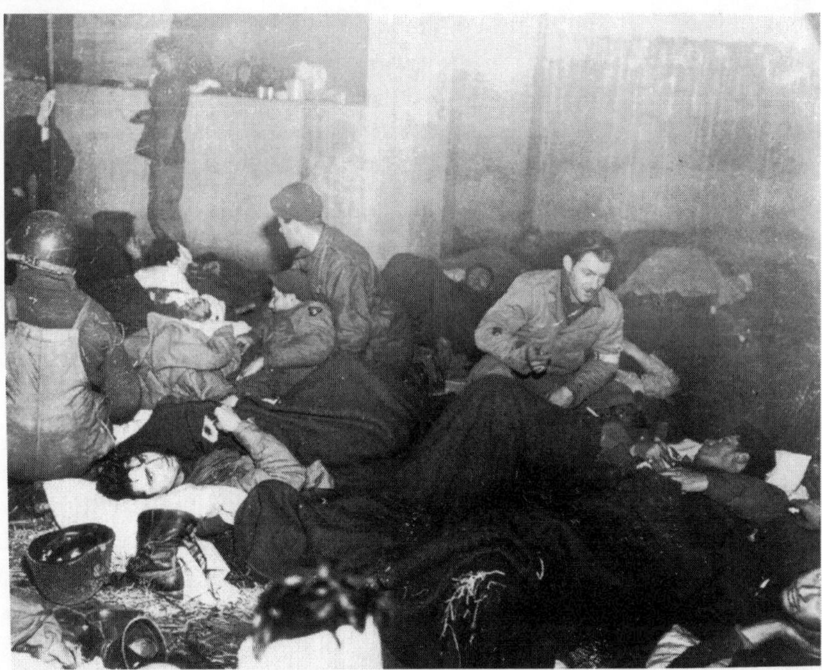

Aid station in Bizory chapel east of Bastogne, photographed by Cleto Leone, medic for the 501st Parachute Regiment. (*National Archives*)

uation possible, the place quickly filled. Some estimated over 250 were housed there, so little space that one could barely step between litters. Poor ventilation soon turned air foul, charged with the stench of human blood and sweat. Doctors worked on wounds under little anesthesia, litters placed between medicine chests as improvised tables, sometimes with only a trench knife and saw—all, according to one battalion surgeon, "under the silent gaze of the Blessed Virgin."[29] Wounded became so numerous that the adjoining girls' school, the Institut Notre-Dame, was taken over. Student Maria Gillet watched the endless stream of wounded and observed one ashen casualty: "Where his legs have been I can see only a shapeless mass of crushed flesh, blood spills onto the floor. My thoughts go to his faraway mother." Those who perished were taken to the courtyard and stacked up under frozen canvasses. In the cellars of the same building, nuns collected civilian casualties and refugees. Conditions turned appalling, with almost six hundred people—civilian refugees and American wounded—packed in. Buckets were used as toilets, there was no bathing and little food—the smell took away any appetite anyway—and shortly lice. The mood was somber. Bastognards observed that many Americans felt it was all over for them.[30]

General McAuliffe now commanded from the town proper. He had moved his headquarters from the small village of Mande-Saint-Etienne on December 19, and chose Bastogne's Heintz Military Barracks. The barracks were constructed in 1934 to house the Seconde Regiment de Chasseurs Ardennais of the Belgian army. It was taken over during the German occupation as a camp for Hitler Youth and reoccupied as headquarters for General Troy Middleton's VIII Corps in October. McAuliffe's move came just in time: Mande-Saint-Etienne was overrun the night of December 19, the same night the 326th Medical Battalion was captured.

Care of the seriously wounded now fell to battalion-level doctors. Medical officers from the 81st Airborne Antiaircraft Battalion, the 326th Airborne Engineer Battalion, the 101st Airborne Division Artillery, and the 705th Tank Destroyer Battalion were called together and placed under Major Martin Wisely of the 327th Glider Infantry as an impromptu team for emergency care. Wisely decided on a second major collecting point at Heintz Barracks—Le Petit Seminaire was, by now, teeming with soldiers and civilians. Two buildings at the rear of the compound were empty and unused. Neither was ideal, but they were serviceable. A partial roof covered one, a former indoor shooting range—warmth would be provided by indoor fires—and across the way was a second building, also deserted, which had once been used as a riding stable. Some medical supplies had been scavenged from an abandoned army medical depot. Yet conditions remained crude. Wounded were laid in rows on the sawdust floor and covered with what blankets could be found. Medics and doctors made some attempt to segregate the less seriously wounded from the more critical injuries. Nonbattle casualties, mostly trench-foot cases, were moved into a separate building. Against the back wall were laid those who would not recover—the "expectant" cases.[31] Serious injuries simply suffered. Major surgery was not an option. No one was surgically trained, and surgical instruments beyond the basics did not exist. Those who died were taken away to a separate space for graves registration, their space quickly filled by new arrivals. Blankets, litters, morphine, plasma, and surgical dressings soon reached critical levels. For that reason, the dead were stripped of everything usable. Battalion surgeon Prior witnessed the scene on his visit there with Major Douglas Davidson, acting division surgeon, just before Christmas:

> There on the dirt riding floor were six hundred paratroop litter cases—I cannot recall the number of walking wounded or psychiatric casualties. These patients were only being sustained as were mine. I did see a paratroop chaplain (armed with a pistol and shoulder holster) moving among the dying. . . . Gas gangrene was rampant there, aided and abetted, I'm sure, by the flora on the dirt floor.[32]

Prior was shocked. "I returned to my Aid Station very depressed," he recalled. It seemed the situation there was just as desperate as his own aid station. He later wrote: "In regard to the care of the wounded in Bastogne, I have always believed, and still do, that this did not constitute a bright page in the history of the Army Medical Department. . . . This decaying medical situation was worsening—with no hope for the surgical candidates and even the superficial wounds were beginning to develop gas gangrene."[33]

Adding to the hardships, the weather turned stormy on December 20. Temperatures plummeted and snow arrived, falling in some places to a depth of one foot. In Dr. Prior's aid station, the unusually cold temperatures caused plasma and blood to freeze. Transfusions did not happen, and hypothermia in men depleted of blood was a constant concern. Among those in the field confined to their foxholes, trench foot produced burgeoning numbers of nonbattle casualties, rendered ineffective with painful, swollen, gray toes and feet. In a town without electricity or running water, every activity of daily living was a challenge. Prior's team foraged for meat, jam, and vegetables from every private dwelling and cellar. Snow was melted and boiled for drinking and cooking and washing the wounded. Champagne, stored in abundance, also proved useful, for any number of reasons—including bathing and shaving. Local physicians to help out were nonexistent. Most had been Nazi Party members and had fled or, if Jewish, rounded up and deported. In his aid station, the number of patients climbed. At one point it held over one hundred, thirty of whom he considered seriously wounded. As the supply of morphine diminished, the moans of the suffering rose, day and night a steady cacophony of misery. Even decades later he remembered: "One of the worst sounds of course was the moaning, crying, and groaning of the wounded. I think that took more out of me than anything. It went on night and day. The pain that was being caused to these folks and here we were with practically no morphine—inadequate morphine—to control the pain."[34]

His was a growing frustration that those with head, chest, and abdominal wounds, let alone with creeping soft-tissue gangrene, were unable to get proper treatment. Even with proper surgical instruments, Prior lacked the training to do complex surgery. Chest and abdominal cavities were beyond his capabilities, and there was no one to give anesthesia anyway. Without repair, these men would surely die. And in the meantime, they lay in agony. His Belgian nurses were indispensable for this, lending a kind touch, a gentle presence. Yet the aid station took on the quality of Dante's Purgatorio, sinners purging themselves through immeasurable torments while awaiting Paradise.

"The second echelon medical setup collapsed completely," recalled Captain Bernard Ryan, battalion surgeon for the 506th Parachute Infantry. He observed that the seriously wounded were brought back to Bastogne and treated wherever shelter and warmth could be found, sometimes in ones and twos in individual dwellings.[35] One of his most depressing experiences was making rounds on his men during trips to town and seeing so many in need of surgical treatment. Troubling to witness was one of his good friends, Captain Richard Meason, who had suffered a bullet wound to the abdomen. He lay on a litter "with a full-blown acute peritonitis" from bowel perforation—untreated, a condition almost universally fatal. His pain was excruciating, any movement complete agony. Yet nothing could be done except penicillin and sulfadiazine. Surprisingly, the captain hung on to eventually be evacuated and operated on.[36]

Despite these Spartan conditions, the defense of Bastogne was solidifying. General McAuliffe had masterminded his perimeter by placing troops three to four miles out. To the southeast was the 327th Glider Infantry, directly east was positioned the 501st Parachute Infantry, to their left the 506th Parachute Infantry straddled the Houffalize road, to the northwest was the 502nd Parachute Infantry, and covering the broad western sector was the 420th Armored Field Artillery—infantry and tank forces led by Lieutenant Colonel Barry Browne. In reserve were various ad hoc groups of tanks, tank destroyers, and infantry, many belonging to Combat Command B of the 10th Armored Division and Combat Command R of the Ninth Armored Division. Stragglers from other units, including from General Cota's decimated 28th Division, were rounded up, given some rest and warm food, armed, and used as Team SNAFU. By the night of December 22, the ring was intact.

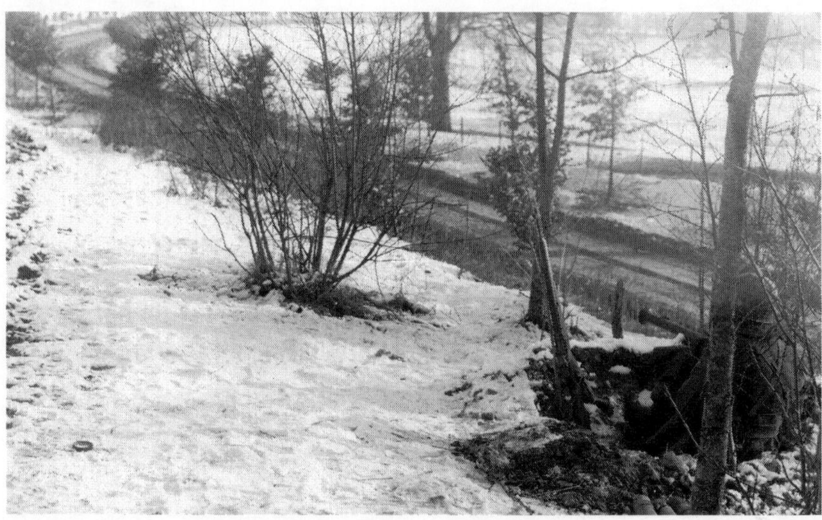

Soldiers of the 101st Airborne Division, armed with bazookas, on guard for enemy tanks on the main road leading to Bastogne, December 23, 1944. (*National Archives*)

But McAuliffe's men took a terrible beating. From all quarters of the perimeter, Germans probed and struck. Shelling was incessant, and attacks by Manteuffel's seasoned infantry unpredictable. Individual soldiers in their icy foxholes waited it out. For each it was a private affair, anticipating those three or four or six figures to emerge from the woods and the killing to begin. Before long, shouts of "Medic!" were heard, and there were scrambles to reach slumped forms. The gray-coated figures fell, but they kept coming, seemingly endless, and the hunkered Americans used clip after clip in their Garands hoping the supply of German fodder would soon end. But it was the shelling, just as in Anzio, that affected men the most—the uncertainty of where the next round would land, totally helpless. One veteran described it: "Being shelled is the real work of an infantry soldier, which no one talks about. Everyone has his own way of going about it. In general it means lying face-down and contracting your body into as small a space as possible. In novels you read about soldiers . . . fouling themselves. The opposite is true. As all your parts are contracting, you are more likely to be constipated."[37]

Yes, death was close, very close. It sat on their shoulders like patient buzzards. It nipped at their courage and sapped their vitality. It overtook many, silently or with great fanfare as if to boast of its permanence; a living horror for those who watched its rampage, disassembling friends and comrades. Infantryman Donald Miller remembered: "People didn't crumble and fall like they did in the Hollywood movies. They were tossed in the air and their blood splattered everywhere. And a lot of people found themselves covered in the blood and flesh of their friends."[38]

And when it was all done, the survivors gazed out at the bodies lying in heaps, the wind blowing their camouflaged white blouses, the snow dusting their grim, maroon faces. Many wondered at the sense of it all, such wasteful handling of precious humanity.

Generals Eisenhower, Bradley, and Patton had met in Verdun on December 19 to discuss strategy against this new German Ardennes offensive. The agreement was that Patton would shift his armored units to the north and attack the base of the bulge. "[T]he enemy must never be allowed to cross the Meuse," was Eisenhower's insistence. By then, though, the major objective for Patton's troops was the relief of Bastogne. It was clear that this would be a pivotal battle, and the 101st was in danger of being surrounded and wiped out. His 4th Armored Division was already on the way. "Destiny sent for me in a hurry when things got tight. Perhaps God saved me for this effort," Patton wrote in his diary—maybe a bit prematurely, as his armored units had to fight bitterly to break through."[39]

The struggle for Bastogne's crossroads occurred in salient outposts, villages with names like Foy and Marvie, Assenois and Villeroux, Senonchamps and Longchamps, Bizory and Mande Saint-Etienne. Squads and platoons of infantry, handfuls of Sherman tanks and tank destroyers confronted legions of German Panzers. It was out there, in farm fields and hillocks and forests, that American blood was spilled. Aid stations set up in farmhouses or any structure with walls and a roof, maybe even in a timber-and-dirt-covered foxhole near battalion headquarters, housed just one doctor for an entire battalion. Medics risked their lives bringing in the wounded, often directly in the line of enemy bullets. Such was the case of Private Everett Padgett, a medic with the 401st Glider Infantry outside of Mande Saint-Etienne. Seeing a group of stricken soldiers exposed in front of him, he donned a helmet with large red crosses and wiggled out to bring them in, shots smacking the snow around him, only to find that two had holes in their heads and were lifeless and the third so close to death that any attempt to move him would be immediately fatal. He returned empty-handed, his charges left where they lay.[40] Anyone moving at the front—medics or otherwise—was fair game for German snipers. And the task of moving men half frozen and half alive out of harm's way, perhaps a mile or longer, involved more risk. Ingenious methods were devised. Corrugated metal sheets torn from shed roofs became improvised toboggans on the snowy terrain.

THERE WERE COUNTLESS STORIES of skirmishes and the casualties that followed. Just outside the tiny town of Foy, off a road barely a bridle path, the 3rd Battalion of the 506th Parachute Infantry, the "Band of Brothers" outfit, tangled with Panzergrenadiers—in a clump of trees called Bois Jacques (Jacques' Woods). Tank cannon proved particularly deadly—and plentiful. Contact with tree branches prematurely detonated shells, with metal and wood slicing into those below as lethal rain. Sergeant Sam Hefner recalled that one tree burst showered some of his men underneath. He heard a cry for help, so he crawled over. Two men lay immobile, one already dead, the second face down "with a huge gaping hole at the base of his spine," paralyzed. They were able to slide him back to safety and onto a jeep, supporting his limp legs and cracked back. He lived, but spent the rest of his life in a wheelchair. Veterans would have those stories in a thousand places and a thousand moments across Bastogne. Private Ralph King, manning a machine gun, suddenly started to scream. His buddy, Gene Johnson, ran over to find King's left shoulder torn away, exposing bone. He dragged him out and sat him against a tree. "Medic!" Johnson called, but they were slow to arrive. King kept looking at his shoulder but turned paler and began to fade, the beginnings of shock. Johnson, aware King might be dying, slapped him across the face, shouting, "Don't you dare pass out on me. Don't you dare!" Medics finally took them both to Heintz Barracks. Even there, Johnson, wounded from fragments in his scalp, remembered, "It was bitterly cold . . . and the only thing that kept us from starving was bullion soup."[41]

In all these firefights, Bastogne's defensive ring held. McAuliffe had a plan, and it worked to precision. His reserve units, patched-together armor and renegade soldiers, were thrown into breeches when needed. And his artillery, plentiful in that American way, fired at will to the German's rear, pounding troops, disrupting any attempts to mount an attack. There was a supreme confidence in this band of GIs. And it bewildered their Teutonic foes. Disbelief was probably a leading reaction when General der Panzertruppe Heinrich von Lüttwitz received McAuliffe's response to a demand for surrender on December 22. "NUTS," was the terse reply.[42]

On the other hand, German attacks were piecemeal. Ferocious in spots, they lacked overall coordination and were beaten back by Bastogne's garrisons. But it all consumed supplies. Yes, Americans love their artillery, but stockpiles were diminishing. Soon gun batteries were told not to fire "until you see the whites of their eyes."[43] Even small-arms ammunition was scarce at times, and in those lonely outposts, those foxholes and trenches, paratroopers were urged caution. Be frugal. Be deadly. And food for hungry men, where was it? Ingenious doughboys scavenged the countryside and warehouses. An abandoned VIII Corps bakery was discovered, loaded with flour and coffee and sugar, even Ovaltine. Collected supplies were managed centrally and distributed according to need. Priority went to the wounded, of course, but pancakes became a staple of the GI diet. Medical supplies dwindled to a trickle, with morphine syrettes even becoming a rarity—and irreplaceable. For men deprived of surgical attention, for wounds of bones and bellies, pain relief was paramount—the most elemental of care.

It was all not enough. The lifeline of besieged troops is resupply—ammunition, food, water, fuel, clothing, and medical supplies—and Bastogne's garrison was no different. Basic sustenance was key. At Bataan it could not happen, and the results were tragic. At Anzio, the only sustaining fortune was ready access by sea. For Bastogne it had to be by air. All roads had been sealed. And air supply, like the sea, is at the mercy of the weather. Skies had been soupy over Bastogne. Heavy clouds, fog, and poor visibility made flights hazardous and air drops pointless. Precision targetings were critical so that material could be retrieved by friendlies and not fall into enemy hands. For this task a group of highly trained and motivated paratroopers of the 101st Airborne, called "Pathfinders," were selected. These men were strictly volunteers, former members of the 506th Parachute Infantry, that swaggering bunch who cut their hair into Mohawk style for the Normandy invasion. Their job was to land—hopefully in friendly territory—and set up "Eureka" beacons that would transmit a signal to C-47s equipped with "Rebecca" receivers, a radio link, even in overcast skies. These would guide transports of the 50th Troop Carrier Wing, 9th Troop Carrier Command, into Bastogne and pinpoint parachute drops of material.

Pathfinders took off in two C-47s in the early morning of December 23. Two "sticks" (ten-men groups) were flown into Bastogne while twenty-one C-47 Skytrains of the 441st Troop Carrier Group loaded with supplies circled over France. Their drop zone was to be a gently rolling farm field between Bastogne and Senonchamps. At the start, the weather was horrible, dense low-lying clouds almost hugging the ground, conditions so bad even the birds were walking, as the saying went. But both sticks of Pathfinders landed well within the American perimeter, directly on target. Eureka beacons were turned on, activating Rebecca receivers, and in came the Skytrains. The formation approached at nine hundred feet, hoping to surprise any German gunners and foil antiaircraft batteries. Just before they reached Senonchamps, the clouds suddenly parted with unlimited visibility. Flying right down the Marche-Bastogne roadway into the Eureka beacon, they passed over a Panzer column. Machine guns opened up and one plane, the lead, was shot down, but the rest made their precision drop. Two more resupply missions were flown that day, totaling 264 aircraft. Of those, 253 arrived over the drop zone and released 334 tons of ammunition, rations, and medical supplies in parapacks.

The next day, Christmas Eve, 157 C-47s followed their Pathfinders in dropping more supplies.[44] Invaluable medical material recovered (almost 100 percent of dropped supplies were taken in) included whole blood, Vaseline gauze, litters, blankets, atropine, tetanus toxoid, pentothal sodium, distilled water, syringes, and sterilizers.[45] But, just as fast, they were greedily drained. For example, the 26,406 K rations delivered were only enough to supply Bastogne's troops for a little more than one day.[46] By Christmas Eve little was left. Even countryside scavenging had come up empty. And on Christmas Day, all planes were grounded by the weather. Christmas was a K-ration day, for those lucky enough to have K rations.[47]

The two days after Christmas, though, saw massive air drops. On December 26 and 27, 420 C-47s delivered hundreds of tons of supplies on target. In addition, ten gliders of the 440th Troop Carrier Group carrying three thousand gallons of petrol gingerly touched down without raising a spark. It was a good thing they did: each glider was crammed with three hundred gallons of gasoline in jerry cans lashed together on the floor just behind the pilots, making them veritable flying Molotov cocktails. On December 27, fifty gliders of the 439th and 440th Troop Carrier Groups set out, full of much-needed ammunition and more petrol. But this time the Germans were not sitting idle. With the familiar drone of aircraft and winged silhouettes against baby blue skies, dreaded 88-mm Flugzeugabwehrkanone cranked skyward and rhythmically blew death into the air, soft puffs of black smoke belying a more sinister purpose, pulsing shards into tender metal wings and fuel tanks and fuselages. One glider disintegrated in midair, a direct hit on its cargo of TNT. Others dove sharply to the ground after their release, pilots veering right, left, up, and down to evade flak. Fourteen of the accompanying C-47s were hit and shot down, and 39 of the 218 crew members did not return: seventeen were killed outright, one died of his wounds, and twenty-one were captured. Of the fifty-eight crew members of the 440th Troop Carrier Group's thirteen C-47s that participated in this run, thirteen died, a mortality figure of 22 percent.[48] The 440th suffered over 40 percent of its casualties that day.[49] This was hazardous duty for aircrews. Skytrains were slow, unarmed, and sluggish, easy prey for German gunners. But they sustained Bastogne. It is likely that without those flights, Bastogne's defenders would have been outgunned, starved, and overrun—a costly tragedy and embarrassment for the United States. General McAuliffe understood. He later communicated: "I would like to express to you and your command the admiration of all of us in the 101st Airborne Division feel for the grand job of air resupply. . . . Needless to say, Bastogne could not have been held without that excellent support."[50]

Meantime, by Christmas Eve over three hundred battle wounded and some 280 non-battle casualties, mostly trench foot or frostbite, had crowded into the stark facilities at Heintz Barracks.[51] Not all, of course, made it there. Countless casualties were cared for in homes, barns, and buildings around Bastogne, many by Bastognards. Prior had collected another one hundred at his little grocery store on the Rue de Neufchateau. Most had "minor" wounds—gunshots, fragment injuries of arms and legs. But many—a sizable minority, perhaps even 30 percent—suffered much more serious injuries. Some of these survived without immediate surgery—no vital organs affected. Others did not. Even limb wounds—torn, avulsed muscle and bone—were subject to infection, including gas gangrene. Those chewed up arms and legs began resembling what the Germans of the First World War called Trichtergelaende, or cratered land—human counterparts of the fissured, creviced waste of no-man's land. McAuliffe was keenly aware that without surgery the lives of his wounded were in jeopardy. He called at the barracks hospital once, saw them lying on straw, some still bleeding, many even without bandages, and vowed never to visit again. It weakened his resolve to witness so much misery.[52]

Some had already died. Colonel Barry Browne, leader of Task Force Browne, was one. On Christmas Eve, atop one of his 105-mm self-pro-

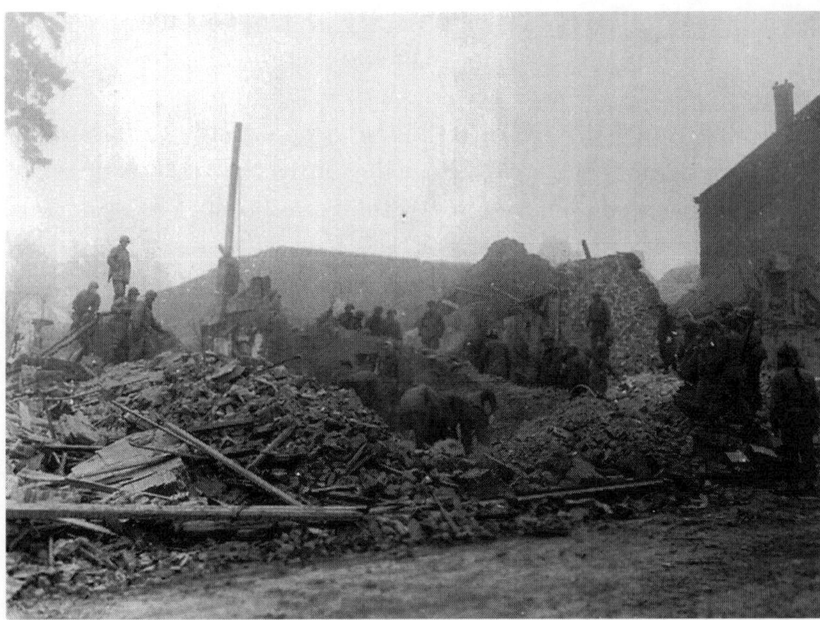

Dr. Jack Prior's first aid station on the Rue de Neufchâteau in Bastogne after the bombing on Christmas Eve, 1944. (*National Archives*)

pelled howitzers near Senonchamps, Browne was struck in his lower back by an airburst. He was hurriedly taken back to Bastogne. Urgent surgery was needed because of probable internal injuries. But there was no surgeon. And there would be no evacuation. He lingered for too long but mercifully succumbed on Christmas Day.

These were pitiful conditions. Amazingly, the acting division surgeon, Douglas Davidson, confident that his paratroopers could withstand anything, had turned a blind eye. Maybe he felt that help was on the way, that Patton's tanks were at the gates, or, conversely, that help in any form was a forlorn wish.[53] Jack Prior had appealed for some type of evacuation during his December 23 visit, but heard Davidson claim that any relief by a surgical team, in or out of Bastogne, was virtually impossible. Prior had even sent ambulances loaded with the critically wounded out on a mission of mercy, hoping the Germans would let them through. In fact, they did. Donald Addor of the 10th Armored was one of those. He made it to Paris and an amputation, his leg irretrievably gangrenous. Had he not, he surely would have died. More needed to go. Finally, on December 26, Major Wisely, chief at Heintz Barracks, received official permission to negotiate passage of the most gravely wounded through German lines. The Germans agreed but postponed evacuation to the following day. By that time, Patton's tanks *were* at the gate.

No, Christmas 1944 was not "Merry" for the men stationed in and around Bastogne. The Luftwaffe paid the town a visit on Christmas Eve. Bombs fell on Prior's aid station at the Sarma. Planes banked, came around, and strafed the rescue workers. Thirty wounded were trapped and died in the building as it collapsed, most burned to death. One Belgian nurse also died attempting to remove injured. Dr. Prior, narrowly escaping himself, was livid. He believed the raid was intentional. Survivors pulled from the wreckage were moved to Heintz Barracks, adding to the swelling mass of humanity.

The Luftwaffe were not the only Germans active that Christmas. Panzergrenadiers launched a major thrust Christmas Day around Champs and Longchamps, hoping to rupture the American ring. Generalmajor Heinz Kokott, placed in charge of capturing Bastogne, threw elements of the 15th Panzer Grenadier and 26th Volksgrenadier Divisions into the attack. Probes had told him the Americans were weak in this sector. On the contrary, crack paratroopers—Glider Infantry and the 502nd Parachute—were there, entrenched and determined. Headquarters of the 502nd had been set up at the Rolle Château,[54] a sprawling complex more like a Hollywood movie set than a tenth-century castle. Officers looked out over gentle sloping hills covered with pine forests, small lakes, and running brooks. The snow added to the scenery, making it look like a winter wonderland. Many had just returned from Christmas Eve Mass in the chapel. Stables on the premises held an aid station where wounded sprawled on blankets and beds of hay. Christmas morning would not be so idyllic. Danger lurked in those forests. In fact, a number of Panzers and infantry did pierce the perimeter south of Champs and drove all the way to Hemroulle, a command center for the 401st (327th) Glider Infantry. Stubborn paratroopers, though outnumbered, squashed the attack, driving Panzers north and south. Some appeared over the crest of the hill approaching the chateau. Fearing they would be overrun, Davidson instructed Lieutenant Henry Barnes, a medical evacuation officer, to care for the more seriously wounded in the stables. The casualties who were able, the lightly wounded, those who could hold a rifle, were put on the firing line. In Barnes's aid station, the noise of explosions and gunfire panicked the wounded, and he had all he could do to simply calm the men down. Other officers began burning medical books so that the Germans would not know how many men the unit had lost. Barnes later recalled: "Here it was Christmas morning in a Belgian chateau with a room full of wounded, and outside all hell was breaking loose. I glanced at the wounded, smiled comfortably. . . . The shooting was just outside the wall and the sound of grinding tanks could be heard."[55]

At the last minute, the tide was turned. All eighteen German tanks that had rolled past American lines were destroyed along with the Grenadiers who accompanied them. Hellcats of the 705th Tank Destroyer Battalion belched murderous canister fire on German infantry and aided in knocking out a number of German Mark IVs. But the Germans came perilously close to engulfing American units that day. At one point, Lieutenant Barnes even overheard German commands issued from a tank just outside his aid station. One American officer, peering out of a door with his revolver in hand, stood face to face with a 75-mm tank cannon not fifteen yards away. "This is no place for my pistol," he said to his buddies as he closed the door. At the end of the day, Colonels Steve Chappuis and Patrick Cassidy of the 502nd, weary from a hectic day of battle, sat down to their Christmas dinner of sardines and crackers. General McAuliffe, breathing a sigh of relief but frustrated that Patton's tanks had not yet arrived, sent a message to General Middleton: "We have been let down."[56]

Yes, "show me a hero and I'll write you a tragedy," wrote F. Scott Fitzgerald. And once again it played out at Bastogne with the story of Renée Lemaire and her war-sister Augusta Chiwy. Renée and Augusta, two literal angels of mercy resolutely labored amid so many fallen and forsaken troops. They were recruited by Jack Prior, desperate to find help to care for his wounded tankers. His usual cadre of medics had been decimated during the retreat from Noville. He had literally bumped into the women on the streets of Bastogne.[57]

Both had been residents of Bastogne. Both were nurses, home for the holidays and soon trapped in the melee of December 16. One, Chiwy, was the product of an illicit affair by her father and a Congolese woman while he was stationed in the Congo in the 1920s. Brought to Belgium at six and promptly discarded by her father, she was raised by his brother, a local physician, and his wife. Dr. Chiwy had funded her nursing education in Louvain. It was there that she now worked, at l'Hopital Sainte-

Elisabeth, called by her maternalistic nuns "*Mon petit ange noir*" (My tiny black angel). She stood barely five feet tall. But Chiwy was a chocolate fireball, with sparkling eyes, boundless energy, and a quick wit. And now she reveled in her homecoming, bouyed by the familiarity of Bastogne, of her uncle and aunt—Mama Caroline she called her. Lemaire did not see herself as what she truly was, what locals would call *tres elegante*. Rather, it was a sweetness for the disadvantaged, those in need of companionship and conversation, that compelled her to visit the sick and old and lonely. Yes, she was also a Bastognard. Her father, Gustav, ran a hardware store on the Rue du Sablon—the main thoroughfare—and her family lived upstairs. She, too, had been attracted to nursing and had been schooled in Brussels, where she now worked as a visiting nurse. At age thirty, Lemaire was a ravishing beauty, with dark cascading hair and a shy demeanor, quiet, private. But an intense compassion brewed inside her, all the more a subtle exquisiteness. Like most dutiful daughters, she came back to Bastogne for Christmas. The Brugmann Hospital where she did much of her work, had given her permission to spend the holidays with her family.

But then that Saturday when the drumfire began on the western front, all changed. Cannonading was felt more than heard, like tectonic shifts in the very fiber of the earth—unsettling to all Bastognards. There was no leaving. Captain Lee Naftulin had been looking for anyone with medical training to help out at the aid station. Word of mouth had led him to the Lemaire's home. Naftulin approached Renée's father, Gustave, who then introduced him to his daughter. She agreed to talk. He took her to meet Jack Prior, who was unshaven, drained, but relieved he had found a willing nurse. Prior spoke with a weariness, with a disbelief, without comfort. She heard of his shot-up men, how they winced in pain. Might she lend a hand, he asked. It was such a request, almost pleading. No Army medics remained, they were all done in by the Germans. There was a sincerity about him, his tone subdued, spoken from a deep sobriety that comes in the presence of unrelenting suffering. She could not refuse. And Renée had directed him to Augusta Chiwy's residence. Augusta had already volunteered to work in the cellars of the School of the Sisters of Notre Dame de Namur on the rue du Sablon, which were filling with Bastognards seeking shelter from the bombardments. (Her uncle volunteered as well.) Both Augusta and Renée, sensing the weight of the moment, began their work on December 21 at Prior's aid station in the Sarma store on the Rue de

Neufchateau. Naftulin was drawn to Renée. In those few days before Christmas he would spend any free time he had with her, even escorting her through the streets of Bastogne on her errands. According to biographer Martin King, "he was besotted with her."[58]

It was a selfless service they offered. There was nothing enticing to stay in that war-torn town. The danger was palpable. Their family members may have already left. But there they were, among the tattered inmates of Prior's makeshift hospice. Chiwy even joined the doctor on field trips to retrieve wounded, out in the rolling plains west of town, careening along cowpaths, barely evading the occasional mortar burst. As they ran to fetch the wounded, their figures in the snow were sure to draw fire from Germans hidden in a copse of trees, behind barns, in trenches indistinguishable from the normal anatomy of farmland. But there was not even a close call. Maybe it was her small size that saved her, Prior mused. But she retorted, "Oh, so they're not going to see a black face in white snow? They're just bad shots."[59] It was risky business regardless. Any citizen caught aiding Americans was sure to be summarily executed. Back at the Sarma, she would help him with his surgery—what there was that he could do. With little light in the basement, it was hard to tell clean wounds from gangrene, and it was often too late. Using cognac as anesthesia, there were even one or two amputations done. Renée Lemaire was less ambitious, more inclined to the softer side of nursing. She cleaned and bathed her patients, changed dressings, emptied pots full of excrement. Inglorious chores they were, but those for which nurses are beatified, that elevate the esteem of the sick from intolerable disgust to dignified resignation. Yet with little surgical training and few surgical supplies, Prior was handicapped. A shelter from the weather and enemy fire was the most he could provide—or so he thought.

December 24 had brought some respite. Those usual noises of combat had temporarily subsided. Only scattered injuries had arrived. Renée had decorated the stark quarters with a Christmas tree from her father's hardware store, adorning it with K-ration tinfoil wrappings and even some surgical scissors. In fact, Chiwy and Prior were about to share a bottle of champagne to celebrate Christmas Eve. They had slipped from the hospital to a vacant building next door. It was then that familiar rumblings were heard, those distinct, purposeful rumblings that could only mean bombing runs. No American planes made sounds like that. Shortly, explosions tossed them off their feet and filled the room with smoke, dust, and darkness. It was one of those blinding moments when minds think of nothing but the instantly racking contortions inflicted by a force far greater.

Chiwy remembered a "boom," and all the windows were blown out. The explosion blew her through a kitchen wall, but despite this, she was miraculously spared. Prior was thrown to the floor but was also uninjured. He rose to his feet and stepped outside to the whine of a second German plane as it flew over and strafed the area. Where his aid station, the Sarma, had been was a gutted, flaming structure, the entire three-story building eviscerated by the blast and teetering on collapse. Sergeant William Kirby, a member of the 20th Armored Infantry, was posted just across from the aid station, about thirty or forty yards away. Renée Lemaire, whom he had met a few days before, went back into the structure to try to help wounded get out. As she pulled victims from the collapsing building, she yelled in broken English, "Help, help, water, water." Some say she pulled six soldiers out. Kirby then saw an incredible act. "She was safe and sound out of the building but decided to go back in and help." It is likely at that point the structure, weakened by the explosion, completely gave way. She never returned. Dr. Prior recalled, "My men and I raced to the top of the debris and began flinging burning timber aside looking for the wounded, some of whom were shrieking for help." He and his men pulled a few from the wreckage and then "the entire building fell into the cellar." It is probable that this was the instant Lemaire ran back in.

Chiwy joined Prior in digging through the rubble in search of survivors. One boy was caught and pinned by a beam. As fires licked nearby, he screamed, "Shoot me! Please shoot me!" They were able to cut him free. It was "just a pile of bricks," Chiwy recalled. They dug deeper using their bare hands and soon uncovered the bloodless, alabaster face of Renée Lemaire. As they tried to pull her free, they bared a gruesome sight: Lemaire had been cleaved in half by crushing beams. Death had come in a blinding instant. Captain Gordon Geiger, who had escaped the building, watched the whole thing. "My doctor was there [Prior] and he sat down and cried like a baby."[60] They removed her body from the wreckage, and he fetched a white parachute, like the ones she so dearly wanted for her wedding dress, wrapped her upper torso in it, and took the remains to her parents. "The woman was a heroine and a saint. I am an eyewitness to these above facts," testified William Kerby[61]. Thirty young American men, already wounded and lying in the cellar, also died that night.[62]

Prior's surviving patients were moved in with the other casualties housed at the Heintz Barracks. Chiwy continued her service until the Americans pulled out. Then she slipped into obscurity. Augusta Chiwy did not return to nursing for twenty years, so traumatized was she by those events. The siege of Bastogne was a topic she never addressed until decades later.[63] It was even longer before she was found and her work recognized. But Chiwy's response was typical of one so selfless. "What I did was very normal," she said at a ceremony in December 2011 honoring her. "I would have done it for anyone. We are all children of God." And then, at age ninety, Chiwy was finally conferred the Civilian Award for Humanitarian Service by the American ambassador to Belgium, Howard Gutman.[64] Martin King, her biographer, labeled her "*L'Infirmirere Oubliee*" (the Forgotten Nurse). When asked years later by King what she most remembered about the siege, tiny Augusta Chiwy replied in a most unsaintly moment, "the corpses being stacked up outside the aid station. And the smell of death and blood and piss."[65]

And so they receded into the annals of history, these two angels of mercy. They delivered a different message, dispensing like sweet laudanum tinctures of hope and faith to an imperfect world.

15

Airborne Surgeons

Christmas Eve brought more snow and more cold. Germans fired shells at GIs containing colored pictures of little girls wondering where Daddy was—along with an invitation to walk across no-man's land to surrender. It was equally grim for the wounded. They stared at the colorless ceilings of their hospitals and aid stations. Some lucky ones got a shot or two of cognac. Lieutenant Phalen told the story of an entrepreneurial radioman who was able to bring up Bing Crosby who soon filled the room of his aid station with "White Christmas" juxtaposed with silent rows of miserable, lonely men. One doctor commented, "By God, if you saw that in a movie you'd think it was the corniest scene since Sonny Boy died," referring to that tear-jerking song sung by Al Jolson in *The Singing Fool* in 1928.[1]

General Omar Bradley, at 12th Army Group headquarters in the city of Luxembourg, took an urgent message from General McAuliffe on Christmas Eve that surgeons were badly needed. A number of casualties were in critical condition, especially those with abdominal wounds. Despite a distant Patton's assurance of relief, there could be no more waiting. At Third Army headquarters in Luxembourg, Lieutenant Ancel "Gordon" Taflinger and his squadron commander, Major Wendell Bennett, were contacted by their commander, Lieutenant Colonel Murray. The request was simple: could they fly a surgeon into Bastogne? Lives of soldiers depended on it. A light observation plane, the two determined, might be able to breach German air defenses, land, and deposit a surgeon. Both men volunteered to fly the mission, but twenty-nine-year-old Taflinger was selected by Murray. Taflinger seemed well qualified. He was an air liaison officer with the 14th Liaison Squadron at Third Army headquarters and, it so happened, General Patton's personal pilot. A Major Howard Serrell, one of the surgeons from the 4th Auxiliary Surgical Group, had volunteered to make the trip. Plans were finalized. A small, flimsy-looking but durable Stinson L-1 Vigilant, a two-seat, single-engine observation plane of the Army Air Corps, was picked. It was unarmed and thin skinned, but, with a wide wingspan, able to land and take off on short fields. There was only room for two in the cockpit. It would be the pilot and the surgeon—no surgical technicians, basic surgical kits shoved behind their seats. Taflinger knew the plane well. He had flown surveillance countless times spotting for artillery, observing, dropping supplies, and ducking antiaircraft fire all over France. On Christmas Day, an L-1 was sent from Nancy, France, eighty miles due south, landing on the fighter strip at Luxembourg City. It was there, on that barren tarmac, that they met, Lieutenant Taflinger and Major Serrell. After refueling, Serrell loaded his stuff—instruments, some penicillin, and a supply of ether—and the two took off in late afternoon. Taflinger flew in at six thousand feet, but it was tricky. German antiaircraft batteries bristled around the perimeter. His only hope was that they would not want to waste ammunition on such a puny target. But aware of the risk, Taflinger had written Nicole, his seventeen-year-old French lover, leaving his belongings to her. He wrote that he loved her, as if it might be the last time she heard those words from him. She waited in Nancy for his return.

Tall and imposing, with dark, slicked-back hair and a stern demeanor, Howard Serrell commanded a room. His no-nonsense façade, deep-set eyes, and desire for precise, decisive solutions made him the quintessential surgeon. His nickname, "Buck," hardly seemed fitting for an otherwise cosmopolitan figure born near Montvale, New Jersey, in 1905. Few were so convinced of their life's passion as was Buck Serrell. His was a gripping intellect, intensely inspired. Dartmouth and Cornell Universities seemed proper preparation for so learned a scholar, and the surgical profession the logical conclusion for a man absorbed with a curiosity of anatomy and the catastrophic derangements of illness. It was with focus and intense consumption that he engaged a demanding residency, welcoming opportunities to lose himself in the complexities of patient care and the intricacies and intimacies of the surgical suite. So it was no surprise that Buck Serrell melded perfectly to community practice in Greenwich, Connecticut, and encountered a nurse, Margarita Noble, "Migi" to her friends. She was shockingly gorgeous. But there was a kindness about her that resonated with him, as if drawing from him that same benevolence. And of course the new, talented surgeon was a magnet in his own right. No less for Migi. More so, she saw a gentleness in him to which few others were privileged and that arose in a caring manner for those less fortunate. They clung to one another and were soon married.

But then war came. Perhaps a genetic thread of service captured Serrell's attention. A great-grandfather, General Edward Serrell, must have instilled it. Commander of the 1st New York Volunteer Engineers in the Civil War, he had no hesitancy to answer President Abraham Lincoln's call. Now a similar crisis was upon Buck. Indeed, this great crusade stirred something inside, something patriotic, humanistic. While some sought physician deferments, that was not in Buck Serrell's character. Duty bound, maybe, one can only conjecture. A private man at the core, Serrell seldom shared his motivations. There was little doubt that the skills of the surgeon would be sorely needed. War and surgery are inexorably linked, the care of the wounded almost exclusively a surgical domain. When he departed Greenwich in November 1942, Serrell left not only a thriving practice and a devoted wife but two small children. In later years, they had only sketchy pictures of their father's exploits, hardly aware of the adventures that enfolded him. Major Serrell was assigned to the newly formed 4th Auxiliary Surgical Group. Critical cases would be the focus—patients so ill that any movement would be hazardous. Yes, this would be another perfect fit: front-line surgery on desperately injured men. Serrell was off to Lawson General Hospital in Atlanta, the assembly point for the 4th Auxers.

It was not until late April 1944 that his surgical team deployed to England and the sobering business of war began in earnest. On those windy, cold June days, men from the "Fighting Fourth" trickled into Normandy, funneling through Utah Beach, Major Serrell among them. All members had reached the continent by July 19. They were temporarily attached to General Bradley's First Army, itching to break out of Normandy. Teams were dispersed to various units—field and evacuation hospitals—Serrell's team included. Casualties were plenty and experience bountiful in a perverse sort of way. By August he was with Patton's columns romping across France. It was there, entering Belgium and Luxembourg—wide-open countryside ideal for Patton's armor—that the numerous evacuation hospitals were set up for the final push into Germany. The 4th Auxers bore the brunt of surgical work. For the Reich's last stand, casualties were expected to soar. Twenty-four general teams were beefed up with six orthopedic teams, six shock teams, four neurosurgical teams, four thoracic teams, and four maxillo-facial teams. Howard Serrell was part of Team Four. All teams were part of the twelve evacuation hospitals of Patton's Third Army. So it was in Luxembourg City on Christmas Eve that circumstances brought Buck Serrell and Gordon Taflinger together, and the plot was hatched to put him into the small, besieged town of Bastogne.[2] What in those moments entered his mind? One can only speculate. Buck Serrell had never flown before, the chance of crashing was real, obliteration by flak and death palpable possibilities. It was almost certain he would either arrive alive and intact or quite dead. A sense of heroic purpose must have gripped him.

Indeed, Buck Serrell was a good choice. Off Omaha Beach on June 7, 1944, on the SS *Naushon,* there had already been need of him. An LST had taken his first casualty there, fresh from the fighting.[3] And then began a seemingly uninterrupted cavalcade of damaged soldiers. Chest wounds, abdomen wounds. Countless laparotomies and thoracotomies to stop bleeding, plug holes, sew up riddled intestines. Men with these injuries were dying slowly. Serrell stood in the way. His training, his focus, his steely judgment saved them. There were deaths, of course, shock so severe that no amount of plasma or blood or surgery could bring them back. Later, during the Allied assault on Brest, he and his team were swallowed by casualties, sometimes operating on four or five patients a day. This was a professional union—a mission, a calling—and Serrell knew it: devastation wrought on the human frame that only his skills could correct.

In their flimsy plane, Serrell and Taflinger headed for Arlon, then vectored straight into Bastogne, flying at a paltry one hundred knots. Two Thunderbolts accompanied them, reassuring partners in this crazy affair. Once near Bastogne, flak appeared. Taflinger deftly picked his way through the soft black blossoms. Finally, ground lights appeared, and he swung his plane around, put it in a steep dive, pulled up expertly at the right moment, and feathered to the ground. A 101st Airborne jeep rushed over to snatch the doctor and his kits. After Serrell was picked up, Taflinger pointed his Vigilant around, revved his engine, and took off. Almost to the point of stalling, it was a vertical climb, gaining altitude to avoid more flak. He made the trip home to Luxembourg alone, no fighter escort now.[4] But home he went. He heard a cry of relief when he knocked on his Nicole's door.

The scene greeting Serrell on Christmas afternoon was unimaginable. Casualties were stacked, almost on top of each other, in that riding stable—a large, warehouse-sized building, he would describe—at the back of Heintz Barracks. Some were across the way in the shooting gallery, equally miserable. Not sixty patients as reported but more like six hundred. "It was a frightful and terrible sight," he wrote in his diary. The scent of gangrene was unmistakable. The hall reeked of neglect. It was with some consternation that Serrell chose the gangrene cases first. Belly wounds and chest wounds were time-consuming. Sad though it seemed, in looking around, the most good for the time and material he had should be directed to "dirty" wounds, those most prone to gangrene. Debridement and amputations could be done quickly, moving from one patient to the next. "Triage at first impossible," he remembered, the number of cases absolutely overwhelming. Here the clock was the precious commodity—how many could be saved in the time allowed? A small chamber adjoining the riding stable, unheated and with only one dangling light bulb, served as Serrell's operating suite. Patients were carted in, wounds undressed and cleaned with soap and water. With scalpel and scissors and whiffs of ether, Serrell trimmed away putrid, bruised tissue until bleeding could be seen, a sign of viability. In some, the only recourse was amputation. More ether, a circular incision through healthy tissue, tying bleeding vessels, then out came the saw. Rasping through bone—that familiar seesaw requiem—and off came the limb. Dressings were applied, and on to the next one. Within twenty-four hours, twenty operations had been completed.[5]

Around 9:00 AM on December 26, two pilots, Captain Ray Ottoman and Lieutenant Al Kortkamp of the 96th Squadron, 440th Troop Carrier Group, took off in a C-47 branded *The Trusty Township* from their home base near Orleans. In tow was a CG-4A "Waco" glider. In that cockpit were Lieutenant Charlton "Corky" Corwin Jr. and the flight officer—a "Blue Pickle," as they were called from the shoulder insignia they wore—Ben "Connie" Constantino.[6] Neither man knew their mission; it had been labeled "secret." Once at the fighter base at Etain, the intrigue cleared. That Waco glider would soon be filled with surgeons and supplies and flown over Bastogne, almost due north. Cut loose at that point, it would descend to the earth, hopefully in one piece.

Two surgical teams had been chosen for the mission. All were volunteers. From the 12th Evacuation Hospital in Nancy came Captain Henry Hills (orthopedic surgeon) and Captain Edward Zinschlag (general surgeon). They were joined by surgical technicians John Donahue and Lawrence Rethwisch. From the 4th Auxiliary Group, Major Lamar Soutter (general surgeon), Captain Foy Moody (general surgeon), and Captain Stanley Wesolowski (anesthetist) stepped forward. They were accompanied by their surgical technicians, Clarence Matz and John Knowles. The entire operation was clandestine. An entry in the 12th Evac diary for December 25 cryptically mentioned only that Captains Hills and Zinschlag and Sergeants Donahue and Rethwisch were going on a "special mission." That night, Christmas night, "a special surgery team [Soutter, Moody, Wesolowski, Matz, and Knowles] spent the night."[7]

Robert Soutter was upper-crust Boston. His rearing was distinctly Boston Brahmin. Harvard College—a Hasty-Pudding member and irregular contributor to the *Harvard Lampoon*—Harvard Medical School, Boston Children's and Boston City Hospitals. Then a busy orthopedic surgery practice and part-time faculty member at Harvard. Being a staunch Massachusetts Democrat, there was no other choice. He saw that his offspring, Lamar, had it no different. Curly haired, brainy Lamar, horn-rimmed glasses and all, spent adolescence at boarding school in New Hampshire and Harvard College. Then, like the old man, it was on to Harvard Medical School, with an insatiable hunger for the frontiers of science. But again, maybe less cerebral than it might seem. Some might have called him a party animal in college. After graduation, a restless—maybe bored—Soutter struck out for adventure. There followed a stint on a Woods Hole research vessel, the *Atlantis*, sailing across the Atlantic from Copenhagen, a trip fraught with hazard: mechanical troubles, a disabled captain, and bouts of seasickness. Then, in medical school, a wilderness adventure from Alberta, Canada, to Fort Yukon in Alaska, a one-thousand-five-hundred-mile trek by land and canoe. After graduation, he was off on an expedition to the North Pole, sponsored by the Smithsonian Institution and the Field Museum of Chicago.

Taken by surgery, Soutter picked Presbyterian Hospital in New York for training. At the time, the aristocratic Alan Whipple was chief of surgery, already stunning the surgery world with his groundbreaking operation for pancreatic cancer. His was a premier department that was revolutionizing surgical education. There was a conviction, he broadly announced, that residency training should be standardized, insisting on a requisite number of years to gather proficiency. Hammered home were the importance of instruction, supervision, and repetitive skills. And there was a cadre of faculty to corral and fortify young trainees: Hugh Auchincloss, William Parsons, and Arthur Blakemore.[8] Soutter flourished there. Fluent in German, he cared for victims of the airship *Hindenburg* disaster and even accompanied the pilot, Max Pruss, home to Frankfurt after his recovery. Yes, Lamar Soutter was a man of destiny. Certainly his boss, Dr. Whipple, thought so: "Soutter has been one of the best men we have had in a long time—thoroughly capable, reliable, industrious, and absolutely trustworthy."[9] After Soutter married Norah Goldsmith in 1940, the couple moved back to Boston, where he completed more training in chest surgery at Massachusetts General Hospital. He stayed on there, a Harvard faculty member like his dad, developing a landmark achievement: the first blood bank in New England. But within a year war had been declared, and Soutter was called to service. He entered the army, and by virtue of his stature was assigned to the 4th Auxiliary Surgical Group. Once in Europe, Patton's Third Army absorbed the teams. Adventure engulfed Soutter now, as he cared for the victims of embattled Metz while Patton pounded away at the city. There was no dearth of intensity, always a new casualty waiting, more blood to be spilled. But even that was not enough. A call went out for volunteers to reach surrounded Bastogne, and incredibly, they would be airlifted, as it turned out, in gliders. He volunteered. Perhaps it was that incredible energy, that restlessness, always wanting to excel—maybe prove himself—that made him do it. A close friend later wrote, "He was willing to take risks. And he had a dogged determination." Or, as his wife put it, "Taking risks . . . might well have been his personal credo." Whatever the reason, Soutter was the first to volunteer and now found himself climbing into that canvas-and-plywood glider on a frigid morning in December 1944. He was thirty-five.

There was to be at least one fighter escort, but the navigator for *The Trusty Township,* Lieutenant Robert Mauck, had concerns. The exact location of the landing zone was not clear, and they were headed into very unfriendly territory. The margin for error, the buffer between American and German lines, was slim indeed. Back in the glider, Constantino and Corwin were not a little apprehensive. And the grainy photograph of the drop zone they were handed just before takeoff was no comfort. Landmarks were still blurry. And there were few provisions for safety. Before takeoff, Corwin advised the medics, perched atop their equip-

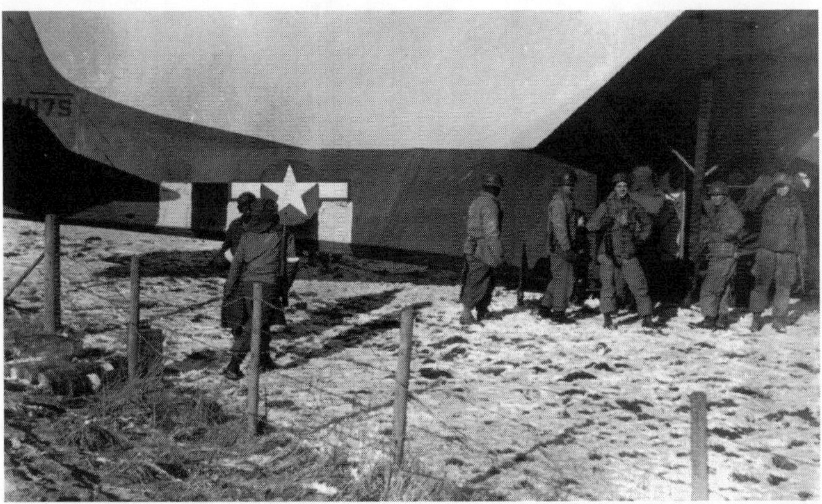

Glider used by airborne surgeons to reach Bastogne on December 26, 1944. (*National Archives*)

ment, to grip the metal tubing when it was time to land. There were no seat belts—and no parachutes. None of the men had ever been in a glider. Soutter reluctantly handed off his brandy flask before takeoff—he wanted to minimize weight. As they boarded, all read the sign on the glider's emergency exit: *Is this trip absolutely necessary*? At 2:45 PM, *The Trusty Township*, glider, crew, and surgeons pulled up from Etain's runway, edged to the north, and began their journey. The roar of the towing C-47 engines and pounding of wind drowned out all conversation. Each man was left to his thoughts—perhaps the last he would ever have.

A pinpoint ground fire was seen. The smudge pot? There was supposed to be a smudge pot lit. When *Township*'s Ottoman put on the green light, Corwin was unconvinced. Too far out, he thought. In an instant, there was that familiar jolt as plane and glider separated. Too late now. They were at three hundred feet, and the towplane banked for the return home. In fact, Corwin was right. The spot of light was a building aflame, hit by German artillery. The landing zone was still three miles away. Spectacular maneuvers and a higher airspeed carried the glider in. Even terrain and a snowpack cushioned the landing almost one hundred yards from American lines. "The prettiest sight in the world were those docs gliding in," said one sergeant with the 101st Airborne. They came to rest in no-man's land so effortlessly that crew and occupants hardly sensed it. GIs called out from the woods, doors flung open, and glider men exited, bolting for safety. Rifle cracks could be heard, Germans a stone's throw away. After taking stock, paratroopers and surgeons went back and unloaded the six hundred pounds of supplies. It was a full hour before trucks arrived. Soutter, Hills, and Zinschlag left immediately for the barracks. The others stayed to load up a second truck.[10]

Midafternoon, the surgical teams arrived at Heintz Barracks. Buck Serrell, in blood-stained fatigues and drawn features, greeted them. Shaking hands, he introduced his group of four exhausted battalion surgeons. Then it was on to a summary orientation. "Soutter, Moody, and a team from the 12th Evac came in by glider the evening of the 26th," Serrell's diary recounted. The new surgeons were struck by the rawness of the place, by the tell-tale smell of blood and sweat—and more. By their count, the large riding hall held almost 150 patients (Serrell's estimation of six hundred might have been a slight exaggeration). In the entire space there was only one light and no heat. Men were lying on litters and straw pallets, packed one next to another. Others, the walking wounded, had been cleaned out, sent to the shooting range across the promenade. But there were many, Serrell had surmised, in cellars, basements, any shelter in town. Only God knew their condition. Dr. Henry Hills was appalled at the sight. He recalled that distinct sickly smell of gangrene, of festering wounds. Many were due to frostbite and trench foot, doughboys exposed too long to frigid temperatures and sodden boots.[11] "Some of the wounded had been there for days. It looked like the Atlanta railroad station scene in *Gone with the Wind*," Hills recalled.[12] There to help were Jack Prior and nurse Augusta Chiwy, their bombed-out aid station in ruins. Prior functioned as an anesthetist, Chiwy and fellow Belgian nurses Andrée Giroux and Blanche Dombier-Hardy served as surgical assistants.

Like Serrell had done, first priority was given to those with dirty wounds, to forestall infection and gangrene. Surgeons stepped through the maze of bodies, selecting ones most susceptible. Three more operating tables were set up in Serrell's small cubicle. The five glider physicians divided into two surgical teams. Two anesthetists—Captain Zinschlag and a volunteer from the 10th Armored Division, Captain Reed—each took two tables and alternated back and forth. Work began by early evening and went right on through the night. Most were amputations, gangrene too far advanced to salvage limbs. Some wounds had gone nearly eight days without treatment. Stockpiles of blood had been expended. One large store was shattered earlier by a shell burst, absolutely coating ceiling, walls, and floor in crimson. "The place looked like a slaughter house," Dr. Phalen remembered.[13] But plasma was plentiful—and needed. After a few hours rest on December 27, the surgeons were back at it, operating again throughout the night. In total, over fifty operations were completed in the first twenty-four hours alone. Only a few died, but to Major Soutter, they were too many.[14] "We did what we could do, and, of course, we lost many," he told a reporter years later.[15] What struck deepest was the near panic of his patients at screeching dive bombers. "[T]he sound of the wounded screaming as they listened to incoming bombs was the worst thing he ever heard," Soutter's son recalled his father saying. On one occasion a blast blew the door in, and plaster from the ceiling showered the patients. Lights went out, but for the surgeons there was hardly a pause. As if practiced a dozen times, surgery continued by flashlight. Of course, in the grime and grit of their operating space, sterility was left to the imagination. Surgical gowns and drapes were nonexistent.[16] All knew, though, that as bad as things were now, they were sure to get worse if men could not be evacuated. A minority of the cases had lingering internal injuries, and a critical decision had been made not to do major chest or abdominal surgery.[17] Patton was expected soon, but their wounds could not wait indefinitely. Sepsis—massive infection—would take them sooner or later. In fact, on December 27, Patton's tanks did arrive. The next day, the 1st Platoon of the 60th Field Hospital sped in and relieved Buck Serrell and Soutter's teams. The surgeons had worked almost continuously for forty-eight hours. But their departure was decidedly less dramatic than their entrance, bused out in the standard GI issue deuce-and-a-half.[18]

For Buck Serrell, there was no rest. Even after his marathon performance in Bastogne, the following day he was back at work, repairing a soldier from the 35th Infantry Division whose belly had been sliced open by a shell fragment. New Year's Day brought four more cases and strafing runs by German planes. All this was dutifully scratched in his diary but none was disclosed to family members, at least not his son. "Dad was a man of few words," Howard "Chip" Serrell Jr. said. "I never heard him speak of any wartime experiences." He only knew of the Silver Star awarded to his father from a newspaper article which surfaced years later. "Dad was truly beloved by his patients. . . . He knew how to reassure and calm them down, much as he did in Bastogne." Dr. Serrell returned home to Greenwich, Connecticut, where he resumed his thriving surgical practice until retiring in 1978. Howard "Buck" Serrell, hero of Bastogne, died peacefully in 1985.

16

Relief

On Christmas Day, as Major Serrell and his pilot were loading for Bastogne, the skies over the town were cloudless and a crystal winter blue. "A clear cold Christmas," General Patton wrote in his diary, "lovely weather for killing Germans."[1] His men were churning north, tanks and armored vehicles of Combat Command R of the 4th Armored Division. Patton had assured Eisenhower he could do it, on even a slimmer timetable than he thought possible. Coming from the south, colliding head-on with the German Seventh Army guarding the southern shoulder of their Ardennes offensive had cost Patton's divisions horrific casualties and precious time. But the obstinate Patton insisted on frontal attacks, again and again, day and night, in order to break through to Bastogne. Icy roads, cold, and snow compounded the situation, making slow going for metal-treaded tanks. With progress grinding to a crawl, his men would not give the embattled troops of Bastogne a present on Christmas Day. There was no breakthrough. Patton's troops were still kilometers south, battering Germans outside of Lutrebois and Assenois.

"At 1400 [December 26] Gaffey [Major General Hugh Gaffey, commander of the 4th Armored Division] phoned to say that if I authorized the risk, he thought that . . . Colonel Wendell Blanchard [commander, Combat Command R, 4th Armored Division] could break through to Bastogne by a rapid advance. I told him to try it. At 1845 they made contact and Bastogne was liberated. It was a daring thing and well done," Patton wrote in his diary.[2] Sherman tanks of Lieutenant Colonel

Creighton Abrams's 37th Tank Battalion, firing to the right and to the left and straight ahead, blasted their way through the tiny village of Assenois just outside of Bastogne and made contact with paratroopers of the 326th Engineers who were manning that sector. "The relief of Bastogne is the most brilliant operation we have thus far performed and is in my opinion the outstanding achievement of this war," the not-so-humble Patton later wrote his wife.[3] The slim corridor was quickly shored by follow-up troops and armor. Knowing the desperate straits of the wounded, just behind the armor came a fleet of ambulances escorted by light tanks intent on ridding Bastogne of its fallen. That very night the first cases were sent out. Twenty-two ambulances and twelve trucks took 260 of the most critical to the 635th Clearing Company at Villers-devant-Orval, about forty miles away, near the French border. The ambulance attendants, mostly African American, handled the litter cases with extraordinary care and compassion. One of the injured, Lieutenant Robert O'Connell, remembered it well: "Many of our 101st men were in poor shape from their wounds. I remember how these black soldiers picked us up and carried us with words of encouragement. 'You're going to be all right now—I'll take care of you men.'"[4]

The 635th Clearing Company had been alerted to the arrival of casualties, they thought, through a truce arranged with the surrounding Germans at Bastogne. As it turned out, all that was not needed. Patton had cleared the way. Patients were unloaded, sorted, and distributed to nearby evacuation hospitals. Ambulances and trucks returned to Bastogne, reloaded, and made a second trip, arriving back later that night. A total of 652 patients were evacuated before midnight.[5] Convoys continued the next day, a steady stream of battered men heading south. A reporter for *Stars and Stripes* saw them pass: "The convoy of wounded came out of Bastogne in a slow trickle. . . . The day was beautiful if you like Belgium in the winter time. . . . The wounded sat stiffly in the trucks. . . . The dust of the road had made their hair gray, but it did not look strange because their faces were old with suffering and fatigue."[6]

The more seriously wounded identified at Villers-devant-Orval were transferred to the 107th and 39th Evacuation Hospitals and the less critical to the 103rd Evac. People at the 107th Evac had been on the move. The thunder of the German offensive on December 16 sent them high-tailing back to Libin and the Château Roumont, former home of the 102nd Evac. They were uprooted from those plush surroundings on December 21. News had reached them that Bastogne had fallen, the 101st

Airborne were surrounded, and Nazi patrols were observed a few miles down the road. "Clear out in 10 minutes," was the order. Off they went to Carlsburg, setting up in the Saint Joseph's school. They were there less than twenty-four hours when reports filtered in that German paratroopers had broken through and were looting and killing. Once again they packed up, this time for Sedan, France, just over the Belgian border. The hospital moved into L'Ecole de la Textile du Nord, a building formerly occupied by Free French fighters. Despite warnings of German troops within twenty miles, doctors and nurses were simply too exhausted to care, and the hospital stayed put. According to reports, around one thousand two hundred patients arrived over the next few days, most fresh out of Bastogne via the Villiers clearing company.[7] Many came wrapped in parachute silk, tablecloths, civilian blankets and comforters, anything that could provide warmth. Nurse Ruth Puryear alone supervised the evacuation of four hundred wounded from Bastogne—three days across rutted roads to France.

The 39th Evac had set up at Virton, in southern Belgium in a Catholic girls' school, another named Saint Joseph's, on Christmas Eve. On December 27, they were notified of the relief of Bastogne and received the portentous message: "Take as many cases as you can without limiting the number to one hundred. Then send cases to 107 Evac."

That same night, 148 Bastogne wounded arrived directly from Villiers. The men were filthy, in pain, their wounds soiled and dressings stained with blood and pus. Yet spirits were surprisingly bright. One nurse wrote, "Despite the large number of casualties and severe injuries received, their [the paratroopers'] morale seemed extremely high."[8]

A number of burn victims were among the casualties. Armored conflict around Bastogne, particularly with the thin-skinned American Sherman tanks, had produced a share of ghastly burns. American tanks that many cynical troopers called "Ronsons" after the popular cigarette lighter, were prone to ignite violently after a shell hit, the skinny armor too easily penetrated. Men inside would roast to death or tumble from hatches in various stages of incineration. Those not picked off by enemy infantry suffered the anguishing fate of scorched victims. And all listened to the howling raves of men trapped inside. For any who survived, doctors knew burns would be the nemesis of wound care. Denudation of skin, shifts of body fluid, and infection laid low many victims—sepsis and organ failure often their fate. Early cleansing and coverage is critical. If not, the penalty is sure to be infection.

Those men of the 60th Field Hospital who relieved Serrell, Soutter, and the other "airborne" surgeons had raced up from Oermingen, France, and entered Bastogne through Patton's corridor. It was Edward Churchill's model of the mobile surgical hospital—surgical teams of 4th Auxers, beds, and all the support people necessary. Hospital records from those Bastogne days reflected that: "Surgical and shock teams have enabled the field hospital to function as a surgical unit, caring only for non-transportable cases. . . . The surgical teams should have two surgeons . . . capable of performing the heaviest type of extremity, abdominal, and chest trauma."[9]

Arriving with the 1st Platoon were the standard surgical and shock teams: two surgeons, Major Samuel Karlin and Major Pratt, along with the shock team of Captains Albert DeFuria and Charles Bates—all 4th Auxers. In another whirlwind effort, they managed ninety-four casualties, even operating on critical abdomen and chest cases—all this in just two days before they were relieved by men from the 495th Collecting Company and Company A of the 92nd Medical Gas Treatment Battalion. The "gas men," more familiar with chemical warfare casualties, found themselves wading through triage and emergency treatment of battle wounds. Before midnight December 31, Company A saw eighty-nine more patients. New Year's Day the gas men were gone, moved to Cobreville, south of Bastogne, where their work continued. "[S]econd echelon medical evacuation for the [101st] division . . . performed under the adverse weather conditions of snow and extreme cold," the records explained. A total of three thousand two hundred patients would pass through.[10]

WAR CORRESPONDENT MARTHA GELLHORN visited Bastogne on December 29, coming on the heels of Patton's tanks. The so-called southern corridor, the Assenois corridor, was, in her words, an avenue of "death and destruction." The landscape was littered with burned-out vehicles and tanks; burned and gutted houses; bloated, dead cattle; and dark clumps of human bodies. "The American dead had been moved inside the smashed houses and covered over," Gellhorn noted. And the woods were full of dead Germans; those young grenadiers who had tried to storm American fortifications now lay strewn about in frozen heaps. But she was told, in no uncertain terms, that the struggle for Bastogne was not over. "The front, north of Bastogne, was just up the road and the peril was far from past," she reported.[11] Certainly, the men in Bastogne understood that. December 30 saw the most concentrated bombing and strafing attack of the siege. Many more civilians hit the road, convinced that fleeing the embattled town was the only solution to survival. And they might have been right. German cannon continued to blanket the place. On January 5, a random artillery shell hit a truck full of mines and stiffened dead bodies parked in front of Le Petit Seminaire. Thirteen men from the 501st Demolition Platoon were killed, mingling their parts with those of the already deceased. The only identifiable remains were the arm and head of one of the enlisted men.

Snow and more snow added to the miseries of the besieged. By January 3, it was waist deep, and the cold was bone chilling; some of the lowest temperatures on record were logged: -20 degrees Fahrenheit. By New Year's, almost as many nonbattle casualties had assembled as battle wounds, with frostbite and trench foot now endemic.[12] Equally disturbing were reports of dysentery. In the cold it was impossible to clean mess kits or abide by usual measures of sanitation. But it was impossible to tell actual numbers. Innumerable wounded and sick were treated outside official collecting points, in the myriad aid stations, houses, barns, and chateaux around the perimeter. And the exact number of dead would not even be known, not for a while. Bodies frozen in death and covered in snow scattered through the woods and dales were not to be found for weeks. And it was simply too dangerous to retrieve the corpses. It was now a landscape of milky snow dotted with dark forms and streaks of crimson. And every now and then a sudden, blinding, orange blast. For poet Louis Simpson, then a private in the 327th Glider Infantry, it was his vision of a white hell:

At dawn the first shell
landed with a crack.
Then shells and bullets
swept the icy woods.
This lasted many days
the snow was black.
The corpses stiffened in
their scarlet hoods.[13]

The Germans were hardly finished with Bastogne. Unable to penetrate Patton's southern corridor, they pounded from the north the tiny hamlet of Foy along the Houffalize Road, and clashed with paratroopers around Champs and Longchamps. January 3 and 4 were particularly bloody days as Panzers, in rare coordinated attacks along the northern rim of the perimeter, threw the weight of their armor and infantrymen against thin American defenses. Shells uprooted trees, sending whizzing pieces of shrapnel everywhere. Paratroopers, enduring ground-trembling artillery barrages, curled in their foxholes, then rose as if from the dead to mow down charging infantry. The toll on both sides was appalling. In the 2nd Battalion, 502nd Parachute Infantry sector around Longchamps, Company F lost forty-seven men, Company D forty-eight, Company E fourteen, and Company I ten. To the northeast, attempting to take Foy, one veteran of Company E, 506th Parachute Infantry, said, "Every replacement that came into the platoon got killed in that town."[14] Of January 3 Leonard Rapport wrote, "It was a day productive of fear, frustration, and bravery."[15] Medics crawled from wounded to wounded, bandaging, splinting, and dragging victims back to safety. Johnny Gibson, a medic with the 506th, recalled one soldier sitting in the snow with a leg missing below the knee: "The man's foot and part of his leg were still contained within his boot . . . lying on the ground no more than 20 feet away. Although the casualty was pale and suffering from traumatic shock, he was still able to support what was left of his leg with both hands. . . . I bent down to dress the mangled stump but the man refused treatment . . . but asked me if I would be kind enough to collect his severed leg."[16]

Gibson turned the casualty over to a group of passing troops and medics and, as he walked away, could still hear the soldier arguing about his leg. From the foxholes and gun pits deep in the forests around Noville, evacuation to an aid station a few hundred yards away was a trying experience. Major Bob Harwick, commander of the 1st Battalion, 506th Parachute Infantry, could not forget his wounding in the Fazone Woods, just west of Noville. "[W]hen I saw the mess in the center of my chest, I felt a rush of emotion, anger, frustration, and perhaps a little regret."[17] He said a prayer for his daughter Bobbie—she might soon be without a father, he surmised—and waited for the medics. His ride back to the aid station was an unforgettable experience. The road, essentially a logging track through the woods, was crisscrossed with deep frozen ruts from Sherman tanks, making a corrugated, jolting journey. Shells were exploding all around, some so close he instinctively covered his face. At the forward aid station at Luzery, he was examined, tagged "FOR EVACUATION," and transported back to Bastogne and out to an evacuation hospital. And fortuitously so. The first-aid encampment at Luzery, well within range of German cannon, came under fire, making it a disagreeable place to linger. Captain Jim Morton, commander of 3rd Battalion, 506th Parachute Infantry's Headquarters Company, had been wounded and transported there. He felt the shelling was as bad as at the front: "When we reached the forward aid station it was under mortar fire. . . . Doc Feiler [Captain Sam "Shifty" Feiler] happened to mention that he was having trouble locating the morphine in the dark so we told him to forget about pain relief and just get us the hell out."[18]

Medic Johnny Gibson himself was wounded. A tree burst sent shrapnel tearing into his back. When he exhaled, he could hear bubbles springing from the wound. "I thought I might be a goner. It felt like my entire right lung was ripped open and exposed. I felt the blood run down my spine," he remembered.[19] Morton and Gibson were sent back to the regimental station in Bastogne lashed to a jeep, where the surgeon, Major Louis Kent, Chaplain Father John Maloney, and medic Miller inspected the group. Morton was informed that his left foot was nearly severed at the ankle and would need to come off. Gibson got a chest tube and an operation; shrapnel had ripped through his right lung and diaphragm and lodged in his liver. He survived to be evacuated to Paris; had Patton not arrived, he might not have.

American lines held. Replacement troops helped, inexperienced and untested but warm bodies anyway. They streamed through the Assenois corridor along with ammunition and supplies and fanned out across the perimeter. But moves to drive the Germans out were failures. Attacks were met with blistering counterattacks, paratroopers advancing, stalling, and pulling back. New replacements fell before comrades even learned their names—some in combat only hours. Battalion surgeon Captain Bernard Ryan would not forget the experience around Foy and Noville: "Blood trails . . . marked in the snow where our wounded had dragged themselves. . . . Never have I lived through such a nightmare. All night long, shells screamed into the woods. . . . It was nearly impossible to evacuate the wounded. . . . Through the whole night we heard the screams of the wounded and the moans of the dying."[20]

Towns and villages were destroyed. Foy, the scene of so much back-and-forth fighting, was leveled, its church gutted, the distinctive spire obscenely amputated: "Foy is the scene of utter desolation and ruin. No building has escaped the savage artillery fire. Scores of American and German dead attest to the bitter fighting in this vicinity. Many dead horses and cattle litter the streets . . . as yet no civilians have been seen."[21]

But the beleaguered men of Bastogne—the "Battered Bastards," they called themselves—soon got help. Of course, "help" was a term they disavowed. The paratroopers were quite sure they could single-handedly beat the Germans, thank you very much. Their main request: bullets, beans, and bandages. Allied strategy to reduce the "bulge" from the Ardennes offensive was to pinch it at its base. Coupled with the abscess of Bastogne in its belly, the German thrust soon lost vitality, strangled from the outside and withering from within. From the north, General Hodge's First Army initiated a counteroffensive on January 3, and to the south Patton's Third Army wreaked havoc on German Panzers and Volksgrenadiers, relentlessly muscling them backward. By January 11, there were unmistakable signs that the Germans were heading east, "an orderly and leisurely withdrawal" it was described.[22] Others found them a beaten, dejected line shuffling toward certain defeat, caring little whether they were killed or captured. On January 14, paratroopers finally captured Noville, the town where they had been bloodied earlier in December and again over the first days of January. Grenadiers retreated in haste. They left most of their wounded for the Americans to deal with. On January 16, patrols of the First Army made contact with men of the Third Army near the Ourthe River, completely collapsing the German salient. The Ardennes offensive was at an end, an utter German disaster, countless lives spent to dispel the rantings of a lunatic fuhrer.

The people of Belgium also paid a dear price for the seesaw capriciousness of war. Across the Ardennes, in countless tiny hamlets, the targets of artillery and bombs from both sides, ruination abounded. Homes were destroyed, livestock killed or, if wounded, bellowing in pain. Half-starved dogs roamed the countryside, feasting off half-dead cattle. Water was poisoned by white phosphorus or decaying remains. And worst of all civilians—including women and children—maimed or killed by stray shells, bullets, and mines, were now gone, homeless, or useless. So tragic, they were sometimes the targets of air attacks, their forms in the snow indistinguishable from combatants. Others were the victims of Nazi brutality, or simply in the wrong place at the wrong time during battles and fortunes that they cared almost nothing about.

After the relief of Bastogne, evacuation hospitals ramped up for the influx of casualties. The American counteroffensive swamped available beds, supplies, and personnel. For the 102nd Evacuation Hospital in Huy, the week of December 21 was its busiest. Admissions jumped to five hundred or six hundred per day. In this hospital alone, some estimated nearly one-fourth of the casualties of the Ardennes offensive passed through during bitterly cold weather, snow, and ice. Inside, shifts were extended. Few had time off. And patients arriving were in pitiful shape, the trauma affecting mind and body alike: "Officers, nurses, and men worked 12 hour shifts day after day and night after night. Still the patients came in shot to pieces, frozen, and sick. Most were fed up with seeing men blown to bits before their eyes, but many were just homesick and frightened."[23]

They came in droves. On Christmas Eve, 513 were admitted. Chaplain Ren Kennedy wrote of "a line of ambulances at the front door waiting to unload and another line at the back door waiting to take them to a general hospital." Christmas Day saw 667 more admissions, 575 evacuations (out the "back door"), and 150 operations waiting to be done due to a backlog from the day before. By that evening there were still 70 queued for surgery. On December 26, the grimy paratroopers from Bastogne began arriving, 378 that day, and twenty-five operations. To many of the personnel, this was no longer the patriotic "adventure" it had promised to be. It was becoming sad, grueling business.[24]

At the 103rd Evacuation Hospital in Longuyon, south of Bastogne, five hundred casualties, many from Bastogne, were admitted in its first twenty-four hours of operation. Paratroopers were surprised to see nurses this close to the front. "They shouldn't be up this far. It's too dangerous for a woman," one soldier commented. The nurse to whom he directed his comment, Captain Beth Veley, smiled. She was already a veteran of Bataan and Corregidor. Her gold identification bracelet proudly bore the initials "B.B.B."—The Battling Bastards of Bataan. Nurses became the backbone of medical care. In white turbans, white masks, and white surgical gowns, they were the unfailing companions of surgeons in the operating rooms. Some even functioned as on-the-job-trained anesthetists.[25] On the wards, often in oversized fatigues, they toiled tirelessly, starting transfusions, giving medication, changing dressings, bathing, walking, and all the nameless plebian activities doctors ignore and patients crave. Yet their femininity was indispensable. It spilled onto the splinters of fractured souls and soothed their torment. A sympathy emanated that resisted fatigue as if stimulated by misery alone and found only in those who catered to the most basic needs of humankind.

No less than surgeons, they, too, faced the stark brutality of war and the rows of disassembled men. Lieutenant Mary Ferrell was a nurse in the shock ward at the 101st Evac Hospital—the "Chamber of Horrors," she called it. She remembered that the halls reeked of "gore and sweat and human excrement." Nurses saw these young boys, arms and legs missing, sometimes three of four; severed spinal cords, meaning permanent paralysis; open bellies; open chest wounds. The dying often did not die quickly. They lingered, moaning, gasping throughout the day and night. In those cases, prayers were not for recovery but for a merciful, speedy end. "Sometimes I think maybe it's a good thing their mothers can't see them when they die," Ferrell added.[26] But it was women whom these boys longed for, surrogate wives and mothers. Someone who would spend time sitting, touching, smiling. Someone who would be there at the end.

Among the worst were the amputees. Land mines were everywhere it seemed, planted by both sides to channel infantry and armor along targeted routes. For soldiers who survived, the explosions tore at lower limbs, mangling and shredding tissue, bruising and devitalizing muscle and bone. Often there was outright loss of foot or leg. For what remained, the combination of cold weather, mud, and neglect produced wounds that inexorably led to infection and the need for amputation. At the 128th Evacuation Hospital in Verviers, Belgium, nurse Marte Cameron walked into the operating room one evening in late December to find eight patients lying on makeshift operating tables—sawhorses supporting litters—with one or two legs in the air in preparation for amputations. It was a chilling sight to see so many boys facing a lifetime of indignity, who would struggle to maintain a presence as worthy of their manhood as before.[27]

Captain Harry Fisher, captured at Wiltz on December 19 and singled out because he was Jewish, saw the battles around Bastogne from a unique perspective. Taken away by German troops and feared shot, Fisher, on the contrary, was quite alive and had been put to work as a doctor. He soon found himself as part of a Verbandplatz—a first aid station. His particular station was at Bras, not too far from Bastogne. There he witnessed the Panzer Lehr, of which he was now an unwilling member, attack Company I of the 501st Parachute Infantry around the hamlet of Wardin. Company I, completely outgunned, was almost wiped out. Almost fifty men were lost, and the survivors scattered. Fisher thought many more fell. He took care of some of the paratroopers brought by his captors to his aid station. One soldier, blazing away at a German Tiger tank with his machine gun, was hit by an 88-mm shell at fifty yards. He was still conscious when Fisher saw him, but with a huge gaping hole in his abdomen. "That fellow had what it takes," Fisher said. "He lived twelve hours"—longer than one could have imagined with a large part of his midsection gone. All in all, it was a night emblazoned in his memory: "There were over a hundred casualties that I saw myself. . . . I'll never forget that night. I was trying to take care of a hundred casualties in one of those two-by-four Belgian basements. Most of the casualties had to stay outside in the rain."

When the Americans began shelling the house, the Germans decided to evacuate—in a hurry. Fisher remembered that most of the wounded were left behind. Later, in another aid station in another bombed-out basement, in the village of Marvie, he took care of another American hit by a German grenade. "I counted over a hundred separate wounds," he remembered: "The poor fellow was so cold he couldn't move a muscle. All he could do was nod his head. He died in a couple of hours. What a miserable way to die."

He recalled toward the end: "No blood, no plasma, no instruments, no decent bandages. And a steady stream of casualties. It was killing. I never worked so hard in my life."

Captain Fisher remained in captivity, eventually shuttled to Germany with other prisoners, including some 3rd Auxiliary doctors. He suffered abuses, privations, and hunger, but he survived to be liberated in March 1945.[28]

For the 101st Airborne, the fight around Bastogne drew to a close January 17, a day as miserable as most, snow and rain clear through. George Koskimaki, then a T/3 with the 101st, seemed numb to the whole predicament—even the good news. A month at Bastogne might do that to a man. He wrote in his diary: "The division is being relieved today. We are to go into Corps reserve somewhere to the rear. It is cold and snowy."[29]

And on that day, the day before their scheduled departure, a few more would die and a few more were maimed—parting shots from a tenacious foe. The division was to move to the south, to the province of Alsace. A brief ceremony was held January 18, medals were given, and the town mayor, Leon Jacqmin, presented the flag of Bastogne to General Taylor. A placard was raised in the town center reading, "Bastogne, Bastion of the Battered Bastards of the 101st." As for the "Battered Bastards," some moved into a convent, the first shelter in a building since they arrived, and were serenaded by girls brought in by the nuns and teachers. Some got their first shower in weeks, even with hot water—they refused to get off the trucks unless it was. Others took off jump boots for the first time since their arrival at Bastogne to find their socks disintegrated. Trench foot was rampant; unlucky ones endured amputation of both feet. Regarding their new assignment in Alsace, they were told it would be an inactive part of the line. "[B]ut hadn't they told us the same thing before Bastogne?" a few chuckled.[30]

The official tally for the 101st Airborne paratroopers was 482 killed or died of wounds, 2,449 wounded, and 527 missing or captured. Of those supporting units, Combat Command B of the 10th Armored, the 705th Tank Destroyer Battalion, the 755th and the 969th Field Artillery Battalions, an additional 117 dead, 422 wounded, and 134 missing or captured.[31] Many comrades had been left in the frozen fields around Bastogne or hobbled into hospitals around the bulge. Some units were obliterated. Private David Webster on Company E, 506th Parachute, summed up the feelings of most survivors: "When I saw what remained of the 1st Platoon, I could have cried; eleven men were left out of forty."[32]

In Third Army hospitals in December, where most of the casualties from Bastogne ended up, almost eleven thousand five hundred men were admitted, nearly one-third of whom suffered nonbattle wounds from frostbite and trench foot.[33] More than two-thirds of battle casualties bore the stigmata of high explosives, so prodigious was the use of artillery and armor by the enemy. The Germans were enamored with it, the Americans not far behind. The trusty rifle—Garand or Mauser—accounted for less than a quarter of battlefield wounds.[34] Enormous amounts of blood had been transfused—by some accounts 529 units of fresh whole blood and 5,382 units of stored blood. And eight thousand bottles of plasma had been added to it. Hemorrhage and shock were still the big killers: half of the 314 men who died in the hospital perished from it; many more succumbed on the battlefield, unable to summon help or trapped in aid stations.

There are always sad closings to any war story—on the heels of victory comes tragedy. Bastogne and the Ardennes were no exceptions. The 424th Infantry, the sole surviving regiment of the ill-fated 106th Division, found itself attached to the 7th Armored Division and had taken up defensive positions around Manhay after the loss of Saint Vith. On the counteroffensive in early January, the 424th had attacked from the north, outside Trois Ponts through Spineux and Wanne, battering the shrinking neck of the German salient. It was here, on the night of January 13, that Jarret "Jerry" Huddleston Jr., son of an Anzio hero, found himself under heavy artillery fire, attempting to rescue a battered company of fellow soldiers. Suddenly an airburst lit up the sky, probably enemy tank fire. Men dropped, among them Jerry Huddleston. When reached by an aid man, he refused care, insisting that others be treated first. When he finally agreed, it was too late. Jerry died on a litter somewhere in the Ardennes woods. The Huddleston family—like many Gold Star families—lost two members to this war.[35]

Part 4

Chosin

"When a cold wind catches men in the winter out on the mountains, it frequently means death to them."

—W. R. Carles, *Life in Corea*, 1888

17

The Hermit Kingdom

THE NATIVES CALLED THEIR LAND CHOSON, A TERM MEANING "morning calm" or "fresh morning." They were a proud but mistrustful people, and their geography lent itself well to a policy of isolation, an inaccessibility that in the words of the nineteenth-century chronicler William Elliot Griffis would "insulate her from the shock of change."[1] But Westerners had intruded, through the gateways of neighboring China and nearby Japan, and had bastardized the name to Corea, taking the Japanese title Korai given to one of the dominant states of the peninsula in the ninth century. The "Coreans" were justified in their distrust. The inhospitable peninsula had been a backwater nation carved up over the centuries by China and Japan. These two powers, over time, had considered the mountainous terrain a buffer zone against aggression, each desiring possession.

More recently, the Russian Empire loomed ever larger to the north. Like Poland, Korea was used as geographic leverage by one or the other as they sought to dominate the Asian mainland. After the Russo-Japanese War of 1904–05, US president Theodore Roosevelt, as "peacemaker," benevolently offered Korea to Japan in the Treaty of Portsmouth. This was done despite the fact that Korea had made a treaty with the United States in 1882 saying that America would come to Korea's aid should it be attacked. It was no secret that Roosevelt admired the Japanese, as they were industrious, organized, and disciplined, much like Americans. Korea represented little more than a bargaining chip in dividing Asian spoils between the two combatants. Japan lorded over its "protectorate" for the next four decades. But in 1910, all pretense of it being a protectorate disappeared, and the country was unabashedly annexed. Japan appeared to have nothing but disdain for its new colony. All that was Korean was suppressed, even the language. The Japanese intended to obliterate any semblance of Korean culture and independence. As a result, the occupation dismantled Korean self-governing and any political process. Of course, Korea proved to be of value to the Japanese for launching further intrusions against the Chinese, their real archenemy. Imperial Japanese troops spilled out of northern Korea and into Manchuria in 1931, quickly pushing out the reluctant forces of Zhang Xueliang and occupying the rich and fertile farmlands, renaming it Manchukuo. In 1937, Japan invaded China proper, bringing Russia into the mix. While Soviet premier Joseph Stalin pledged support to nationalist China (under American favorite Chiang Kai-shek), his pledge was, in typical Stalin style, insincere, and he eventually backed Communist strongman Mao Tse-tung and his "people's" movement.

The Soviet Union belatedly entered the Pacific war six days before the cessation of hostilities (August 8, 1945). Its troops quickly overpowered the Japanese forces in Manchuria and streamed into northern Korea, rounding up six hundred thousand prisoners. The Russian bear sat gluttonous at the bargaining table to divvy up the spoils. At the Moscow Conference in December 1945, Korea was partitioned as a trusteeship among the United States, the Soviet Union, Britain, and the Republic of China. However, it was the two superpowers, Russia and the United States, that would provide a protectorate for the country, facing off at the agreed-on thirty-eighth parallel. Soviet troops quickly expanded their occupation of the north, establishing a seat of government at Pyongyang. While Koreans were clamoring for independence, it was not to be. Once again, Korea would not be united as a country but would be ruled by two very different types of tyrants: one, a young unknown, the gullible and malleable Kim Il Sung, and the other an aging, cerebral, but vehemently anti-Communist, Syngman Rhee. There would be no unification. Joint US and Soviet commissions in 1946 and 1947 failed to make any progress in the process. The Soviet Union, intent on expanding its Asian empire and recognizing the value of a Communist buffer in Asia, was ill-inclined to listen to such nonsense from the United States. And Americans, finally finished with the Asian menace after the defeat of Japan, could care less about another Asian country.

As David Halberstam put it, "Without the threat of global Communism, America cared nothing about Korea."[2]

On August 15, 1948, the Republic of (South) Korea was established with Rhee as the new president. The American military government ended. Over the next eight months, fifty thousand US troops were withdrawn, leaving a skeleton force of five hundred officers and men as military instructors to train the new Republic of Korea (ROK) defense force. This would strictly be a policing army, deprived of any substantial armament for fear of antagonizing North Korea and its Soviet guardians. There was the added fear that Rhee would use a strong military to encroach on nearby Formosa and the regime of Chiang Kai-shek, whom he hated. In contrast, Communist dictator Kim Il Sung made no apology that his force of sixty thousand regulars, equipped with captured Japanese and new Soviet weapons, was a "superior army," routinely rattling his saber at compatriots just south of the thirty-eighth parallel.[3] Yet, Rhee's government turned a blind eye to Koreans, so long under the thumb of foreign domination, and their desire for social reform. Dissatisfaction was fermenting among leftists and Communists, whom Rhee could not appease or control.

Kim was the quintessential Soviet puppet. A former guerrilla fighter in China, he was identified as a durable, dependable Communist leader and ready to acquiesce to his Soviet masters. Stalin felt he was the ideal man for North Korea, not individualistic or popular and ready to be molded as the Soviet leader saw fit, complying completely with Soviet mandates. He was received by his compatriots with dismay; they had hoped instead for a seasoned, charismatic leader. The awkward, monotoned Kim ruthlessly seized control in dictatorial fashion, exactly as envisioned by the distant Stalin. In fact, he was described as being much like Stalin, completely paranoid about his subordinates and pitiless in his desire for absolute dominance. North Korea employed the Soviet model, and socialist mobilization fueled the state's economy. There was rapid, expansive land reform, the beginnings of industrialization, abolition of social barriers, and state-directed production, education, and health care. And Kim desperately wanted a unified Korea, a desire communicated time and again to Stalin, who, eventually, in biblical Pontius Pilate fashion, washed his hands of the affair, giving tacit approval, and encouraging the young tyrant to seek the support of a closer ally, Communist China. In fact, one Korea was a desire shared by most Koreans, South and North. A divided country was unacceptable.

By 1950 North Korea had become a powerful force for unification and had developed the political and economic stability to test the mettle of its southern countrymen. Premier Kim had developed his army, now richly supplied with Soviet technology, for a singular purpose: crossing the thirty-eighth parallel, occupying the South, and dismantling the American-led Republic of Korea. It was consistent with his hagiographic delusions that two hundred thousand South Koreans would rise up and welcome him, providing grassroots support for Communist unification of both countries. Beginning in early 1950, his army swelled with the incorporation of thousands of troops returning to North Korea after serving in the Communist Chinese armies overrunning China, most by then battle-hardened veterans. In June 1950, Kim began positioning his forces just north of the thirty-eighth parallel, and on June 25 they flooded across, spearheaded by Soviet-made tanks and over one hundred Soviet-made planes. Seoul was their sumptuous target.

Word of the North Korean incursion quickly reached President Harry Truman. With Soviet domination of Eastern Europe and much of Asia, the threat of a worldwide Communist conspiracy was clearly on the minds of many Americans. Of most concern was expansion into Western Europe. And Truman, despite his Midwestern ethos of honesty and candor, had become hardened in his years of dealing with Stalin, a man who was quite comfortable avoiding those qualities. Truman had come to believe that Stalin respected only strength; the weak he would trounce underfoot. It had fallen on the Soviet Union and the United States to define the new order imposed after the collapse of the Axis powers, with war-weary Great Britain and France licking their wounds. Reluctant to acknowledge the end of colonialism in Asia, the United States continued to bolster half-hearted and usually corrupted attempts to maintain control of Western-style governments in Southeast Asia. More vividly, it saw the Soviet Union as dedicated to global dominance, worrying over expansionistic tendencies in Europe and even the Middle East. So with bona fide aggression across the thirty-eighth parallel, Truman suspected the unfolding of the plot, directed by Stalin himself, perhaps the eastern tentacle of a worldwide effort to grab more of Europe or the oil-rich Middle East (Iran was thought to be the likely target). A stand had to be taken. Truman noted in his memoirs: "I remembered how each time that the democracies failed to act, it had encouraged the aggressors to keep going ahead. Communism was acting in Korea, just as Hitler, Mussolini, and the Japanese had acted ten, fifteen, and twenty years earlier."[4]

In fact, and it was unclear to American leaders at that time, Soviet support of former colonies vying for independence in Asia was the only option. Young revolutionaries in Asia had been rejected by Uncle Sam, who was still unconvinced that a new order was here to stay and was reluctant to offend allies who were the former colonial masters. It was nationalism that fueled Communist partnership; nationalism and the corrupt governments shored up by Western powers that had created a caste system guaranteeing the subjugation of peasant classes. Of little comfort to these idealogues was the bitter fact that Communist states were run by iron-willed dictators no different than the abusive tsars and emperors of antiquity.

Despite a United Nations resolution condemning North Korea's aggression, Truman was livid. "By God, I'm going to let them have it," Truman boldly announced to Louis Johnson, his secretary of defense.[5] It was clear that the nascent South Korean army was not fit to provide much resistance, so American involvement was inevitable. With the massive June invasion, ROK forces were quickly routed and retreated south. At first, Truman threw air and naval support at the South Koreans, but all knew, without saying, that American ground troops would be necessary if the South was to be rescued. Truman ordered General Douglas MacArthur, then in Japan, to immediately tour the peninsula and appraise the situation. MacArthur was a man Truman secretly loathed ("Mr. Prima Donna," he referred to him as). Nevertheless, MacArthur had the respect and admiration of the public and had taken on the rehabilitation of the Japanese as a personal crusade and passion. He was one who proclaimed to know the "Oriental" mind-set like no one else.

Douglas MacArthur had been magnanimously appointed supreme commander for the Allied powers at the surrender of Japan. Efforts by Stalin to carve out a piece of Japan were flatly rejected by Truman, who was intent on maintaining American control over the Japanese mainland. It fell to MacArthur to transition the Japanese from the devastation of war. Nipponese imperialistic aspirations had cost the lives of one million two hundred thousand men and over six hundred thousand civilians and utterly destroyed over two million homes. Many cities and industrial areas were flattened by Allied might. And in reconstruction, MacArthur had done a marvelous job. The industrious Japanese immediately took to him and took to the streets, cleaned the rubble, and, with US aid, returned their homeland to a livable, vibrant country. As far as American presence, MacArthur downsized the garrisoned Eighth Army, relegating its soldiers to a lackluster and slothful existence, one that soon stripped them of combat efficiency—and a good deal of weapons and material. As for nearby South Korea, also under his jurisdiction, he cared little; his preoccupation with Japan was total.

Yet MacArthur's whirlwind tour of South Korea in June 1950 was sobering. Seoul, the capital, was already in enemy hands. Rhee and his cabinet had slithered south, and the whole ROK Army was rolling backward before the North Korean surge. MacArthur wired Washington: "The South Korean forces are in confusion. . . . It is essential that the enemy advance be held or its impetus will threaten the over-running of all of Korea. . . . The only assurance for holding the present line and the ability to regain later the lost ground is through the introduction of United States ground combat forces into the Korean battle area."[6]

He was convinced that the North Korean's momentum would carry them straight through to the port city of Pusan on the southern tip of the peninsula. South Korea would be swallowed in their wake. That was enough for Truman. Despite his worry of provoking a wider conflict with China, and at the behest of the Joint Chiefs of Staff, he agreed to liberal mobilization of ground forces under MacArthur's command in a memorandum dated June 30. MacArthur now had free reign to "utilize Army forces available to you . . . Subject only to requirements for safety of Japan in the present situation which is a matter for your judgment."[7]

In Japan, ready ground forces of the Eighth Army at MacArthur's disposal were four understrengthed and poorly equipped units: the 7th, 24th, and 25th Infantry Divisions, and the 1st Cavalry. Most had only two battalions per regiment instead of three and were woefully short of heavy weapons and armor. It had been one of those inevitabilities of peace. The US Army was dramatically downsized at the end of World War II. The public and Congress were eager to get men out of uniform. Pax Americana was at hand. Truman had opposed demobilization, but even MacArthur had fed the frenzy by glamorizing his successes in the occupation of Japan. So placid was the Far East now, he argued, that troop strength could be reduced by more than half, down to two hundred thousand. By 1948, the army's entire strength was down to half a million, and MacArthur's command totaled less than one hundred fourteen thousand. Three of MacArthur's four divisions were down about six thousand men each. The 25th Division, due to the full-strength 24th Infantry—an all-black outfit—actually had all three regiments. Yet four field artillery batteries, four antiaircraft batteries, one hundred antitank guns, and most of the heavy armor had been stripped away by enforced budget cuts. Even more disturbing was the lack of training, command, and esprit de corps. The hardened edge and superb officer corps of World War II had vanished. Garrison duty promoted complacent attitudes, spotty field exercises, and inexperienced leadership. Turnover of personnel—almost 40 percent annually—fostered slackening morale and brittle unit cohesion. It was into this pot that MacArthur had to dip to furnish Truman's infantry for Korea. The first up was the 24th Infantry Division, stationed closest, on the island of Kyushu. The division was 15,965 strong but combat green and led by officers, commissioned and noncommissioned alike, who were fill-ins from other units. Two remaining regiments were in deplorable shape—the 34th and 21st Infantry—but they were ably led by General William Dean, a seasoned combat veteran and the only division commander who had any knowledge of the mountainous terrain of Korea. Victory in World War II for the rank and file, though, had created a culture of arrogance. Green doughboys, most of whom had never seen combat, boasted, "As soon as those North Koreans see an American uniform over here, they'll run like hell."[8]

The Eighth Army Medical Corps was in even worse shape. Out of an authorized strength of 346 doctors, attrition, cutbacks, and disinterest mustered only 156 in the summer of 1950.[9] A visit by Deputy Surgeon General George Armstrong on the eve of the Korean conflict found that "the Medical Service in Japan is fine; they are not short of doctors." As a consequence of this outlandish report, the number of hospitals was shortly reduced. Major General James Bethea, former surgeon for the Far Eastern Command, of which the Eighth Army was an integral part, cringed at the governmental slashing that soon followed: "The outlook for medical service within the FEC [Far Eastern Command] during the year [1950] presents a grim picture from a personnel standpoint. Commencing in January 1950 and increasing each month through June 1950 the losses of Medical Corps officers will be extremely heavy."[10]

Yet the public was fed a different perception, even early on in the war. By September 20, before the American Hospital Association convention in Spokane, Washington, military leaders—army, air force, and navy—pitched that "United States medical care in the Korean conflict is better and faster than it was in World War II."[11] In reality, not only quantity but quality suffered. Young men who would provide medical care now were, for the most part, not seasoned surgeons nor military officers. They were all too often pulled from residency training and teaching hospitals. As for lack of skill, the chief of surgery at Walter Reed Army Hospital in Washington, DC, had a fix for that. "There's only one way to learn good surgery and that's to get bloody wet," he claimed.[12]

18

The Ascent

Douglas MacArthur was gloating. His ill-equipped divisions had taken a thorough thrashing in July as North Koreans pushed poorly trained and poorly armed ROK and American boys down the peninsula, finally corralling them into a rough quadrangle called the Pusan Perimeter—not quite the Korean ass-kicking envisioned by field commanders. It was then that a stroke of brilliance—MacArthur's stroke—entered the picture in the form of landings up the western coast near Seoul at Inchon. A whirlwind offensive had retaken Seoul and linked up with allied units busting out of Pusan. They had the North Koreans on the run. And on the Americans surged, across the thirty-eighth parallel and into Pyongyang. There was no stopping there—MacArthur smelled victory. It was on to the Yalu. On the west side, the Eighth Army stormed north, briefly hassled by some Chinese troops. On the west, X Corps—1st Marine Division and 7th Infantry Division—landed and began a willy-nilly trek toward the Manchurian border. MacArthur boasted American supremacy. But some would say fortunes are parceled out in equal measure—good and bad. Crowning successes are offset by stupendous blunders. MacArthur's fortunes were racing toward that equilibrium.[1]

It was a reckless decision, fraught with danger and against better military judgment. It was a move spurred by General MacArthur's delusional notion that Korea was his for the taking and that Communist China, on the other side of the Yalu River that separated North Korea from

Manchuria, dare not cross it in any strength. Yes, there had been butchery north of Pyongyang at the end of October. Elements of the U.S. First Cavalry Division had been encircled near the small hamlet of Unsan and almost wiped out. Chinese troops were clearly involved. But MacArthur blamed it all on Chinese "voluntary personnel" who literally stumbled onto American units when they only meant to harass forces of South Korea. The Chinese were just a rag-tag bunch of irregular guerrillas as poorly trained as he mistakenly thought the North Korean army had been months earlier. In an impulsive note from his headquarters hundreds of miles away in the Dai-Ichi Building in Tokyo, MacArthur stiffened. "I recommend against hasty conclusions which might be premature [that Chinese troops were massing]," he wrote to the Joint Chiefs of Staff on November 4, 1950. In other words, on to the Yalu.[2]

MacArthur would not pause. North Korea was low-lying fruit, and he was going to pluck it. He had Washington in his pocket and exhorted his troops to advance, as if some Roman emperor given free reign by his senate. To the Yalu. Bring the war to a rapid end, he roared. For the troops "Home by Christmas" was the scuttlebutt. Once again, morale soared. In the western sectors, the start date for the new offensive was set for November 24. In the east, X Corps wound their way through mountain passes for the edges of Manchuria, the 7th Division snaking along the coast from Iwon, 150 miles north of Wonsan, and Smith's 1st Marine Division trudging up toward the Chosin (Changjin) Reservoir[3] to soon link up with comrades to the west. The dividing line between the two armies was the Taebaek mountain range of central Korea. The stopping point would be the very border of Manchuria.

But the winter of the North Korean mountains hit with full force. Siberian cold swept in, snow and ice covered what footpaths there were. All hunkered down under layers of quilted cotton and wool. Each side would face a common enemy now: the weather. Tactics were framed to a large extent by frigid temperatures, cold enough to frostbite naked hands hoping to squeeze jammed triggers. Tanks were useless; artillery limited in mountain terrain. It was guerrilla country, combing hills, entrenched in high ground, mobile, lightly armed. Fighters quick to maneuver, outflank, encircle. Horrid weather, precipitous terrain, few passable roads, and long supply lines, were perfect conditions for the Chinese. Peasant soldiers and toughened veterans, they were used to stern conditions. Endless masses of minions whose welfare meant almost nothing to their commanders were sent into the hills to stalk Ameri-

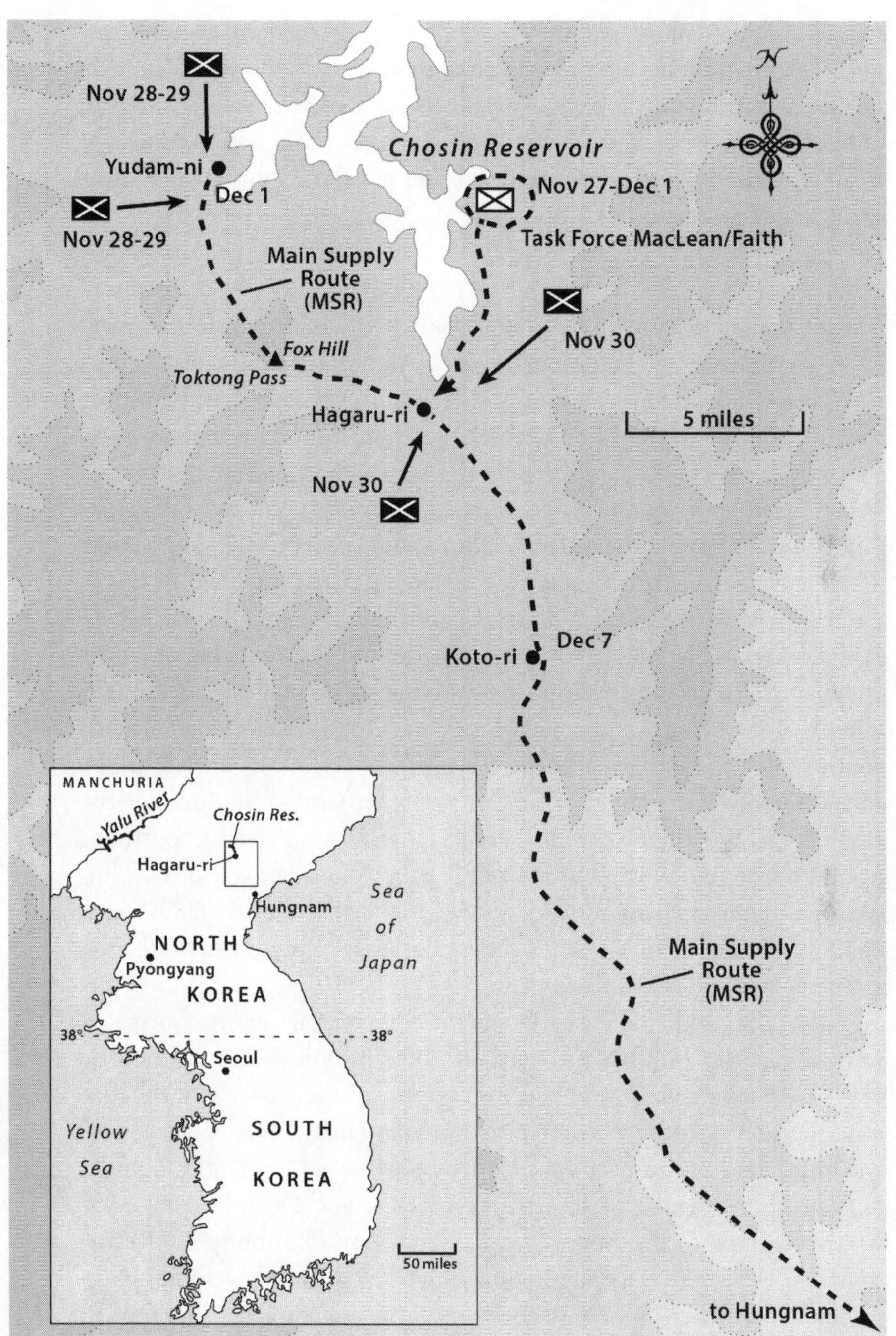

Map 4. Chosin Reservoir area, November-December 1950.

cans—Peoples' volunteers, they were called. Ruthless officers sent lines of infantry, barely armed, in blind charges, hoping that some would succeed in falling on GIs. For the Americans, on the other hand, it was one of the most ill-conceived offensives on record, and only the courage and fortitude of individual soldiers and Marines saved the United States from a disaster of monumental proportions.

THE NORTHEAST REGIONS OF KOREA were alien country indeed. Craggy summits with perilous passes etched across almost perpendicular inclines rose above hidden valleys and rutted roads. It was surly terrain, terrain meant for concealment and ambushes. There were only two passages from the northeast coast of Korea to the Yalu River and Manchuria. One began at the port of Iwon and tracked north through the villages of Chori and Pungsan, up through Kapsan to the border town of Hyesanjin. The other passage, to the south, originated at the port town of Hungnam, a thriving community called the third-largest city in North Korea. It sits on the coastal plain of the Songchon estuary, which flows from the mountains east of the Chosin and Fusen Reservoirs and eventually empties into the Sea of Japan at Hungnam. Opposite Hungnam, on the south rim of the estuary, was the town of Yonpo and its airfield. Eight miles inland was the larger community of Hamhung. A vital transportation center, the town bestrode rail service to Wonsan to the south and Sonjin to the northeast, leading into Russian Vladivostok. Surrounding was one hundred square miles of agricultural districts, almost an endless expanse of emerald rice paddies. These flatlands were probably the most spacious in all of North Korea.

Along the east bank of the Songchon, a gravel road and narrow-gauge railroad ran past Hamhung toward Oro-ri eight miles beyond. The road was wide enough, but just barely, for two-way traffic. At Oro-ri, the road crossed the Songchon and then paralleled the Hungnim River up toward the hills. Here the ground was still flat and the road level, although serpentine, following the twists and turns of the river. The route snaked on to Majon-dong in the Sudong Valley and then Chinhung-ni twenty-seven miles distant, both small villages set in a distinctly agrarian background. But then lanes headed up and narrowed, climbing by switchbacks, cut precipitously into the face of looming mountains, cliffs on one side, deep chasms on the other. The trail must climb two thousand five hundred feet in just eight miles to reach Koto-ri atop the

Kaema Plateau, called by some "the roof of Korea." This coiling roadway up and over was named Funchilin Pass. The terrain here was almost devoid of vegetation, the route bumpy, the landscape resembling arctic tundra. In the midst of the pass was the so-called Gatehouse, controlling the waters of the Chosin Reservoir, one lane passed over giant pipes propelling water downhill to hydroelectric plants.

From the hamlet of Koto-ri, the slender road, a dirt-gravel path of varying widths now, followed the Changjin River, comfortably tucked away in a gentle valley, as it snaked north to empty into the Chosin Reservoir. The Chosin Reservoir lay at an elevation of 3,510 feet. The Chosin and neighboring Fusen Reservoirs fueled three large hydroelectric systems clustered in the mountainous eastern regions of North Korea, furnishing energy to the entire region as far away as Hungnam and including bordering parts of Manchuria. Central to this system were the Changjin and Pujon Rivers, tributaries of the Yalu. During the Japanese occupation, as early as 1927, with creation of the Fusen Reservoir, building of the Pujon River (Fusen) Power Plant was begun. In 1933, Nippon Chisso, with the support of the governor general of Korea, established the Changjin Power Plant by constructing the one-hundred-fifty-foot-high Kalchon-ni Dam across the Changjin River. Four of these vital power centers were near the Chosin Reservoir and two at the Fusen (Pujon in Korean) Reservoir.[4] But in November 1950, the Chinese learned that the power plants at the Fusen Reservoir had never been fully completed and were not operational.

Eleven miles north of Koto-ri was the village of Hagaru-ri, near the southern tip of the Chosin Reservoir. While not by any means a metropolis, it was certainly more developed than the gritty hovels of Chinhung-ri and Koto-ri. At Hagaru-ri, the road sent branches to either side of a crooked finger of reservoir, which almost kissed the town, separated by just a mile of marshland. On the east side the road, hardly wide enough for two trucks to slip by side by side, wound through wasteland bordering the reservoir overshadowed by mountains towering to eight thousand feet toward Sasu-ri, across the Paegamni-gong estuary to Hudong-ni, then bending east, rising and skirting a hill mass named Hill 1221 by the Americans. On to the Pungnyuri Inlet, frozen over in winter, the tiny roadway—hardly a cowpath by now—hugged hill masses rising on both north and south, across the Pungnyuri-gang and up into the mountainous wilds of North Korea. From there the path led to Changjin and to the Yalu.

From Hagaru-ri on the west side the roving passage ascended up through the four-thousand-seven-hundred-foot Toktong Pass and then descended through deep, dark gorges into the valley of the Munon-ni River. Steep walls of hills cradled the road as it entered the hamlet of Yudam-ni, touching the western finger of the Chosin Reservoir, situated in a broad valley ringed by menacing, distant massifs. Yudam-ni was only eight air miles from Hagaru-ri, but with all the hairpin turns, the road distance became fourteen miles. These now were mountainous regions, desolate, foreboding, frigid in winter, snow covered, barely compatible with vehicular traffic. Without the warmth of fires and shelter from subzero winds, human survival in the elements was doubtful.

The entire seventy-eight mile stretch from Hungnam to Yudam-ni—to be called the Main Supply Route, or MSR—was the only road available for movement of troops, armor, and supplies and for evacuation of casualties to the rear as Marines and soldiers advanced on the Yalu. It was a precarious path, with innumerable chokepoints, bridges, and streams, ideal for flanking enemy troops to encircle, cut off, and annihilate intruders. Bordering hills peering over the lonesome roadway were perfect locations for hiding troops and ambushes. Inhospitable terrain, tortuous access, and the weather made any attempt to roost and fortify impossible. One must either advance or retreat.

In late October, with only a hint of frost in the air, the 1st Marine Division had landed unopposed at the harbor of Wonsan on Korea's northeast coast. Wonsan was one of the best natural harbors in Korea. A hub of sorts, it offered the best natural route from Seoul over the mountains. To the north and south, Wonsan's rail system and roads connected the ports of Hamhung and Pusan. MacArthur had at first intended the Marines to wheel west from Wonsan and pinch North Koreans against the Eighth Army at Pyongyang. But Pyongyang fell on October 20. Now MacArthur aimed X Corps at the Manchurian border. From Wonsan, then, Marines would drift north toward Hungnam and Hamhung. They were to move out via the Chinhung-ni–Koto-ri–Hagaru-ri corridor, turn west, reach the Kangge–Huichon road, cut Chinese supply lines, and attack from the rear any Chinese troops threatening the Eighth Army.

By November 2, the 7th Marines, trucked from Wonsan to Hungnam, had relieved ROK forces on the Hungnam–Hamhung–Sudong road. Days later they collided with Chinese forces intent on feeling out Leathernecks in the Sudong Valley. Following a sudden, nasty little firefight, the Chinese melted away. Marines marched on to Hagaru-ri. Another change of orders (almost a daily occurrence now from MacArthur's fickle headquarters), Operation Order 20-50, issued November 9, directed the entire 1st Marine Division to shift north and congregate around the Chosin Reservoir. From there, Marines would push farther north to Yudam-ni and beyond. The 5th Marines set out for Hamhung and were slated to relieve ROK forces to the east of the Chosin Reservoir, and Colonel "Chesty" Puller's 1st Marines were given the ignoble duty of patrolling the rear areas of the Hamhung–Chinhung-ni corridor. By November 10, in subzero weather, the 7th Marines reached Koto-ri with no opposition, and by November 14 they were in Hagaru-ri. By that time the 5th Marines had reached Koto-ri, and the 1st Marines impatiently stomped around the Chigyong–Hamhung area. Once Colonel Ray Murray's 5th Marines entered Hagaru-ri they were to turn right and bolster the eastern flank of the Chosin Reservoir. The 7th Marines were marched north, past Hagaru-ri, on toward Yudam-ni. A few days later, Puller's 1st Marines packed up and moved up the Sudong corridor just south of Hagaru-ri, bringing up the rear guard. By then all 5th Marine battalions were east of the reservoir.

Then new orders appeared on November 25 issued by Lieutenant General Edward "Ned" Almond as X Corps Commander, implementing MacArthur's general operation plans. According to Almond's Operational Order No. 7, the 1st Marine Division was to advance north and westward, seize Mupyong-ni, and advance "to YALU River, and destroy En in Z [enemy in zone]."[5] In detail, the 5th Marines were marched back to Hagaru-ri and told to back up the 7th Marines attacking up toward Yudam-ni. In their place would be a thrown together a Regimental Combat Team of 7th Division soldiers. The 7th Division commander, General David Barr, put Colonel Allan MacLean in charge of two battalions of the 31st Infantry, a battalion of the 32nd Infantry, a tank company and field artillery, and antiaircraft batteries. By early afternoon, November 27, many of MacLean's troops were in place, and the Marines pulled out to Hagaru-ri. "Team MacLean," as it would later be called, had barely arrived, strung out, poorly organized, and more or less sitting ducks. Their days of infamy would soon begin.[6]

So, on November 27, the jumping-off date for Almond's final push to the Yalu, the 7th Marines were in Yudam-ni, the 5th Marines strung out behind them, moving forward to attack west of Yudam-ni, and the 1st Marines patrolling Hagaru-ri to Koto-ri. Only one battalion of the

1st Marines was garrisoned at Hagaru-ri itself, a critical supply point for movements north and west. Little did they know, divisions of Chinese troops were all around them, hidden in those Korean hills. The trap was in place.

THE 1ST MEDICAL BATTALION of the 1st Marine Division[7]—all five companies—had completed unloading hospital equipment and medical supplies at Wonsan by October 31.[8] With the redirection of the Marines to the Hungnam–Hamhung area, Companies A, C, and E were hurried from Wonsan to Hungnam. Company A, the division hospital, deployed just west of the town in what had been a civilian hospital, supposedly reserved for the army. But once the navy and Marines moved in, there was little choice but to let them have it, especially after that wicked skirmish near Sudong and Chinhung-ni. In twenty-four hours, the hospital admitted 261 patients. And before long, 450 beds were full of Leathernecks. Companies C and E, assigned to support the 5th and 7th Marines, moved up to Hamhung. Men of Company C found a small building with chopped-up rooms—not great for a hospital but all there was. The men of Company E fared better. They rummaged through a modern, two-story building to set up their clinics and surgical spaces. With rooms for triage, emergency treatment, and operating, the area looked more like a mobile surgical hospital than a sick call infirmary. After the 7th Marines clashed with Chinese on November 6, a detachment of Company E under Lieutenant Commander Charles "Ken" Holloway was dispatched to Chinhung-ni as a forward surgical team. With no heated modern buildings there, they holed up in pyramidal tents and foxholes.

Companies B and D stayed at Wonsan. The 1st Marines were still there. A bunker near the airport holding thirty cots was their hospital; for surgery there was a parked trailer nearby. At least there was quick access to the beach, and not far off shore the USS *Consolation*. After several days, when the 1st Marines moved over to Hungnam, Company B up and left its tiny bunker fighting North Korean ambushes the whole way. Company D moved to near Hamhung by the middle of November.

Navy doctor Ken Holloway was more a Marine than a sailor. The thirty-one-year-old had graduated from the University of Texas, served as a destroyer medical officer during World War II, and completed one year of a surgery residency at the Virginia Mason Clinic in Seattle, Washington. Forced into a more lucrative general practice, he bored quickly and jumped at the chance to rejoin the navy in 1949 to complete his surgery training. On July 1, 1950, while he was finishing a hernia repair, an operating room technician poked his head in the door and read the order for Lieutenant Commander Holloway to "proceed immediately" to Camp Pendleton, California, and the 1st Marine Provisional Brigade. A little over one month later, on August 7, he walked off the USS *Pickaway* (APA 222) onto the docks of Pusan, South Korea. In Holloway's unit, Medical Company C, or "Charlie Med," were three orthopedic surgeons, two general surgeons, two internists, two dentists, and a number of corpsmen. "It was a very mobile unit," he wrote, "generally located a few miles from the front lines, and equipped to offer major surgery to casualties who could not be safely evacuated without treatment."[9] During action around the Pusan Perimeter, he worked with surgeons of Lieutenant Colonel Kryder Van Buskirk's 8076th Mobile Army Surgical Hospital (MASH)[10] in the village of Miryang, beefing up his surgical acumen. All in good time, his "Gyrenes" landed at Inchon in September, and Holloway saw over a thousand casualties over the next several days.

By the time of the Wonsan landings, Holloway was in command of Company E—Easy Med. And now he headed up a small detachment of doctors to be sent with the 7th Marines as they struggled up the MSR into mountains around the Chosin Reservoir. Section I it would be called. Emergency surgery was the role, right behind front-line Marines. Already in those pyramidal tents not far from Chinhung-ni, he and his men had treated over a hundred badly wounded Marines and shipped many back to Hamhung. Some were even operated on in a special surgical trailer, cramped and close but sufficient for minor wounds. Most then left by truck or cracker-box ambulance, a few by helicopter, heads and feet sticking out the sides.

Like so many Korea-era surgeons, James Stewart had been intent on learning his surgical profession as a resident at the Touro Infirmary in New Orleans. It was August 1950. For men like Stewart, the navy was an irresistible source of supplemental financial support for the meager salaries of postgraduate programs.[11] He was now four years into his training, one of internship, one of pathology, and now two of surgery. That was when all went south. He received orders for activation and deployment—now. His limp appeal fell on deaf ears. It was time to pay the piper for those cushy monthly supplements. One month later, Lieutenant Stewart was wading ashore at Inchon with the 1st Medical Battalion, E Company, looking for "782" (combat) gear and a weapon—all strange stuff, as he had no basic training, no indoctrination, nothing.[12] Onboard a ship to Wonsan, he met Lieutenant Peter Arioli, who, after some perfunctory checking, anointed Stewart an "official" navy surgeon.

Now at Hungnam, he was in even deeper, picked for Section I, Ken Holloway's forward surgical team. The boy from New Orleans busied himself with digging latrines and foxholes and working in that "deluxe" surgical trailer. Instead of Dixieland, the sounds of recoilless rifles and hand grenades rang in his ears. Action around Chinhung-ni had been an eye opener all right, for everyone. Stewart had a line of injuries waiting but could fit only one at a time in his trailer. Corpsman William Davis, 1st Battalion, 7th Marines, was stunned by those first few days of combat. "We'd had firefights and casualties before but we never had anything like this before," he recalled. Bad wounds were especially disturbing; there was so little that could be done in the field. Davis remembered one platoon sergeant hit in his midsection:

> He was lying on the deck and I went over to him. All I could get was a thread pulse. He was bleeding and I put bandages on him but I didn't think he was going to make it down off that hill. . . . I wrote . . . on his little toe tag that he was KIA.[13]

Staff Sergeant Archie van Winkle in fact survived the chest wound and a shattered arm he suffered while rallying his men to fight off the Chinese. His Medal of Honor citation said that though he was bleeding heavily, van Winkle ignored his own plight for the sake of other Marines.

On November 14, Section I was on the move again, up into the mountains, first to Toksu-bong and then up past Koto-ri to Hagaru-ri. Stewart's surgical trailer was left behind; the path up Funchilin Pass was simply too narrow. In Hagaru-ri, Holloway found a single-story building that once served as the city hall for a population of five thousand. Now walls and ceiling needed to be repaired—there was a large bomb hole in the roof—but there was little time for that. Hospital supplies were moved in. Staff partitioned the large central room into an admitting space for exam and triage, a ward space big enough for almost one hundred patients stacked in double- and triple-decker wood frames, and an operating area for major (one table) and minor (three tables) cases. Stewart remembered, "The engineers built a rack to hold a standard stretcher. That served as the operating table for major surgery."[14] Customary procedure was to strip all incoming casualties of weapons, ammunition, and field gear (except sleeping bags and parkas) in the admitting area. Every-

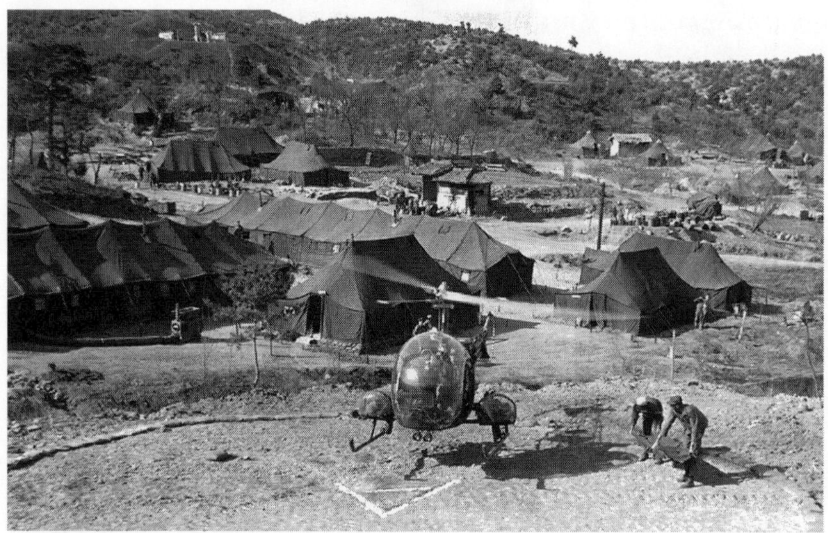

An evacuation helicopter of Marine Observation Squadron 6, carrying wounded Marines from the front lines lands at "A" Medical Company of the 1st Marine Division in 1950. Naval corpsmen stand by with stretchers to unload the wounded men from the helicopter pods and rush them to the operating and hospital tents in the background. (*National Archives*)

one was examined—especially their armpits, groins, and backs. Of course, there was no radiology or laboratory equipment. Diagnosis and treatment were based on examination only. Those in shock were first priority. Their immediate destination was the operating room—more convenient for resuscitation: handy surgical equipment and easier to keep warm. At first, any serious injury, including chest and abdominal trauma, was sent back to the division hospital. Before long, inclement weather and roaming Chinese troops forced immediate surgery. On November 22, help arrived. Company C, headed by Commander Hal Streit, set up its hospital in a schoolhouse just outside of town, another dilapidated building that was weather proofed as much as possible. First casualties arrived on November 26. More snow fell. Temperatures plummeted.

The Korean winter was setting in. By late November, it turned bitterly cold. And in Koto-ri, Hagaru-ri, and Yudam-ni, arctic blasts hit with brutal suddenness. Few were prepared. Colonel Homer Litzenberg, commander of the 7th Marines, wrote: "The doctors reported numerous cases where the men came down to the sickbay suffering from what appeared to be shock. Some of them would come in crying; some of them were extremely nervous; and the doctors said it was simply the sudden shock of the terrific cold when they were not ready for it."[15]

Battalion surgeon Lieutenant Edward Byrne was baffled by the reaction of his Marines: "I noticed when we first moved up on the plateau [Koto-ri] and met . . . our first intense cold that there was a shock reaction among many of our men . . . in a condition similar to what you would see of men under terrific mortar or artillery barrage. There was a marked tremor . . . and in some cases, there was a marked suppression of the respiratory rate."[16]

Frigid temperatures seemed to numb inside as well as out, as if the senses slowed in response. Not everyone had been issued winter wear. For those who had, clothing was layered: skivvies, long underwear, green shirt and trousers, sweatshirt, cold-weather pants, and finally a parka topped with a fur-lined cap and earflaps. Helmets went over that. For hands there were wool glove liners and then thick canvas mittens with a separate trigger finger. Boots were shoepacs—some called them "Mickey Mouse boots": uninsulated rubber on the bottom and leather on top. They came up to the ankles. Half-inch flat felt inserts and socks were worn inside. With subzero temperatures, the problem was that socks absorbed sweat, and sweat turned to ice. And ice froze to skin. Even bundled up, it was hard to stay warm. Dentist Morton Silver with the 5th Marines remembered: "The frigid winds from Manchuria ate into our flesh and froze any parts of our anatomy exposed for a few moments. We tried to erect warm-up tents, but were frustrated by the rock-hard frozen ground. Wooden tent pegs were useless."[17]

Med Company D had moved from Wonsan to Chigyong, following the 1st Marines, and was settled in at Koto-ri by November 25. No buildings in this rickety town were large enough for the company, so up went tents. By then the ground was frozen to a depth of twelve to eighteen inches, and rail spikes and iron bars were necessary to pound into the earth to support canvas. Lieutenant Commander Gustare Anderson, the commanding officer, remarked, "A steady fall of snow, empty stomachs and tingling feet spurred cold, clumsy hands on to greater speed." Within two hours, pyramidal tents and roaring stoves were in place for shelter and warmth. That got the men through a bitterly cold night. The next day, four additional tents were hammered in as the hospital. One was a receiving tent, another a minor surgery tent, a third a supply tent, and a fourth a ward tent. "It is remarkable," Dr. Anderson said, "how sub-freezing temperatures can retard operations, especially when working in tents.

Even normal activities such as dressing and personal hygiene became tedious procedures." It seemed everything froze—blood froze and hemolyzed, plasma froze, normal saline solutions froze. Stoves were fired twenty-four hours a day in hopes of keeping blood from freezing. During surgery, fires continued despite the use of flammable anesthetics. It was just too cold to operate without heat.[18]

Men of Holloway's Section I waged a losing battle with the cold. Rations were frozen, the water trailer froze, medications froze, plasma iced. Favorite meals became slices of bread. They were heated on a wire rack on top of the gas stoves and made into toast. For Thanksgiving dinner, turkey and all the fixings were served on stainless steel trays. Men stationed outside had to eat fast or the food would shortly be frozen to metal. Yet Sunday, November 26, dawned to a clear-blue sky, and the temperature reached almost 12 degrees Fahrenheit. "Everything was quiet and peaceful," Holloway recalled. He walked back to his quarters, took a shower, and put on clean clothes. "I felt just fine."[19]

Robert Shoemaker's one-year rotating internship at Saint Luke's Hospital in Cleveland ended June 25, 1950. He was part of the navy's V-12 program, designed to corral a cadre of professionals like doctors for wartime activities. The extra money earned by his ensign's commission allowed him to get married during an impoverished internship. The newlyweds were bound for the San Diego Naval Hospital for two years of cozy duty. But Korea changed all that. Instead it was on to Camp Pendleton by August to join the Marines as surgeon for the 3rd Battalion, 11th Marine Regiment (artillery). On September 1, he was onboard the USS *Okanogan* steaming across the Pacific. Three weeks later he was at Inchon, and by Halloween he was on his way up the MSR side by side with towed howitzers. Brown rice paddies, scrubby pine trees, and gawking, passive peasants were the only scenery; farther up mountains like the Rockies, poplars, pines, and bushes on hillsides. Here and there were terraced rice fields. By Hagaru-ri, he was bundled tight in cotton underwear, long johns, wool socks, a wool sweater, windproof trousers, wool mittens, ski mittens, a parka, and the soon-to-be-notorious shoepacs. The air was crisp but strangely quiet, as if on purpose sound had ceased, awaiting a cacophonous overture: "At night the moon shining on the treeless snow-covered mountains gave an eerie light that was foreboding. What was going to happen? We all had unanswered questions. Would the Chinese mount a large-scale attack? It was so cold the snow would crunch underfoot and the wind was biting."[20]

Lieutenant Shoemaker picked a simple farmhouse as his aid station, not far from Company E's surgical detachment. And the routine of sick call began. Dysentery crept in, that diarrhea of newcomers susceptible to indigenous bacilli. It was far worse in the cold. The misery of crawling out of warm, sleeping bag cocoons to defecate in temperatures below zero, liquid stool freezing even before it hit the ground, and the inability to wipe with flimsy toilet paper, became a true loathing. Soon, though, that would be a distant irritation. It was November 28. The Chinese Second Phase Campaign was about to begin.

On November 25, General Ned Almond issued his Operational Order No. 7. Marines would drive through Yudam-ni, head for Mupyong-ni, and bolt forward to the mouth of the Tumen River at the Soviet border. MacArthur exuded confidence, blissfully unaware of—or unconcerned with—the Chinese in waiting. The jump-off date was set for November 27.

19

The Descent

On November 26, captured Chinese soldiers claimed there were up to six Chinese divisions in the Yudam-ni area. Yet X Corps and First Marine Division Headquarters continued to be fatally optimistic. Chinese units were withdrawing, commanders insisted. And if they decided to fight, they would shortly be crushed by blistering American firepower. No doubt the drubbing American forces took at the onset of the war escaped their memory. The advance to the Yalu would start without delay.

On a frigid November 27 morning, elements of the 5th and 7th Marines began their attack west of Yudam-ni. Resistance stiffened, and by nightfall gains were modest at best. The Marines settled into an otherwise quiet night, dispersed in the hills around Yudam-ni, and two rifle companies, Charlie and Fox, were strung out on the fourteen-mile road from Yudam-ni to Hagaru-ri, guarding the only link rearward, the vital MSR. By 6:30 PM, Yudam-ni was pitch black. The temperature was already minus 20 degrees Fahrenheit. In darkness, three divisions of Chinese troops had spread out in front of the Marine perimeter. At half past nine, mortar fire erupted, bugles sounded, and whistles screeched. Swarms of Chinese communists in their mustard-colored uniforms and rubber sandals rushed Marine positions. Human waves, some would call them—more accurately, groups of fifty or more—seeming like a sea of humanity. Marine .50 caliber machine guns chattered red hot, pivoting back and forth, dropping Chinese troops. Garands cracked, grenades flew, mortars thumped. But they kept coming. And Marines fell.

In the early hours of November 28, casualties filtered into aid stations, young Gyrenes teeth chattering, pale as ghosts, maroon splotches on olive drab. Doctors worked on them in medical tents way too close. The Chinese were almost at their doorstep. Commanders hurriedly pulled the aid stations back; bulldozers used to dig howitzer positions were turned loose to sink new aid stations. Up and down the MSR Chinese came. Charlie and Fox Companies caught it bad. Charlie Company made it back to Yudam-ni. Air strikes helped, lacing the hilltops with napalm. Fox Company, holed up at Toktong Pass, was not so lucky. Cut off, surrounded, the men were on their own. A relief column from Yudam-ni tried to reach them the next morning but was stopped cold not more than three hundred yards from the Marine perimeter. Even Corsairs from Marine air squadrons failed to break the Chinese hold. Pilots saw the enemy dug in, dotting the landscape, stalking their cornered prey. There was no help for Fox Company this day.

At Yudam-ni, Tuesday morning brought an unexpected quiet. The Chinese had drifted off, no doubt licking their wounds. But they were out there, all around. It was no stretch to realize the Marines were surrounded, isolated. Doctors tallied 29 men killed, 119 wounded.[1] A number were badly hurt and in trouble. They were kept inside tents. The less serious cases—numbering at least one hundred—were laid side by side outside on beds of straw and covered with tarpaulins. Some of the wounded even worked keeping the stoves stoked inside tents. Chester Lessenden, in civilian life a dermatologist from Topeka, Kansas, was a 5th Marine Battalion surgeon. His was one of those aid stations that moved during the night after rounds punched through the tents. Now he looked over his grizzly audience of prostrate patients. Some had that vacant stare of the afflicted, wanting not rescue or reprieve, just relief. Others were painted with the gray of approaching death. And everyone shivered. Lessenden recalled later: "Everything was frozen. . . . Plasma froze and the bottles broke. We couldn't use plasma because it wouldn't go into solution and the tubes would clog up with particles. We couldn't change dressings because we had to work with gloves on to keep our hands from freezing."[2]

It was so cold that he was reluctant to cut away clothing for fear of causing deeper hypothermia that would compound the danger of any serious injury. Safer to leave them stuffed in their sleeping bags. "Actually a man was better off if we left him alone," Lessenden observed. His assistant surgeon, Brooklyn dentist Morton Silver, took any wound from

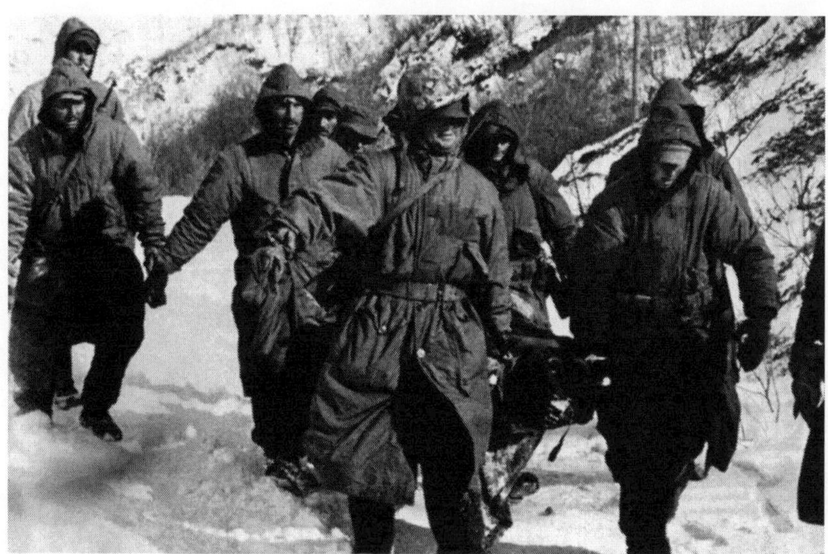

A wounded Marine being carried by stretcher to an aid station. (*National Archives*)

the neck up—including brain injuries. "The truth of the matter was they weren't dead, but they were just as good as dead," he told an interviewer years later. "It was just horrendous to see this. You did the best you could."[3] A "penicillin brigade" was formed, and three hundred thousand units of penicillin were given to anyone with an open wound. Chest holes were plugged, bleeding stopped—sometimes. Not much else to do. Evacuate? One ambulance tried to make it to Hagaru-ri. No luck. The driver, his wounded, and the bullet-riddled ambulance were back in thirty minutes. The Chinese were everywhere. The injured would have to mingle with the dead.

By morning, Bob Shoemaker's aid station with the 11th Marines was one lone pyramidal tent packed with wounded. The bare frozen dirt floor was covered with brown bundles of misery. He and his four corpsmen worked alone on their charges, Lessenden and the others a mile away. One measly stove, the only source of heat, burned out after some idiot ran off with the heating fuel. During that first night, Shoemaker counted seventy wounded brought in, most the victims of small-arms fire. He had no tables and no light. On hands and knees, in pitch black, he went from casualty to casualty. "Much of the specifics of what went on that night are lost to me by a state of confusion related to the sheer numbers of wounded," Shoemaker divulged. Survival was beyond his control. It was disgusting, what little could be done. "The situation was, and still is, a heavy burden to bear."[4] He worked bare handed, sterile gloves unavailable. One clogged airway was opened not with a tracheostomy tube but an improvised wire "C" clamp, cutting through neck tissues with only a local anesthetic. That crazy clamp was strong enough to keep tracheal cartilage apart, a life-saving effort. But for others, the night was their last. By morning, the odor of death and stale blood was strong. One sergeant, wounded by a sniper's bullet, commented that the tent "reeked with the rank odor of an abattoir."[5]

At Hagaru-ri, enemy units attacked from the south and north Tuesday night, November 28, around a four-mile perimeter thinly held by Marines. Yet action at Yudam-ni the day before had put all on alert, and the Marines hunkered down in tight defensive postures. With the rush of a Chinese charge, automatic fire brought them down—in droves. By daybreak it was over. Marine lines had held. In front of them seven hundred enemy bodies, some piled four or five high, were counted. Lieutenant Robert Fleischaker was battalion surgeon for the 1st Marines and right in the middle of it. Among the crop of new Korean-era doctors, he had been called up from training at the naval hospital in Chelsea, Massachusetts, in July. Fleischaker; an even greener assistant surgeon, Dr. George Farrell, fresh from internship; and ten corpsmen were running the battalion's aid station. Korea was the first deployment for either of the two doctors. But the Inchon landings and battles around Seoul had acclimatized them. Now bona fide veterans, they had traversed Funchilin Pass layered in winter gear and arrived at Hagaru-ri on November 27. "A collection of rough wood buildings and mud huts," recalled Fleischaker. In typical military style, though, a suburbia of tents had been added, including Fleischaker's aid station.

During the attacks on the night of November 28–29, Fleischaker and Farrell saw a steady stream of casualties. Even though temperatures reached subzero, plasma and saline somehow stayed thawed—a good thing, as there was plenty of use for it. All during the night, wounded were carried in, and before long, every space in every tent was filled. From one patient to another, surgeons tore open clothing, checked injuries, stopped bleeding, splinted limbs, and gave morphine. Corpsmen busied themselves with intravenous needles and plasma. "It was midafternoon of 29 November before bleary eyed doctors and corpsmen could wash the blood off themselves, and interrupt work for a bite to eat," Fleischaker remembered. He and Farrell had been so occupied during the night that they were not aware of the bullet holes piercing their tent that daylight revealed.[6]

For a few days, Lieutenant Stewart and Section I at Hagaru-ri had been treating 7th Marines casualties as they trudged to Yudam-ni. Many were simple frostbite cases. But the night of November 28 was different. Hagaru-ri was under attack, and wounded poured in. At first, Stewart was absolutely mesmerized by the numbers and found himself lingering pointlessly among litters, worrying on priorities. Then suddenly, an epiphany: this was "mass casualty," and economy of effort was imperative, teamwork a must: "I found myself initially wandering amongst the wounded, doing quick evaluations, trying to read the entries on the attached casualty tags . . . then moving on to the next. A terrible waste of time, accomplishing little! I soon found it more efficient to leave the triage to the other docs . . . and to proceed to render care quickly to anyone who needed my level of care."

Stewart belonged in the operating room. Patients were brought to him, those badly wounded with near-fatal injuries. Corpsmen took care of more minor cases: lacerations, fractures, and frostbite. It proved a memorable night. Small-arms fire smacked against Stewart's building as he labored over one abdominal case after another, "patching or excising or bypassing damaged intestines." A Marine was carried in blue—cyanotic—from a sucking chest wound, gasping, close to cardiac arrest. Frozen clothes were peeled away, and Stewart slammed in a chest tube. With that and a little warming, the boy pinked up, began breathing, and gave a grin—snatched from death. Little did Stewart know—the bullet smacks now merely background noise—but Chinese gunmen came within yards of his hospital until a group of British Royal Marines drove them back over a hill. For Stewart's small detachment, one day rolled into night into the next day. There was always another case to do, another bleeding body to fix. How could he keep them all straight? Well, someone did. Seventeen major operations in ten days was the grand total. Standing room only was how Ken Holloway remembered it. Over one hundred beds filled. "We were trapped with no way to get in or out of our little enclave," he wrote.[7] There was no easy day at C Med either. Too many shattered boys to count. Fortunately, anticipating a bloodbath, on November 28, a surgical team with Commander Byron Bassham and Commander D. M. Pino of A Med were choppered in to help save shot up and half-frozen American troops.[8]

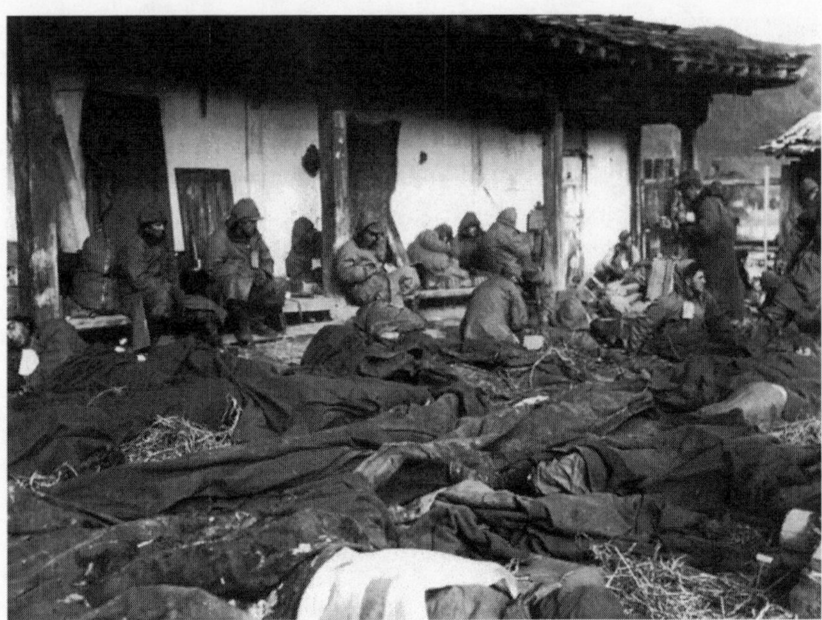

Wounded Marines waiting for evacuation at Yudam-ni. Some would be taken by helicopter, but the majority were trucked out during the breakout to Hagaru-ri. (*National Archives*)

Back at Yudam-ni, November 30 saw more wounded. Aid stations were consolidated—tents taken down, put back up. Almost six hundred casualties were moved. The rows of damaged humanity steadily grew. So many would not be saved. Henry Litvin, battalion surgeon for the 5th Marines, recalled one poor officer with a bullet hole in the side of his helmet, breathing but not conscious. "I removed his helmet and his brains spilled out like oatmeal onto the snow. . . . I remember putting the helmet back and saying 'Move him over there.'" He was dead by morning.[9] And Marines wondered when it would end. Could they hold out? For doctors, tending the wounded was therapeutic. There was nowhere to hide anyway, the ground so frozen foxholes were impossible. Litvin credibly summed it up: "No matter how scared I was, and believe me, I was scared, when you did your job you weren't helpless. . . . I didn't sit there like a shaking lump of jelly. Work was a great thing for the doc—it overcame his terror."[10]

Nighttime produced a special brand of terror: a favorite time for Chinese attacks. Aware of their predicament, doctors worked by flashlight;

anything stronger would draw fire. And their tents were well within range. "The unwelcome darkness fell upon us like a lethal cloud," Morton Silver wrote.[11] He had his sidearm—they all did—but it would hardly be enough if the Marines gave way.

Marine Observation Squadron Six, called VMO-6, flew single-engine OY-2 Sentinels and Sikorsky HO3S-1 helicopters. Their mission: aerial reconnaissance, search and rescue, and medical evacuation. For medical transport, the Sentinels could carry only one patient, but modified Sikorskys held up to three litters. A durable craft, the helicopter was powerful, stable in the air, and required little maintenance. By November 28, anticipating trouble with General Ollie Smith's Chosin-based offensive, Sentinels and Sikorskys were put on the rough tarmac at Hagaru-ri. Once the Chinese opened up on Marines at Yudam-ni, helicopter flights commenced immediately, resupplying the garrison and evacuating the wounded. There was even a Sentinel landing on December 1, jeep lights used to illuminate the Yudam-ni airstrip. Over four days, from November 27 to December 1, fearless pilots choppered 109 badly wounded Leathernecks out. Not a few Sikorskys were clipped by small-arms fire in the process.[12] One was brought down near Toktong Pass trying to rescue a critically wounded Marine on December 3, killing the pilot, New Jersey native, twenty-seven-year-old Lieutenant Robert Longstaff.[13]

"The weather conditions presented the most cruel of all the problems we faced," wrote Ken Holloway. "The cold bore down relentlessly. It reduced efficiency. It numbed our thinking and judgment. It inflicted crippling frostbite on many thousands who did not have adequate protection." Horrible frostbite it was, mostly feet. Shoepacs and sweat had iced socks to feet and toes—literally frozen to their boots. Change socks? That was laughable. Chinese marauders were keen on any above ground activity. Gyrenes were stuck in foxholes and bunkers for hours and days. When boots were finally removed, doctors had to dissect wool from blistered flesh. Soles of feet were raw meat. Gray-white tissue underneath meant dead tissue, maybe amputation. Warming was the only hope. Inside, ten stoves blasted continuously. Now eighty-octane gasoline for fuel; heating oil had frozen too. Yet even then, the temperature barely rose above freezing. One benefit of the frigid weather: seldom were patients hemorrhaging when brought in. Wounds were frozen. Few had ever seen that: pink, coagulated blood over bullet holes—the perfect hemostatic plug. Some likened it to a bouquet of rosy cotton candy.[14] But with warming, watch out: blood thawed and bleeding started.[15]

On its summit at Toktong Pass, Fox Company herded fifty-four wounded together. For shelter, two tents were propped against the hillside. There were no doctors, only corpsmen—but damn good ones. No matter. There was little to do but change dressings (by candlelight), bundle sleeping bags for warmth—with men stacked side by side—C rations, and morphine syrettes. Of course, morphine froze in syrettes. Before injection, corpsmen thawed them in their mouths. Plasma was worthless, frozen solid. Men died for lack of it, simply bled out and died. Nothing could be done. Thank God for those helicopters, though. Pilots got through, dropping food, medicine, and ammunition and taking a few critical boys out. Forty-three wounded Marines were airlifted in brazen sorties by the ungainly Sikorskys of VMO-6.[16]

General Smith sensed disaster. His Gyrenes were tough, but cut off the MSR and, sooner or later, men would wither. There had to be relief—and a way out. The MSR was crawling with the enemy. Nothing was getting through to Hagaru-ri. And Koto-ri looked like one big parking lot: trucks, men, and supplies jammed up, needing to get to Hagaru-ri. The road had to be opened. Smith gave the task to Chesty Puller and his 1st Marines. Colonel Puller put together a hodgepodge group—British commandos, some of his 1st Marines, and armor—under the command of a rugged, seasoned Brit, Colonel Douglas Drysdale—some 900 men, 141 vehicles, and 29 tanks. Task Force Drysdale it would be called. They would barrel through and clean out the Chinese. Jump off was the morning of November 29. It was a disaster; slow going on the MSR—a rutted, narrow roadway—and a well-placed Chinese ambush saw to that. In a spot called Hell Fire Valley, the column was chopped into three pieces by the enemy. The forward section fought on to Hagaru-ri, the rear section stumbled back to Koto-ri, and the middle section was almost annihilated, with the Chinese capturing most left alive. A few hid out and somehow made it back. Final register: 162 killed or missing and 321 wounded—over 50 percent casualties. Med Company D at Koto-ri was ready. Dozens of wounded from Task Force Drysdale and Hell Fire Valley arrived later that day.

At Yudam-ni, things had been quiet for two nights. But the Marines were outnumbered and outflanked. The weather was brutal, dead were unburied, and wounded were everywhere. It would be foolish to push ahead, but equally stupid to stay put. Marines were not squatters, they were movers, and by God they were going to move somewhere. Back down the MSR to Hagaru-ri seemed a good idea. Plans were made. One

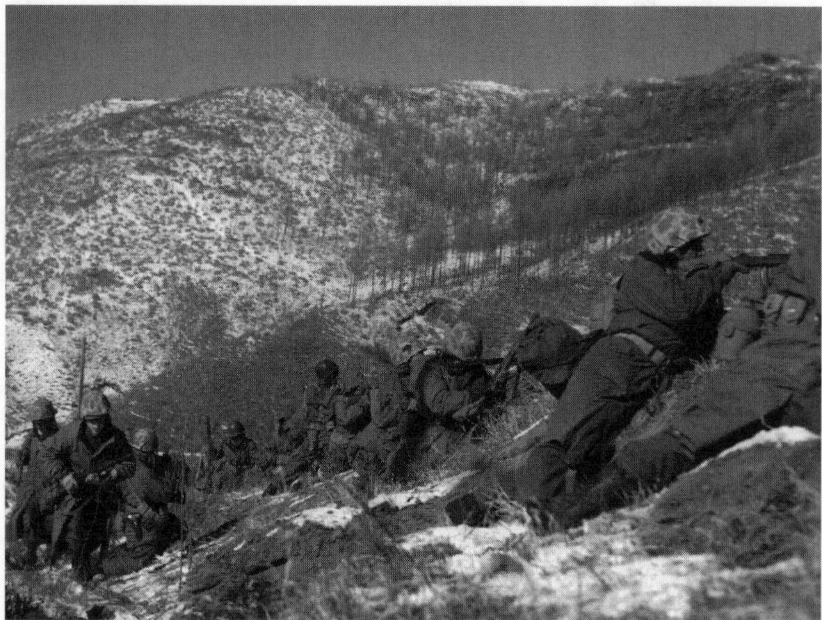

The role of Marine rifle companies during the breakout to Hagaru-ri was to take the high ground on both sides of the MSR in order to keep the Chinese from overwhelming the American convoys. (*National Archives*)

battalion would set off across the mountains to outflank the flanking Chinese and rescue Fox Company. A motor convoy would then leave Yudam-ni loaded with serious casualties, big guns, and a lone Pershing tank. Anyone who could walk and carry a gun would flank the column, spreading out over the surrounding hills. The dead would be left—eighty-five frozen corpses buried in scratched-out graves and covered with frozen clods of dirt. There was simply no place for them in the convoy.

Early morning December 1, the Marines set out. More than 850 wounded packed every available truck and jeep, some even strapped to the hoods of vehicles. Gyrenes combed the hills, driving off Chinese soldiers eager to ambush. At a creeping pace, the column inched along. Like some morbid holiday parade, others crowded Yudam-ni, waiting for their place in line. Dr. Lessenden dawdled all afternoon and night to begin the journey. "[P]oor kids lying on litters on trucks and trailers and we didn't have enough stuff to keep them warm," he later wrote his father. In fact, none of his patients moved until the next day.[17] As the column snaked its way toward Hagaru-ri, doctors and corpsmen walked up and down, checking the wounded. Mostly it was a matter of keeping them warm. Christ, it was cold. Cold enough to freeze the balls off a brass monkey, Leathernecks said. And headway was agonizing. Every so often the column stopped. Shooting started as Marines cleared another roadblock, beat off another ambush. A few hundred yards and the whole process repeated. While trucks idled, anyone on foot warmed his hands on exhaust pipes, pounded his feet, and clapped his arms. There was little water available—all was frozen—and almost no food. "Eating snow does not go very far to relieve thirst," one doctor commented. That first day, snow fell and too soon the sun set. And sure enough, here came the berserk Chinese, lighting up the road with star shells and bugling suicidal charges. Marines raced out to meet them, guns blazing. Doctors watched, hovering over their patients, amazed at the unadulterated, cold-blooded courage of these men.

And the wounded? They were swathed in layers of wool and fleece and parkas but their faces were gray and ghastly as if all their suffering had condensed on this one feature to tell those who passed them that misery dwelt within, the struggles of pain and life. Fourteen miles it would be to Hagaru-ri. Each mile stained with blood and the slow dribble of human existence.

Peter Arioli emigrated from Milan, Italy, to the United States at the turn of the century. An engineer, he built a thriving business in, of all places, Hilo, Hawaii Territory—on the Big Island. There he met and wed local socialite—almost royalty—Edith "Queenie" Laakaumokuakama Sharrat in 1915. A year later Peter Jr. was born, the first of four siblings. Theirs was the good life, a life on the water, fishing, boating, the family's forty-foot auxiliary bugeye the envy of the social set. Peter Sr. sometimes even sailed family to the mainland. Peter Jr. was gifted, a standout at Hilo High School, so much so that he was recruited to Harvard University. Crimsons boasted an international flavor, attracting students from "the far-flung corners of the earth." Peter was quite the hit, dazzling Ivy Leaguers by breaking freshman swimming records in the first meet of his life. "Swimming in the islands comes as second nature to the youngsters," the *Harvard Crimson* speculated, noting that Peter probably took to water by splashing with "the natives."[18] He anchored the varsity team. After graduation, young Peter headed for medical school at Northwestern University. Then an internship at the Mare Island Navy Hospital in Vallejo, California, in 1944. As a patriotic gesture—many of his classmates did the same—he joined the navy reserves in 1942. After an internship he served with the 3rd Marine Division after an internship toward the end of World War II. Then it was residency back home at the Kuakini Medical Center in orthopedic surgery.[19] And now, called up for the Korean crisis, Peter was back, a regimental surgeon for the 7th Marines. He did not look the part; his slender frame conveyed a meekness, but it hid an athletic energy. At Yudam-ni, Arioli got word of the planned rescue mission for Fox Company. The 1st Battalion's surgeon was out of action; there were sure to be casualties. Arioli approached the commander, Lieutenant Colonel Ray Davis, and volunteered to go. Hardened veterans were skeptical. Arioli was too soft some thought, slight of build, quiet, shy. He would never make it, they figured.

But off they went, Arioli and five hundred Marines, a procession that extended half a mile, trudging through knee-deep snow up and down mountainsides in pitch black. The wind, especially on ridge lines, was bitter, the footing icy, treacherous. An anaesthetized indifference crept into the men, almost putting them dangerously off course. The morning of December 2, the Marines found the Chinese encircling Fox Company's hill. A brisk gunfight drove them off but dropped some Marines. The dead were buried in the snow, the wounded loaded onto stretchers and canvas fold-up litters and taken along. Arioli was there for the usual first aid: bandaging, splinting, giving morphine, things any medic could do, but there were precious few available. Finally, by midday, the Marines broke through and hooked up with the Fox survivors. Arioli and Able Company, forming the rear guard with twenty-two litter patients, arrived later that afternoon. The wounded were put in the two aid tents with Fox casualties, totaling well over one hundred. Arioli spent the night working on the wounded. Fox's casualties had received little care; some had only Scotch tape covering their wounds. One had monstrous wounds to both legs. He desperately needed out, but the doctor knew that would not happen. The next day, December 3, Peter Arioli finished his rounds, exited one of the tents, and approached Colonel Davis. It was ill timed. Just as he started to speak, a sniper's bullet smacked into his brainstem, dropping him instantly. There was no doubt of the outcome. A corpsman pronounced Arioli dead on the spot. Suddenness of death in combat shocks even hardened warriors. A gentle and compassionate figure had been taken. With respect, but also burdened by practicality, Lieutenant Peter Emilio Arioli Jr.'s body was added to the stack of frozen American dead to be left on Fox Hill. His remains were never recovered.

JUST AS MARINES WERE PREPARING to leave Yudam-ni, Hagaru-ri took a particularly vicious beating. Darkness on November 30 found Chinese overrunning a bridge close to town and lobbing mortar rounds on the hospital. Swarms of enemy seized East Hill, a commanding rise, and threatened to overtake tent settlements. Marine band members, truck drivers, and cooks rose to the occasion, grabbed rifles, and, with the help of a few Brits, shoved them back, but not without casualties. For C and E Med, it was a full house. Blackout made care even harder, almost by touch alone. By morning, E Med had five hundred wounded, and there were more over at C Med near the perimeter—"as many as 400 patients at one time [were crowded] into every available space in all the buildings."[20] And more were coming, army stragglers in horrible shape from east of the reservoir. Tents were confiscated from Marine housing for more space, and the airstrip was finally finished that day. The first two C-47 transports landed on a two-thousand-nine-hundred-foot runway scraped away by engineers. More flights landed later, bringing out 209 banged-up Marines bound for Hungnam, its hospitals now a safety valve for overburdened medical staffs. In two more days, the runway was lengthened to three thousand feet, and over four hundred more casualties were removed—army and Marine—including sixty cadavers, and over a thousand the day after that.[21] At the same time, transports flew in five hundred sorely needed Marine replacements for the icy trip to Koto-ri.

On December 3, forward elements of Yudam-ni Marines reached Toktong Pass—buried in six inches of new snow. By afternoon, ridgerunning Gyrenes of the 1st Battalion, 7th Marines had joined up. The Chinese tried their best, thousands of them, to dislodge the caravan every foot of the way. But Fox Marines had managed to keep the pass open. Wounded from Fox and the 1st Battalion were loaded aboard trucks, and the caterpillar procession continued down the other side. That evening, just after dusk, the first Marines reached Hagaru-ri. No beaten lot would they be. The last few hundred yards were done in parade fashion: Marines formed up, marched to cadence, and sang "The Marines' Hymn."

At the rear of the column, the Chinese continued to flail against the flanks, always a stone's throw away. At night, warming tents with stoves threw off a little heat for the wounded who were moved in and out. The rest shivered. But no one knew for sure what the next hour or day would bring. The gunfire never stopped, flares drifted down, shadows appeared and disappeared. Henry Litvin remembered: "By the time dusk fell, all of us in the aid station were beginning to act like men who were doomed. There was no conversation. None of us ate a bite of anything. It all seemed so utterly hopeless. . . . We were agonizingly aware that the Chinese could swallow us in a single bite."[22]

It was little help that during the day, he could see figures scurrying over hills Marines had just vacated, as if a vacuum of violence sucked them back in. "I felt like I was literally waiting to die," he said. Dr. Shoemaker remembered setting warming fires. This invariably attracted Marines from the hills, who huddled and tried to thaw their C rations. Otherwise it was impossible to stay hydrated or fed. Out on the hills, though, there was no such luxury. One Marine, Ernie Pappenheimer, remembered: "Warming tents? What warming tents? Hot food? What hot food? You know if you built a fire on the front lines, it would give away your position exactly."[23]

Chet Lessenden recalled getting "50 or 60" new casualties at the top of Toktong Pass—Fox survivors. There was no choice but to "kick off" anyone on trucks who could walk and put new ones aboard. Yet progress was halting: cars and trucks—the only sanctuaries for patients—were stalling out in the cold. One of Lessenden's ambulances, loaded with injured, gave out inches from a steep ravine. It was towed the rest of the way. Completely worn out, Lessenden fell asleep that first night out of Yudam-ni, feet planted in the snow, which was taboo in this weather. There was a penalty for that mistake.[24]

It was not until the afternoon of December 4 that the convoy's rear reached Hagaru-ri. Barely able to keep their eyes open, men still straightened up, looked alive, and filed in those last yards. Litvin mustered newfound energy. "[N]o one ever taught me how to march; but I figured if you kept your head up, your shoulders back, and strode forward as if you weren't tired, that was the way to march like a military man."[25] Over one thousand five hundred casualties followed—an estimation; no one knew the exact count. Frostbite, gunshot wounds, broken limbs—some walked and others were carried. Captain Eugene Hering, division surgeon, commented, "The only way you could tell the dead from the living was whether their eyes moved. They were all frozen stiff as boards."[26] Lessenden finally let someone cut off his boots and saw his frostbitten feet. No big deal, he figured. In fact, he recalled setting an example for other men, more or less a yardstick of whose frostbite was bad enough for evacuation. Captain Hering would bring each frostbitten Marine and soldier by. If their feet looked worse than his, they had a ticket out.[27]

Frostbite injuries were so numerous that they were no longer considered battlefield wounds. Some had remained motionless in arctic temperatures for as long as seventy-two hours, strapped to vehicles—even artillery pieces—or crammed into ambulances. Ken Holloway at E Med figured that "90 to 95 percent" of the casualties suffered from frostbite, in addition to their other injuries. Dr. Stanley Wolf remembered "Initially, when we tried to remove their boots, some of their toes would come off in the boot."[28]

The persecuted masses engorged every tent, every hospital like grateful, redeemed lepers. Holloway saw their faces. They were old men now; Yudam-ni and fourteen miles through Toktong Pass had done that. This was a country of old men—or dead men. No foolishness here. Not anymore. Holloway begged all the Marines to leave their pyramidal tents to make room. As far as his hospital building was concerned, Holloway figured: "We worked almost frantically day and night. At one time I estimated that we had as many as a thousand patients in and around the building. We had so many patients lying, sitting, and standing that we could hardly see the floor. . . . The ones who needed emergency surgery, and there were surprisingly few, managed to get it."[29]

Holloway was not alone. Division surgeon Hering was almost manic, energy meter pegged, beating the bushes for more space. Surgeon Stewart remembered: "He seemed to be everywhere at once, always involved in some task. At times he came in and assisted me in major surgery. Next thing I knew he was outside on one end of a litter. . . . When tent space was filled, he was out rounding up more tents to erect."[30]

Now the process of sorting began—a zombie's bazaar of blistered feet, blanched toes, shot bellies, and gurgling chests. Who should be airlifted out and who could make it on foot—and who would not make it at all? No one was sure when the Chinese would strike, but everyone planned to keep going, to Koto-ri and beyond. Stanley Wolf with the 7th Marines heard the call, "Doc, clear the deck . . . multiple casualties coming in." He pitched in with Hering to triage: "[W]e had to make decisions which I have had to live with all my life," he later said: "Here I got a kid with a sucking chest wound and then I have a kid with half of his head blown off. I know if we get [the first kid] to Japan he can survive, but I don't think the other one will make it. If we got snow the planes couldn't get in and they all would die."[31]

Frostbite cases were sent to a separate tent for rewarming. Two large ward tents were eventually needed. Cotton was put between blistered

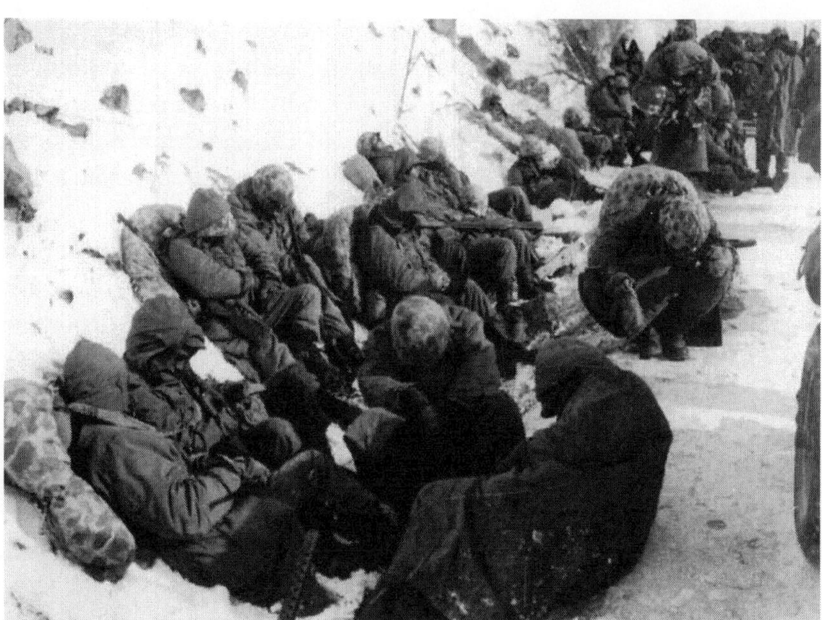

A unit of the 7th Marines takes a break during the arduous trek along the MSR from Hagaru-ri to Koto-ri. (*National Archives*)

toes and a dose of penicillin given. Anyone who could walk was sent back to his unit. Even those who could not walk, if they could carry a gun, were recruited to ride shotgun in ambulances and trucks.

The same day Marines made it to Hagaru-ri, Peking Radio announced, "The annihilation of the United States 1st Marine Division is only a matter of time." And for good reason. Marines were still in the clutches of Communist armies, still outnumbered, and still surrounded. And despite some arrogant nonchalance, a weariness ravaged them. Correspondent Marguerite Higgins was at Hagaru-ri. She looked at Marines who had just arrived from Yudam-ni: "It had been a Korean Valley Forge, and worse than anything in Marine history. The men were exhausted, and the tension among them was all-pervasive. They had the dazed air of men who have accepted death and then found themselves alive after all. They talked in unfinished phrases."[32]

"[D]eeply hurt pride" she called it. For Robert Shoemaker, it was simple depletion. Every ounce of fortitude, every inch of compassion was left on that trail. He found E Company and was handed a two-ounce bottle of LeJon brandy. It was drained in one gulp—and came back up just as quickly, rejected by an empty stomach. Lieutenant Litvin dutifully reported to Captain Hering as soon as he arrived. He then crawled into his sleeping bag and crashed. Chet Lessenden, frostbitten and bone tired, was given a shot of whiskey and a Nembutal by Ken Holloway and found a tent.[33]

One after another, twin-engined Skytrains roared in, flown by the air force 21st Troop Carrier Squadron and 1st Marine Air Wing pilots. Stuffed tents and hospitals decompressed, sending scores of wounded out, those picked by Hering and Wolf. By December 6, a total of 4,312 casualties had left, including 3,150 Marines, 1,137 army, and 25 Royal Marines.[34] "[D]uring this phase of operations the use of air for evacuation was exploited to the utmost," the record read,[35] clearly an understatement. The airstrip never quieted of incoming or outgoing aircraft—under unbelievable conditions. Ice, snow, high altitude, short runways, and Chinese potshots made these adventures noteworthy for air force and Marine aviation history. Air force captain Paul Fritz laid out the challenges: "The cold air was stunning when we opened the side hatch after landing. . . . Conditions at the strip were primitive. The "control tower" consisted of a jeep with a radio in it. . . . After [wounded] were loaded aboard, there was the smell of fresh and dried blood, filthy combat dungarees, unwashed bodies, spent gunpowder . . . all combined into one pervasive stench."[36]

Only one crash occurred. An air force C-47 loaded with casualties lost power on takeoff and came down just outside the Marine perimeter. Miraculously, no one was hurt. Overhead, C-119 "Flying Boxcars" painted the sky with rainbow colors of parachutes – payloads of rations, gasoline, and ammunition "The greatest single factor that influenced the medical service and saved countless lives during this period was the mass utilization of air evacuation by liaison aircraft, cargo planes, and helicopters," X Corps reported.[37] On the ground enormous numbers of supply-laden vehicles vied for Hagaru-ri's primitive roads and parking spaces, a veritable traffic jam. Had the Communists any worthy artillery, commanders whispered, it would have been a massacre.

At Yonpo Airfield near Hungnam, the wounded were met by men of the 163rd Medical Battalion. Critical cases went on to the First Marine Division hospital, Med Company A, the 121st Evacuation Hospital, or the USS *Consolation* offshore. Of the almost one thousand evacuees, only twenty-nine died of their wounds.[38]

The afternoon of December 4, General Almond arrived at Hagaru-ri to meet with General Smith and Colonels Litzenberg and Murray. Hagaru-ri was a liability. There would be a break out to Koto-ri, an "attack to the rear" in Marine-speak. Chinese fighters were lining the route, there was no doubt—it was a gauntlet to be run of unprecedented ferocity. December 6 was set as the breakout day. Hagaru-ri was ominously quiet those two days. The enemy had better ideas.

On December 6, the last sixty-two patients were evacuated from C and E Company hospitals. Hal Streit's C Med housed over one thousand four hundred wounded, including 110 head and face, 66 chest, and 25 serious abdominal injuries. Stewart's Section I processed 1,250 casualties and performed twenty-one laparotomies and five amputations, all in less than three weeks. There had been gripping moments. Simply keeping blood and plasma thawed were major challenges. Sometimes blood froze in the tubing as it was infusing. Once body cavities were opened, steam would rise in the frigid air. Nevertheless, operations began and ended with wood-burning stoves flaming and surgeons and patients bundled, sterility only a minor concern. In the throes of hypothermia, there was little regard for Lister's admonitions.[39] Even head injuries were explored; skull and brain debrided, dura closed. General surgeons took it on. What other choice was there?[40]

The day of departure, all material left behind was torched and burned. Two convoys formed, Division Train No. 1 (escorted by the 7th Marines) and Division Train No. 2 (5th Marines). C Med divided in two. A section went with Train No. 1 and B section with Train No. 2. E Med's I detachment simply walked. Jim Stewart put on winter gear and shoepacs, grabbed a carbine, and joined Train No. 1. Everyone was needed for defense, no exceptions.[41] It was a replay of the trip from Yudam-ni. Stewart remembered "drive a few car lengths then stop for several minutes."[42] Henry Litvin was among the last of Train No. 1 to leave that night. He remembered thinking, "We're dead! All the troops who had been fighting off the Chinese had gone and we were still there. . . . That was a night!"[43] Lieutenant Silver remembered talking to wounded Marines, half-frozen, lying in a field, worried that they would be left behind. When he mentioned it to Colonel Murray, commander of the Fifth Marines, he was told, "Silver, you go back and tell them that if we can't get them out we're not going."[44] Robert Fleischaker stood around for hours waiting to leave. There was plenty of idle time to worry about one's fate. He was toward the end of the column—part of Train No. 2. As they waited beside their trucks and ambulances, he could hear gunfire behind him in Hagaru-ri and farther ahead. They were still there after dark. Fires appeared in fifty-five-gallon oil drums. No one cared if they were beacons for the enemy. It was simply too cold. He did not leave until the morning of December 7. Train No. 1 was already entering Koto-ri.

But not before a brutal night fighting off the Chinese. They were everywhere. Rifle fire, grenades, and mortars in their typical fashion lanced the column. Marines stormed out and the Chinese melted away. Then they reappeared. Bugles and bells and whistles and more gunfire. The fight lasted four hours. At one point, Stewart saw them coming right at him. Carbine up. Click, click. Misfires. Dark forms closing in, he drew his revolver. "I knew my time was at an end," he recalled. At the last minute for some unexplained reason they veered away. Stewart would never know why. Others did not escape. One section of C Med lost a third of its men wounded, one killed. Chinese soldiers actually penetrated a part of the convoy, shooting up trucks and setting fires. Lieutenant Colonel Frederick Dowsett, Colonel Litzenberg's executive officer, was shot in the ankle. Two of his staff members were killed right beside him. A battalion surgeon for the 7th Marines, Lieutenant Robert Wedemeyer, immediately gave first aid to the wounded Dowsett, and the chaplain, Lieutenant Cornelius Griffin, rushed to console other stricken Marines. Chaplain Griffin was picked off, shot in the jaw and shoulder. He would have been killed if his clerk, Sergeant Mathew Caruso, had not shielded him. It cost Caruso his life. Marines dragged Karle Seydel to Dr. Litvin, who was a close friend. But no longer—Seydel had a clean hole in his forehead. "He was a Marine's Marine," Litvin recalled. "It seemed so terrible. I wanted to do something, but his face was gray and he was dead. . . . I have a hard time with his death to this day."[45] The newly injured were tossed aboard anything, strapped in, and told to hold on. In and out of Hell Fire Valley, dead stiff by the side of the road, and on to Koto-ri.

By midnight December 7, everyone had arrived. The eleven miles from Hagaru-ri to Koto-ri cost Division Train No. 1 15 dead and 117 wounded.[46] Division Train No. 2 had it easier, the Chinese more intent on looting Hagaru-ri than bothering Marines. But all told, both trains lost 616 men, including 103 killed or died of wounds and 506 wounded.[47] Stewart was relieved, and still bewildered he had not been cut down. Even more amazing was his ambulance, shot full of holes but no one inside hit. After a trip through the graveyard of Hell Fire Valley, Lieu-

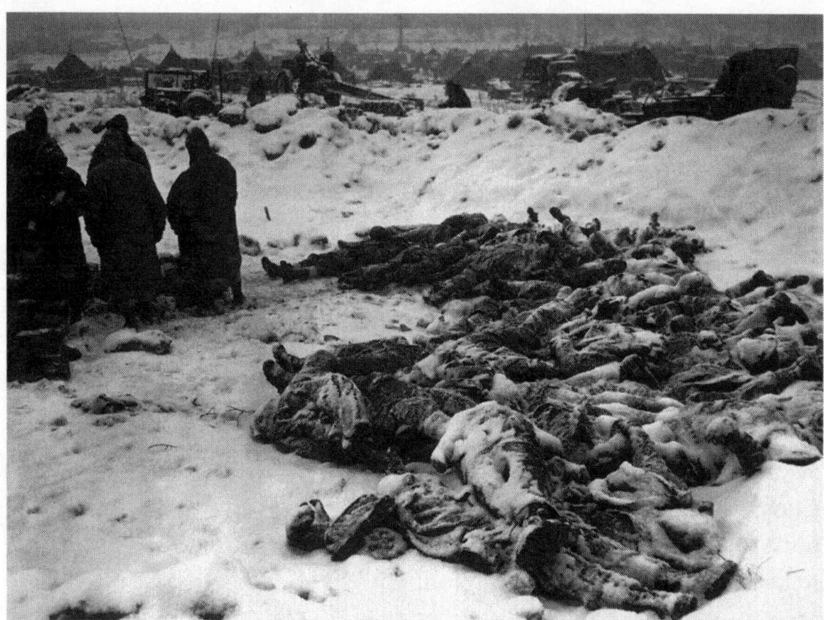

Bodies of Marines and British troops ready for mass burial at Koto-ri December 8, 1950. (*National Archives*)

tenant Shoemaker wrote his wife "the petty things which bob up all the time will be relegated to the proper position of pettiness."[48]

In Koto-ri, members of the army's 185th Engineer Battalion had been at work. Up went squad and pyramidal tents, complete with decks and sides. By December 3, Koto-ri was a genuine tent city. Hospitals and sick bays would hold 250 litter patients. No sooner had they finished than Marine and army wounded surged into the compound, more shivering, miserable refugees—832 in all. D Med doctors—now with Captain Hering and 1st Med Battalion chief Commander Johnson in tow—descended on the huddled heaps. Captain Richard Silvis, a veteran of Iwo Jima and surgeon for the 2nd Marine Division, just happened to be there and eagerly pitched in. Twelve laparotomies were needed, and there was only one death, due to catastrophic liver trauma.[49] But a new crop of criticals had to be flown out. Just in time, the airstrip had been lengthened at the rantings of Chesty Puller. Long enough that now specially equipped TBM Avengers of VMO-6, modified to hold several litters and ambulatory patients, could ferry out. In fact, on December 7, just one

Avenger, piloted by Captain McCaleb, flew eighty-four wounded Marines back to Hungnam in eleven trips.[50] A snowstorm December 8 grounded everything, but the next day a massive effort commenced.[51] TBMs, C-47 Skytrains, even a few Sentinels evacuated almost three hundred wounded.[52]

But there would be no dallying at Koto-ri. Smith wanted his Marines out, and preferably out of North Korea. There was another gauntlet to run, eleven miles down from the plateau, through Funchilin Pass to Chinhung-ni. And there was no reason to think the Chinese would not be ready, bugles and whistles in hand, to pile into hapless Americans. Funchilin Pass would be a chokepoint. A span of roadway directly over the penstocks had been razed. Commanders figured out a plan. The air force dropped off four sections of steel Treadway bridging. Two Brockway trucks, protected by 7th Marine gunmen, would carry the spans. At the same time, 1st Marines from Chinhung-ni would head north to clear the road of Communists. As before, supporting soldiers and Marines would spread out along the flanks and into the hills. They would hunt the Red Chinese before they hunted the Marines. In Koto-ri, there were final preparations; one of the last: bury 117 soldiers and Marines. There would simply be no room on this convoy either.

On December 8, in the middle of that blinding snowstorm, the 7th Marines hit the road south and the 1st Marines left Chinhung-ni. The next day there was perfect weather, clear and bright. Treadway trucks arrived at the pass and laid down their spans. Men and machines gingerly crossed, with only inches to spare. That night was one of the coldest on record. Dr. Holloway remembered it. He wore four pairs of socks, eight layers of clothing, three pairs of gloves, two parka caps, and a steel helmet, "and I was still miserably cold and shivering."[53] His group made the bridge crossing guided by nothing more than flashlights. The Chinese were nowhere to be found. Days of combat had even worn them down. The Devil Dogs were on their way out.[54]

Lieutenant Fleischaker did not leave Koto-ri until the evening of December 10, bringing up the rearguard. After their ambulance inauspiciously slid off the road, he transferred his corpsmen, fellow surgeon Dr. Farrell, and two wounded to a tank that took them the rest of the way to Chinhung-ni and Hungnam. Jim Stewart believed they left Koto-ri sometime after midnight on December 10. "I'm glad I did not see the Treadway bridge. . . . I got inside an ambulance [as opposed to walking across] and said a silent prayer and we literally inched across."[55] Marguerite Higgins remembered that they battled the weather the whole route to Chinhung-ni. "The frost and wind, howling through the narrow pass, were almost as deadly as the enemy," she wrote. Most of the Marines were exhausted. She observed that many "didn't even bother to take cover at sporadic machine-gun and rifle fire. When someone was killed they would wearily, matter-of-factly, pick up the body and throw it in the nearest truck."[56] Lieutenant Litvin, rounding a bend and suddenly seeing flatland, knew they were out of the mountains and out of danger. In fact, at Chinhung-ni his contingent was put on trains—actually open-air flat cars—which took them the rest of the way to Hungnam That was fine with him, anything to get off his feet. By early afternoon December 11, all soldiers and Marines had passed through Chinhung-ni. That evening, they reached the welcomed metropolis of Hamhung-Hungnam.

At Hungnam, A Med had seen the scourges of Chosin. A total of 1,673 patients had arrived, 60 percent (1,010) severe enough to prompt further evacuation. Surgeons did almost fifty major surgical procedures, including laparotomies and amputations.[57] Records showed that only seven died after admission. Many more never made it, hemorrhaging or freezing on the slopes and roadways. Frostbite, though, was endemic. Doctors estimated two-thirds of casualties had it bad enough to evacuate in their own right.

General Smith assumed his Marines would stay in North Korea, maybe man a defensive perimeter around Hamhung and Hungnam. That was not to be. On December 9 General Almond had been told to get X Corps out of North Korea. A huge naval armada assembled at Wonsan and Hungnam Harbors, and over one hundred thousand American, British, and South Korean troops—in addition to a large number of Korean refugees—were loaded aboard. Fresh soldiers of the 3rd and 7th Infantry Divisions set up a defensive perimeter. Grizzled veterans of the 1st Marine Division began loading onto troopships in Hungnam Harbor. By that time, stories of their tortuous passage from Chosin had captivated the American public. Grizzled veterans of the 1st Marine Division began loading onto troopships in Hungnam Harbor. By that time stories of their passage from Chosin had captivated the American public. *Time* magazine had likened the trek of the Marines and soldiers from the Reservoir to Bataan, Anzio, Dunkirk, and Valley Forge. "The running fight of the Marines and . . . Army's 7th Infantry Division . . . was a battle unparalleled in U.S. military history."[58]

On December 15, Marines departed Hungnam for points south. "Ours was a group of men, dirty and unshaven, who universally had weight losses of ten to twenty pounds. I had never realized how grimy and foul a fighting force could be," said Lieutenant Shoemaker aboard the USNS *General Daniel I. Sultan* (T-AP 120).[59] Lieutenant Litvin was immeasurably grateful. During the entire journey from Yudam-ni to the coast he felt utterly hopeless, convinced there was no way they would complete the seventy-mile trip. Now he was in Hungnam and soon aboard a navy ship. "The Navy didn't abandon me. The Navy didn't forget me," he kept thinking. "I walked into a bathroom and started peeling my clothes off. . . . Skin and bones . . . I had lost 33 pounds."[60]

And Ken Holloway had to pinch himself to see if he was really alive. From the frozen wasteland around the Chosin, he was now in a stateroom aboard the *Daniel I. Sultan* with private tiled bathrooms and hot showers. "I ate the entire menu of fresh orange juice, fresh milk, eggs and bacon to order, hash brown potatoes, hot cakes and more bacon with two eggs," he wrote his wife.[61]

20

Massacre to the East

While the Marines' ordeal was playing out west of the Chosin Reservoir, an even more menacing scenario was unfolding to the east. On October 29, as part of X Corps's invasion of North Korea, the 7th Division had landed piecemeal at Iwon, northeast of Hungnam. With some alacrity, if not elan, the 17th Infantry had advanced north to the Yalu River by November 21. There it stood, peering across into Chinese Manchuria. "Heartiest congratulations, Ned," MacArthur cabled to General Almond, "and tell Dave Barr [commander of the 7th Division] that the 7th Division hit the jackpot."[1] Just to the west, a battalion of the 32nd Infantry occupied the town of Samsu, just eight miles from the Yalu. The 31st Infantry roamed a desolate, mountainous no-man's land just east of the Fusen Reservoir. By November 20, General Barr began shifting his 31st and 32nd Infantry to the east to consolidate with his 17th Infantry. It seemed only a matter of days before the entire region could be secured and turned over to ROK forces. Then it was home for Christmas.

The 1st MASH, now veterans of the Inchon landings, came ashore November 9 at Iwon to support the 7th Division. It set up in the hamlet of Pukch'ong, ten miles from Iwon in a picturesque river valley fringed by mountainous terrain. It was a companion to the 2nd Platoon (clearing) of the 7th Medical Battalion, already there. The 1st Platoon (clearing) of the Med Battalion trailed the 17th Infantry marching to the Yalu and settled in Kapsan about forty miles away. The 3rd Platoon was at

Pungsan, midway between Kapsan and Pukch'ong. Yet in the wake of advancing infantry, evacuation was strenuous and jarring, lugging casualties across more than one hundred miles of convoluted mountain trails to even get to the 1st MASH, then another eighty miles to the 121st Evac at Hamhung. Heavy winter weather made it all the more difficult.

Major Oren Atchley, commander of the 7th Medical Battalion, was an early victim of Almond's offensive. He and a detachment of men went hunting for a missing ambulance and its crew loaded with patients traveling from Kapsan to Pukch'ong on November 23. The following day he and his team—now hopelessly lost themselves—were set upon by enemy troops in rocky back roads. Only because Atchley stood his ground and fired on the enemy were his men able to scatter and escape. Two others in the party were killed, and Atchley disappeared. Only two of the five men made it back to the American lines alive. Oren Atchley, missing in action, was eventually declared dead.[2] The sought-after ambulance was never located.

Once Almond had decided to shift all his Marine regiments west of the Chosin Reservoir, General Barr had to muster troops to fill the void east of Hagaru-ri. He cherry-picked units closest to the MSR—his division was scattered all over northeast Korea. A loosely assembled regimental combat team of 2nd and 3rd Battalions of the 31st Infantry, the 1st Battalion of the 32nd Infantry, the 31st Tank Company, the 57th Field Artillery Battalion, a battery of antiaircraft gunners, and a headquarters company were placed under the command of Colonel Allan MacLean, commander of the 31st Infantry. Later it would be known—in ignominy—as "Team MacLean." Tagging along was a detachment of the 31st Infantry Medical Company under surgeon Harvey Galloway.

Colonel Don Faith and his battalion of 32nd Infantry were the first to arrive east of Chosin on November 25. Faith marched his men past Marine checkpoints into the barren countryside, around Hill 1221—an intimidating elevation commanding routes in and out—to forward positions four miles beyond Pungnyuri Inlet. MacLean arrived the next day and first set up his command post in a schoolhouse at Hudong-ni, just south of Hill 1221 but moved some of his officers later to a "jump" command post near Faith's troops. On November 27, a battalion of the 31st Infantry and the field artillery pulled in. The 3rd Battalion never made it, ambushed along the MSR at Funchilin Pass. The column was cut to pieces, survivors lucky to make it to Koto-ri, where they were kept by Puller. At Chosin, MacLean's two battalions were now strung out for eight miles around the eastern border of the reservoir. An entire division of Communist Chinese troops had already encircled them and cut off any escape route. MacLean was trapped.

Just before midnight on November 27, the Chinese struck in force against Faith's forward elements. American lines stubbornly held, but farther south, at the Pungnyuri Inlet, attacks on the 31st Infantry and field artillery batteries quickly pressed in. Chinese soldiers ran everywhere, some firing American-made weapons, circling, running, crouching, shooting through gaps. They pushed on until, like rogue linebackers, they were inside the perimeter looking for quarterbacks. Common infantry—farm boys and shopworkers and college kids—took after them with bayonet-spiked M1s, knives, and bare hands. This was blood sport at its worst, men tangled in pretzels of death. Most stayed motionless. A few crawled away toward khaki tents trailing ribbons of blood. Here and there, pinkish entrails fouled the snow.

Wisconsin native Captain Vincent Navarre was battalion surgeon for Colonel Faith's 1st Battalion, 32nd Infantry. There was no small pride that his battalion had been ranked "Most Combat Efficient in All Japan" a year prior to deployment to Korea. Ferocious in combat, the men stormed ashore at Inchon and accomplished any mission to which they were dispatched. Even the Korean winter had not fazed Navarre, quite accustomed as he was to Wisconsin weather. On the road to Chosin Reservoir, he and his men wisely picked up some fur-lined parkas. By November 27, he had reconnoitered and found a site for his aid station, near Faith's command post on the fringe of the battlefield. Darkness found his station in good order. Navarre was pleased. His stove heater was roaring, boots and parka buckled and zipped.

A flurry of gunfire signaled the Chinese assault. Before long, that night, wounded arrived with horrible tales of quilted men pouring through: "The first was Captain Haynes, slate gray in color with two dangerous wounds. He smelled of powder, his clothes were smeared with mud and snow; and he groaned with pain and muttered about the cold . . . he had obviously lost much blood."[3]

Captain Haynes suffered an abdominal bullet wound and had been stabbed with a bayonet. On his heels were ten or twenty more wounded, some hauled in on litters. The tidy aid station was soon pandemonium. Overflow wounded were put in the nearby Korean house Faith was using as his command post. Litters were lined side-by-side. Haynes and another serious casualty consumed Navarre's attention that night. Haynes appeared hopeless. "In this case and under these conditions, special attention to adequate analgesia took preference. . . . These men needed blood and major surgery," Navarre wrote. "Neither could be had at Battalion Aid Station level."[4] Captain Haynes, thankfully unconscious, died before daybreak.

It was not so fortunate for elements of the medical company winding their way to the inlet where another aid station would be set up.[5] They had passed the command post at Hudong-ni and were heading farther north to the inlet in absolute blackness. Just before midnight, around Hill 1221, Chinese troops stormed the column—a textbook ambush. The Communists had set up a roadblock, and out they came, almost casually walking up and down the line of vehicles, shooting anyone alive. Galloway was in one of the lead jeeps. In an instant, his driver was hit, and then him, shot in the right arm, right leg, and then his head. "Fortunately, I did not lose consciousness and knew just what nerves had been hit and what area of my brain had been hit."[6] His driver somehow recovered and gunned the jeep through the ambush to the inlet aid station. There, Galloway told the battalion surgeon, Captain Sterling Morgan, about the ambush, begging him to send men back to rescue the survivors. With dawn, the tragedy unfolded. Captain Hank Wamble, the medical company's executive officer, was shot in the chest. When brought in, he was barely able to breathe. Morgan worked to stabilize him but without success. He soon died. Captain James Baido, a Filipino dentist from Maryland, was also killed. He had recently told his Aunt Evie he enjoyed his new role as a surgeon, not a dentist. Their remains were never recovered. Some medics and supply officer Clifford Hancock at the rear of the column managed to escape and made their way back to Hudong-ni. Others were systematically executed by roving Chinese.

The Chinese broke off their attacks at sunup. Daylight would surely bring airstrikes, and they feared the heat and flames of American napalm. The perimeter around the Pungnyuri Inlet was sobering. Medic Jim Blohm described the scene: "The area was littered with bodies, Chinese and American. . . . It was a chaos of scattered weapons and equipment; dead bodies . . . litter parties moving wounded to aid tents; litter parties moving the dead to a disposal area."[7]

The temperature dipped to thirty degrees below zero. That day, November 28, General Almond choppered in to visit Colonel MacLean at his forward command post. Faith was there as well. Cut off, yes, surrounded, most certainly. But arrival of the "lost battalion" would fix things, they were sure, Faith was told. Break the deadlock, even resume attacks to the east. Nothing but a ragged bunch of peasants, Almond mused. "We're going all the way to the Yalu. Don't let a bunch of Chinese laundrymen stop you," he told Faith.[8] Soldier on, deploy, and hold the high ground were his instructions. The general then hopped in his Marine helicopter and choppered out. The "lost" 2nd Battalion, 31st Infantry, never made it past Koto-ri.

After sunset, Almond's "laundrymen" were at it again. Attacks commenced around the inlet after midnight. Peppering the American lines, the Chinese were eager to engage the GIs and finish the job. But not that night. Dr. Morgan's aid station was bustling. Lieutenant John Gray remembered the night. Struck by mortar fragments in his thigh, he was brought to the medical tent and saw the doctor "working frantically with stacks of wounded while expressing chagrin at not becoming a Navy doctor," extolling the humane virtues of shipboard medicine. What Gray remembered most were the bullet holes through the tent, speckling Red Cross insignias. And that rounds snapping canvas unnerved workers inside. Gray even saw that surgical basins were full of holes. He'd had enough. Whether it was not to bother Morgan or just that he felt safer with a gun, the lieutenant picked up an M-1 and headed back outside.[9] Inside, days and nights blurred for Morgan. His last letter home for a long while read, "Two days after Thanksgiving the enemy hit again. No kidding ourselves; this was it."[10]

Forward of the inlet, Faith's men were barely holding on. There seemed to be inconceivable numbers of mustard-clothed men, wave after wave. Next morning, MacLean advised Faith to pull back to his position about one mile south and consolidate. One more Chinese assault just might break his line. For Captain Navarre, this meant loading stretcher cases on trucks and collecting walking wounded for a hike back in frigid temperatures. It took hours over snow-covered roads at a snail's pace, but they made it. Settling in a new aid tent, Navarre was assured by Faith that the most serious cases would be choppered out. That afternoon, two helicopters appeared, four patients were loaded in, and off they went. More needed evacuation, but not that day. Marines at Yudam-ni had priority.

It was on that day, too, that Colonel MacLean disappeared. He struck out on the frozen inlet maybe thinking the men firing at him were friendlies. But they were those ragtag "laundrymen," and they cleanly put four rounds in him. He was never seen again.

So now MacLean's troops were in one location. The inlet was their tight perimeter. Tanks from Captain Bob Drake's two platoons tried to break through from Hudong-ni but slipped and slid on icy roads or bogged down in roadside mud. The Chinese took after them with bazookas and even pounded on the tops trying to get in. Somehow twelve of the sixteen tanks made it back to Hudong-ni. Faith, now in command, was clearly in trouble. Nothing was going to get through. Ungainly C-119 "Flying Boxcars" flew over, parachuting ammunition and medical supplies. Strong Manchurian winds blew most outside the perimeter into enemy hands. Navarre pleaded with a helicopter pilot bringing 7th Division chief General Barr for a site visit to come back with more morphine and bandages. It never happened. In the aid tents, officers routinely made rounds urging any of the wounded who could walk and fire a weapon back to the skirmish line. Men were hungry, cold, and drained. They had very little to eat and drink. Water was frozen. There was no using a latrine. Soldiers squatted over helmets and tossed their turds over the edge of foxholes. "Nothing was working out," a private lamented. "We were being shot up bad. We were just in a terrible situation. We were being annihilated."[11]

On November 28, General MacArthur saw the light. Realizing his troops just might be wiped out on both sides of the peninsula, he sent an urgent communique to the Joint Chiefs in Washington: "This command has done everything humanly possible . . . but is now faced with conditions beyond its control and its strength."[12] He insisted on pulling X Corps back to Hungnam and off the coast. Washington promptly approved his plan. Marines were to disengage and leave Chosin, the same for MacLean's troops to the east. That prompted General Barr's visit to Faith on November 30 and his decision to withdraw Drake's tanks and some three hundred infantry from Hudong-ni to Hagaru-ri—a decision that sealed Faith's fate. His men were as doomed as Custer's cavalry at the Little Big Horn.

The Chinese tasted victory. They swarmed over Faith's circled wagons the night of November 30 and December 1. Mortar fire fell like hail around the perimeter, including the aid tent. Shrapnel chewed into Navarre's pants legs, and a detonation was so close it lifted him "a few inches." Still, casualties were pulled, dragged, or carried in, an assortment of moaning misery. A few perished unnoticed, lost in the dimmed recesses of Navarre's private Golgotha. At sunup, carcasses were hauled outside and scavenged for anything useful: coats, boots, gloves, guns, grenades, bullets. Bandages were cut off or unrolled and used again. In a kind of dignified cannibalism, the living were feeding off accouterments of the dead. "The battalion surgeon [Navarre] sat with his hands folded in his aid station. He was physically exhausted and had no medical supplies whatsoever," a patient reported.[13] "Before the night was half through, we were completely out of bandages. Every possible piece of cloth was utilized. I can recall cutting the unused sides and ends of bandages from one man to use on another," Vincent Navarre wrote.[14] For the dead, there was no burial; rock hard, frozen turf made sure of that.

Yet Faith's troops had held. Somehow these wasted men had fired enough rounds and thrown enough grenades and plunged enough bayonets and killed enough Communists. But they were a sorry lot. Smashed and bruised and mangled. Faith thought there might be five hundred wounded. An exact figure was unknown, though likely most were somehow afflicted. But there would be no repeat. This was enough. A breakout was essential. Stay and die, Faith knew, and his men suspected. They had to try for Hagaru-ri.

That next day, orders were issued for the breakout. The monumental task of somehow loading the wounded was first priority. Any existing truck was emptied and then packed with casualties—inside and out, as Navarre found: "The trucks were a fantastic sight. The rears were piled to the tops of the racks, and I mean piled just as full of wounded as could possibly be held. Other wounded were lying across the fenders and hoods."[15]

It took some convincing to coax sapped and gray men to get up and out of the tents. "You want to get outa here, don't you, well we have to get you on that truck," their buddies urged. Of course, Navarre had no problem. His tent was riddled with bullet holes, "more of an 1865 scene than 1950."[16] Medics crammed fifteen or twenty wounded in each truck; every available blanket and sleeping bag was used to keep men warm. Few personal belongings were taken except weapons and ammo. What stayed behind was soaked with fuel and burned. Sterling Morgan remembered, "Nothing was left, I kept only my toothbrush, soap and razor. . . . I even burned some of my clothes."[17] Marine Corsairs howled overhead, driving away any curious Chinese with tumbling canisters of napalm. One fell short, engulfing and incinerating soldiers in the forward elements just as the convoy got underway. That was chilling to watch. "You could see them running all around just ripping their clothes off, just keep on running," according to assistant battalion surgeon Yong Kak Lee.[18] Smoldering survivors, screaming in agony, were thrown into deuce-and-a-halfs with the rest of Faith's wretched remnants.

The nightmare had just begun. Chinese stormed down from the hills, their bolt action Zhongzheng rifles, captured Garands, and burp guns laced the column, firing indiscriminately at troops, jeeps, ambulances, and trucks. Primary targets were drivers, and bullets slapped into cabs, windshields, and windows. Neat bullet holes and starred glass obscured slumped drivers with blown brains. Passengers took their place only to suffer a similar fate. Before long, Chinese soldiers were in their midst, roaming up and down. "When they [the Chinese] reached us they grabbed our weapons, ammo, medical supplies, and food," one infantryman remembered.[19] Simple log roadblocks around Hill 1221 stopped everyone cold. Faith took some men and charged at the Chinese, hoping to force them into the hills. They replied with grenades, one exploding so close to Faith that it sprayed his chest, driving fragments inward. He was barely able to make it back, his vision dimming and voice fading. Like a tragic warrior of Homer's *Iliad*, he was soon overtaken by death, and his spirit departed.

Navarre had no bandages and very little morphine. He could do almost nothing for soldiers limping back from skirmishes. And he was a target himself. He could see the winks of muzzle flashes on the hills. One blasted his right knee, certainly fracturing his tibia, he figured. Blood welled at once. Panicking just a little, Navarre took off his belt and cinctured his leg, pulling tight to cut off blood flow. Someone grabbed him and tossed him into an already filled ambulance. Trying to get around the roadblock, his driver was shot and killed. The ambulance stalled. Then rapid rounds stitched across the sides, drilling neat perforations just above his head. "We have to get out of here, this is suicide," Navarre spit. He and a few others tumbled from the ambulance and took their chances on foot. But his leg gave way and he rolled into a roadside trench, shivering so much he thought he would give away his position.

Along the column, others were doing the same, falling out of ambushed trucks and jeeps. Lieutenant Jerry McCabe, already wounded, slithered out of the truck he was in, hearing screams of GIs being shot by roving bands of Chinese.[20] "A mournful racket," others called it. Bodies of Americans and Chinese lined the roadway, "their blood forming pools from which steam rose into the freezing air."[21] One soldier saw a GI laying on the road with "half his stomach blown away. He cried and screamed for help." The Chinese came by, shoved him into a ditch, and left him there to die.[22]

Those who could pushed on. Around Hill 1221 were the remains of the ambushed medical company; hulks of tanks and vehicles knocked out by enemy fire days before. And there was the body of dentist James Baido, found by one soldier "hit by a shell that took half his head off."[23] At a third roadblock after daybreak on December 2, it was all over. Americans were out of ammunition. The convoy was at a standstill. Those so-called rag-tag volunteers despised by Almond prevailed, striding along the paralyzed column like audacious victors. Dr. Yong Kak Lee recalled: "Patients on the trucks were re-hit by enemy machine guns and hand grenades. Hell couldn't be any worse than this scene. . . . Soon the fighting was over. . . . Deadly quietness because there was not a soul around me. Some trucks were burning red hot."[24]

Chinese troops threw white phosphorus grenades into trucks, incinerating occupants. Others shot drivers who were still alive. Some simply snatched blankets from the half-frozen crammed inside and ran off. Others took potshots at GIs trying to get away—target practice. Medical executive officer Hank Wamble was finished off. Supply officer Brown Sebastian was brought down with a single shot to the head. The Chinese herded captured Americans along at the tip of bayonets, poking fallen forms to see if any life was left. Surprisingly, once gunfire stopped, some Chinese soldiers offered morphine and water to the wounded. It was said later that many of the prisoners were released after a few days.

Escapees in groups of two or three headed south in the direction of Hagaru-ri, many across the iced surface of the reservoir. The Chinese did not pursue; they were happy to pillage the trucks. Dr. Navarre somehow evaded notice by busy Chinese looters, hobbled around, and was finally found by a Korean couple. He was helped to their house and from there put on an ox sled and trundled off to the reservoir. Before long, Marines found his party. Navarre was taken to Hagaru-ri, put on a plane, and flown out, eventually landing on a hospital ship. "I must have been a sight with five day's growth of whiskers and the former, frozen dirt of Korea now warmed to mud over my entire ventral surfaces," Navarre recalled of his stay aboard the *Consolation*.[25] Hardly unusual, its nurses would say. "They were tired of the war," nurse Betty Baker surmised. "They were exhausted. . . . I had one patient who said, 'This is it. . . . When I get home I'm not going to fight another war.' He said it was a terrible war."[26] Indeed, what war is not?

Battalion surgeon Yong Kak Lee also slipped away unnoticed, falling out of his shot-up truck, rolling down an embankment right onto the ice of the reservoir. Unharmed, he took off, reckoning with the stars, until he found Hagaru-ri. Had he been captured, as a Korean native, Lee surely would have been executed. "I ate two trays of food, then slept for 24 hours without realizing that this town [Hagaru-ri] was also surrounded. I felt safe," Lee later said.[27]

From Task Force MacLean, 884 men reached Hagaru-ri. Major Lynch, of the 7th Division staff, counted 559 survivors from Faith's and MacLean's units in combat. The rest were tankers and headquarters soldiers who were pulled out of Hudong-ni. Infantry units were decimated. Two rifle companies in the two forward battalions were left with one officer and thirty enlisted each. An estimated one thousand one hundred troopers of the 7th Division never made it back to Hagaru-ri; they were either killed, died of their wounds, or were captured. "You were one of the few wounded who were removed by helicopter. . . . The whole 3/31 [3rd Battalion, 31st Infantry] was officially wiped out, together with the 1/32 and the artillery battalion," Sterling Morgan later wrote to the evacuated Captain Galloway.[28] Morgan was deeply affected by the whole experience, seeing one after another of his aid men fall. His clan, his fraternity, *his* band of brothers was gone. Wrecked. Too young, too soon, too savage. But on the other side of the world, Harriet Morgan found a letter in her mailbox, after days of silence, a yellow envelope—a telegram. Her heart stopping, she opened it and read: "Am well and fit. Best love from Daddy. All my love Dearest." And there it was, his name—her Sterling Morgan—signed, from Osaka Army Hospital, Japan. She nearly collapsed.

The survivors of the 31st Regimental Combat Team joined Marines at Hagaru-ri, and the 385 hardiest were placed under Lieutenant Colonel Barry Anderson and made part of the 7th Marine Regiment for the breakout from Hagaru-ri.

Nurses of the 1st MASH were there at Hamhung, looking almost as beat as their patients. They had landed at Iwon on November 9 and moved to Pukch'ong to set up their hospital in a vacated schoolhouse. During November, the unit had done 171 surgical cases. Not one had died.[29] As soon as word spread of Chinese hordes at the Chosin Reservoir, the 1st MASH was packed up and moved to Hamhung. It was to this schoolhouse, the MASH billet, that Marines and soldiers from Koto-ri were taken. It was not a glamor spot. Nurses and doctors had been

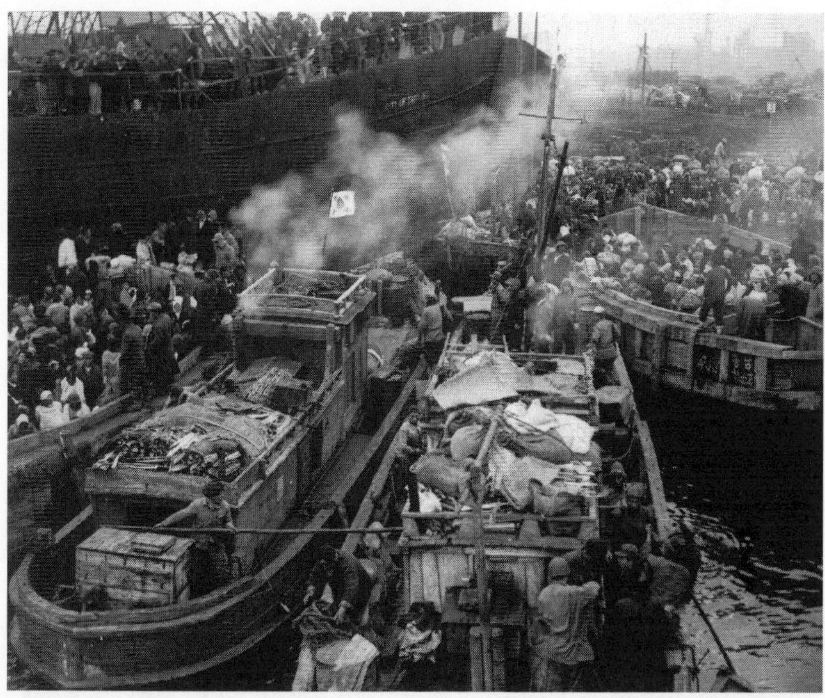

North Korean refugees jam the decks of fishing boats and an LST during the evacuation of Hungnam on December 19, 1950. (*National Archives*)

working without a break, especially now with the new crop of frigid bodies from Koto-ri. "For three days and nights we didn't leave the operating room," Nurse Marjorie Lovelady emphasized.[30] Sleepless furrows lined their faces, the *ennui* of blurred sorrow slumped them, as if no amount of joy could resurrect the banished manhoods entering through their tent flaps. It was they who had rushed to their sides to pump hope and will and grit back in only to find, much too often, it spilled right back out onto a stiff, frozen turf. It was hard to tell who was more wasted. At least one young soldier noticed: "And then this girl—this nurse—took over. Bathed me. Got the anesthetic ready. She looked deader than I did. On her feet for two days, two nights. I was gonna tell her she should have been on the stretcher instead of me. But I conked out."[31]

The 1st MASH did not close until December 13, until the Chinese were just around the corner. There were six operating tables, shifts of surgeons and nurses back and forth, lickety-split—case after case. Then it stopped. The Communists were coming. It was too hot to stay anymore. Tents were broken down, supplies stored, trucks packed. Off to the harbor and on board the Victory ship *Towanda Victory*. Pusan by Christmas.

It was almost a Dunkirk in its magnitude, the evacuation of Hungnam. The navy furnished 109 ships of all types for what was known as Operation Christmas Cargo. Under the watchful eyes of 3rd Division soldiers, Marines and doughboys of the Hourglass Division peeled onto landing craft and gangways, still carrying the filth of Chosin with them—many silent, minds still numbed by the weather and senseless calamities. There was a shuffling of broken hearts. Historian Roy E. Appleman later wrote of this mournful mass: "The cumulative effect of physical fatigue, loss of sleep, short rations, long hours of darkness, subzero temperatures, was a numbness, dullness, lack of alertness and depression of spirit."[32]

Onboard ships, one hundred five thousand troops, seventeen thousand five hundred vehicles, and ninety-eight thousand Korean refugees bedded down.[33] The 3rd Division slipped aboard by Christmas Eve, and the armada headed south. Food and heat, shaves and showers mended physical pains, but for some—maybe all—images would never erase, an inward chill might never leave.

The Korean War dragged on three more years. The fighting finally stabilized around the thirty-eighth parallel in a stalemate more resembling Flanders Fields than America's mighty mechanized warfare. Air and ground forces became mere pawns to the machinations of negotiators posturing around tables at P'anmunjom. Never more would American forces range across North Korea. Marines and GIs died in obscure and despicable hillocks, paddies, and streams of no strategic value, soaking rich Korean soil with blood and frustration. And finally, on July 27, 1953, an armistice, not a peace treaty, was signed, ending the worthless conflict and establishing a demilitarized zone at the thirty-eighth parallel, exactly where the boundaries existed in 1950. Nothing had been gained but anguish and heartache for so many families on both sides. It was truly a waste of youth, energy, and the sanctity of life.

Part 5

Khe Sanh

"You all will soon be in the American history books."
—Col. David Lownds, commander,
26th Marines, Khe Sanh

21

Indochine

VIETNAM IS A COUNTRY OF STARK CONTRASTS. IT IS A PLACE OF RIVERS and a place of hills, of arid highlands and sweltering coastlines, of impenetrable jungles and pristine shores. But all are bathed in the waters of the Song Me Kong (Mekong) and Song Hong (Red River) flowing from Tibet. Tributaries of these two great deltas snake throughout forests and valleys, fertilizing vast flatlands in the north and the south and sending tentacles gripping the Annamite range on their way to the sea. The historian Bernard Fall is said to have characterized all of Vietnam as "two rice baskets on opposite ends of a carrying pole."[1] North and south, the rivers provided the nourishment. They have picked up everything from Yunnan Province in China, through Cambodia, Laos, and finally Vietnam. And even as the brimming, churning waters rush past, full of loosed vegetation and timber, dead tigers and water buffalo, they fail to affect the still ponds of endless rice fields, seething in cultivation. "Everything flows towards the Pacific, no time for anything to sink," wrote author Marguerite Duras.[2] Rivers are what defined the people, at once swirling and placid, a duality not unlike the Vietnamese spirit, an impatience and a lassitude, incandescent passions and quests for tranquility, a taste for war and a taste for peace. And the Central Highlands provided the fulcrum on which held the balance of either teetering end.

Nestled between the civilizations of China and India, it was given the name Indo-China by Danish geographical pioneer Conrad Malte-Brun in 1813. These fertile delta regions were home to a diverse group of peoples defined not only by geography but also culturally, linguistically, politically, and anthropologically. The inhabitants arose from the collision of Austroasiatic, Austronesian, and other proto-Indochinese populations. From those intersections arose the Viet, Khmer, Cham, and T'ai cultures. Each formed a largely peasant society ruled by village micro-oligarchies, though subservient to a bureaucracy of mandarins, responsible for the levy and collection of taxes. This was most developed in the country called Dai Nam (Great State of the South), also known by its old Chinese name of An Nam (Pacified South, generally referring to all of present-day Vietnam). Dai Nam hegemony extended south, enveloping neighboring Cham and Khmer territory in the lower Mekong delta, the Khmer city of Prei Nokor becoming Saigon in 1623.

Yet in the nineteenth century, Dai Nam was fraught with internal disorders, with emperors in the royal seat of Hue often battling hundreds of local uprisings. Coupled with the weakening power of neighboring territories and the ever-present pressure from China, a longtime protectorate of Indochina's economic and cultural (i.e., Confucianism) environment, Vietnam and the Indochinese region were ripe for foreign intervention. In the mid-nineteenth century, this came with the colonial aspirations of France. In order to compete with the widening influence of Great Britain, the French were eager to court favor with China, a huge economic market. The regions to the south bordering China—Indochina—looked to be a suitable entrée. It was Cochinchina, the most southern district, that first felt the boot of French colonialism. An expanded French presence in Indochina, regardless of their military dominance, would never have occurred without the acquiescence of China. And members of the Khmer and Lao royalty, boxed in by the dominant Siam and Viet empires, supported French colonial aspirations; they were willing "protectorates." Even more ominous, through a treaty that proved to be devastating for the royal court in Hue, French colonialists gained extensive holdings in southern Annam. The Vietnamese regions, populous and industrious as they were, could not rally a unified spirit of resistance and soon capitulated.

The voices of hard-liners clamored for the status quo, adherence to Confucian ideology, return of the emperor, and mandarin oversight. Lowlanders in the northern region of Dong Kinh (Tonkin) and central Annam, were the most vociferous. Throw out the French and the Catholics, they demanded. Insurgencies developed into guerrilla warfare. The Can Vuong in Annam, a largely peasant movement led by a few educated "literati," went after the French, intent on establishing a new emperor in Hue. Yet despite a patriotic spirit, such movements lacked cohesion and widespread support and were effectively subdued by French authorities. And the French, intent on bolstering their colonies against the neighboring British in Siam and receiving permission to occupy Tonkin from the Chinese through the treaty of 1884, essentially took over all regions of Dai Nam—Cochinchina to the south and Tonkin to the north—as protectorates and under the direct rule of French authorities. The emperor at Hue remained as a symbolic presence, but his influence was purely at the discretion of the French. French subjugation was detested and opposed, most palpably in Tonkin, and continued well into the next century. The dichotomy between a traditionalist, community-driven economy and culture and a desire for modernization and assimilation of Western values produced internal clashes among Vietnamese factions—and against their French colonists—that were not settled until the exit of American troops in 1973.

The French colonization of Indochina, and of Vietnam in particular, was a bittersweet experience for most Vietnamese. There was, to be sure, some degree of modernization that clearly benefited vast native populations, especially in the fields of health care and education (albeit highly selectively). But the suppression of independence and national unity along with blatant discrimination fueled an already unstable internal faction of revolutionaries that frequently boiled over into armed violence and brutality on both sides. It was not an unfamiliar emotion. For thousands of years, the people occupying these fragrant and fertile lands had rebelled against foreign intruders: the Chinese, Mongolians, and Japanese. Years of subjugation and insurrection fueled a patient intolerance, determination, and insurrection that bled these invaders white, their jungles, mountains, heat, and disease allies in a persistent desire for liberation. France's *mission civilisatrice*, best translated as "civilizing mission," of enlightening "inferior" colonized peoples—the latest imperialistic effort—was opposed by seething radicals, their clandestine maneuvering percolating just below a placid demeanor, intent on ousting the barbarians: "The Western demons will not disturb the kingdom any longer . . . may all the district chiefs and al the village chiefs gather in troops and pursue the pirates [French]."[3]

The Annamites, those peoples inhabiting this exotic land, were indeed a formidable opponent. In the words of Paul Doumer, governor general of French Indochina from 1897 to 1902, they were "beyond doubt superior to all the neighboring peoples. The Cambodians, the Laotians, the Siamese could not withstand them . . . the Annamites make an excellent soldier, disciplined and courageous."[4] This discipline and courage fostered the nationalist movements of the twentieth century that finally gained traction. The literati among the Vietnamese youth abandoned the concepts of Confucianism in favor of the international Communist movement in an effort to erase all vestiges of emperor and authoritarianism. The common field workers, abused by their French and Viet lords, must rise up and seize control of government. Various groups indeed rose and fell, many of the latter at the hands of ruthless French police, until in 1940 one seemed to capture the spirit of social revolution, the struggle of peasant classes against capitalist oppressors. This was the Viet Nam Doc Lap Dong Minh Hoi, the League for the Independence of Vietnam, founded by members of the Indochinese Communist Party under the guidance of a wiry, passionate revolutionary named Nguyen Ai Quoc, soon to be known as Ho Chi Minh. His insurgent nationalistic movement was shortened to the popular name Viet Minh. But it was a long and painful struggle. First there was occupation by Japan, then, at the end of World War II, the Chinese, and finally, a compromise in 1946 by Ho, allowing expulsion of Chinese troops from Tonkin in exchange for continued French presence. In turn, France was to recognize Vietnam as a "Free State," carefully avoiding the term "independence." For Ho Chi Minh it was a negotiated settlement, a compromise, on his long road to national liberty. As for the United States, after World War II, despite unanswered requests from Ho for assistance, there was a steadfast refusal to assist the French military effort and consistent encouragement of meaningful concessions to Vietnamese nationalism.[5]

Ho's Communist leanings were also a deterrent for whole-hearted support of his unification efforts. And his man-at-arms, Vo Nguyen Giap, was the perfect commander, educated, industrious, a student of history. Giap suffused a discipline among peasant volunteers, a desire for selfless service—even to death—tolerance of unimaginable hardships, and pride in the national effort. His was an uncanny understanding of strategy and tactics tailored to the ruggedness of his homeland that once again pecked at the colonialists—a death of a thousand cuts—until their taste for dominance soured like spoiled rice. It would be a people's effort, he said, a movement among all, a total commitment. Much like the great Vietnamese general Tran Hung Dao who repulsed three Mongol invasions in the thirteenth century, Giap perfected the art of guerrilla warfare and counterinsurgency.[6]

But France had no intention of stopping its meddling in Vietnamese affairs. Largely ignoring thoughts of freedom, the French bolstered their troop strength, convinced that the nationalist Viet Minh were preparing for war. Colonial presence and control was focused in the north, the fertile Tonkin Red River delta. Less accessible and hostile were the mountainous regions of the Viet Bac, hostile and teeming with Viet Minh. Negotiations with Ho Chi Minh faltered as the Viet Minh insisted on national independence through the unity of Tonkin, Annam, and Cochinchina. The French, fearful that independence for Vietnam would spell disaster for their protectorates in Laos and Cambodia and an end to their colonial grip in Southeast Asia, poured in troops and military supplies. The Viet Minh must be destroyed. So in 1946, the Franco-Viet Minh War commenced. Driven out of Hanoi, Giap's young troops took to the countryside and sought refuge in the Viet Bac and small villages of the Red River delta. The United States under President Harry S. Truman were hands off, but, in support of France, denounced Ho Chi Minh's Viet Minh movement and supported, instead, a monarchical alternative, the so-called Bao Dai solution.

Now in direct confrontation, the French and Viet Minh squared off. The Viet Minh, no longer a guerrilla movement but a well-trained, well-led, and well-equipped army, were formidable opponents. Finding refuge in the Viet Bac bordering China, Giap shuffled arms, men, and advisers back and forth. Mao Zedong's Communist China seemed an eager supporter. French expeditionary troops under General Henri Navarre tried to raid and disrupt Viet Minh strongholds there but were systematically picked apart. Ho Chi Minh referred to the war as a conflict "between the elephant and the grasshopper."[7] Lightly armed Viet Minh troops created havoc for roadbound French units, ambushing them from the cover of flanking forests and high vegetation. Under the meticulous guidance of General Giap, the Viet Minh had transformed their bands of guerrilla warriors into full-fledged combat units, supplied handily with heavy artillery from neighboring China. Key to their success was the widespread popular support, an almost universal hatred of the French colonialist, and the use of the unpredictable, hostile terrain to their advantage. During the early 1950s, successes on the battlefield seesawed between French and Viet Minh victories. The French held onto Hanoi and Haiphong, the Viet Minh to everything else.

All came to a head in a little-known remote valley called Dien Bien Phu where French paratroopers tempted Giap for a fight in the open.

Giap gave them one, dismantling French fortifications piecemeal in a seven week tour-de-force of massed artillery, strangling antiaircraft fire, and fanatical human wave attacks that whittled away at meager French defenses. Wounds, filth, hunger, and finally empty cannon and guns gave way to white flags of surrender. The capitulation on May 7, 1954, forced an imperative in peace talks at Geneva already underway. Tonkin, Annam, and Cochinchina would be partitioned into North and South Vietnam at the 17th Parallel. France would forsake North Vietnam and soon would leave Indochina altogether. Ho Chi Minh was half-way there, unification within his grasp. Now it would be America's turn. Having funded the majority of the war for the French in the later years they would step in to bolster a corrupt and inefficient government of South Vietnam, sucked into another Asian mess that held absolutely no value to it, only the delusional specter of a Communist world takeover.

22

Khe Sanh Village

WHILE THE SIEGE OF KHE SANH WAS NOT A REPLAY OF THE FRENCH meat grinder of Dien Bien Phu, the overwhelming worry on the part of American commanders was that it would end as tragically. As events unfolded around the Marine combat base in remote Quang Tri Province, the similarities with French entrapment at Dien Bien Phu became painfully obvious. At the highest levels of government all recoiled at the thought of an American garrison annihilated by a bunch of peasant warriors—among other misfortunes an embarrassment of American might. Even President Lyndon Johnson would say at the height of the siege, "I don't want any damn Din Bin Phoo."[1]

The tiny village of Khe Sanh served as headquarters for the Huong Hoa District, a remote, rural area of Quang Tri Province not quite forty miles west of the village of Dong Ha to the east and only twelve miles from the Laotian border. The area is mostly rugged and jungled and inhabited more by Montagnards, ethnic highland tribes, than by traditional Vietnamese. Khe Sanh is inexorably linked to the name Eugene Poilane and the Poilane offspring. The patriarch, Frenchman Eugene Poilane ("Papa Poilane" he was called), was born at Saint Sauveur-de-Landemont in the township of Maine-et-Loire on March 16, 1888.[2] His parents were humble peasant stock, frugal, sedulous, their very existence wedded to the soil. Motherless at an early age, Eugene could not be spared for schooling. Plowing, sowing, herding were indispensable to his father, and Eugene came to relish the land, the richness of the soil, the tendings to nature. So enthralled was he that only as a teenager did his formal education begin. Yet there was a restlessness brewing. At age eighteen, he enlisted in the colonial artillery at Toulon. Auspiciously, his unit was sent to Cochinchina in 1909. It was fifteen years before Eugene returned to his homeland. During the Great War, the young man pined for the front, his place in the trenches. Request denied. France's colonial empire needed him more. So he stayed, even after discharge, the vitality and lushness of Indochina absorbing him into its very soul. At the Botanical Garden in Saigon he met the botanist Auguste Chevalier just weeks before the armistice. Chevalier fed the young Frenchman's passion, sending him afield for the forestry service, a *prospecteur*, or field researcher. Poilane traveled throughout Indochina, to the borders of China and Burma, collecting and detailing more than thirty-six thousand botanical specimens.[3]

It was perhaps on one of these forays in 1918, floating up the Quang Tri River until it intersected with the Rao Quan heading north, a distance of almost twenty-five miles, that Poilane stumbled onto the hills of luxuriant greens, "so many different shades like emerald and jade," as one war correspondent later described them.[4] He might have debarked at the point where the Rao Quan flows by a red clay plateau near the area called Khe Sanh. Footpaths used by Mongols, Chams, and Annamites since the thirteenth century led him to the settlement of a French engineer intent on developing the trail that was to become Route Coloniale 9, the east-west track connecting Dong Ha to Lao Bao on the Laotian border. It led to the Col D'Ai Lao, that groove in the Annamite Cordillera affording passage from the inlands of Laos to the lowlands of Vietnam. Folks of the Bru montagnards drifted into Khe Sanh. Indigenous now to the highlands, Bru were mountain people, driven there by Annamites pushing in from the coast. Bru scattered about in villages so remote they could be accessed by footpaths only. Yet lowland Vietnamese had no countenance for them—simple and stupid they were called. Such antipathy one day bordered on genocide.[5] But Poilane saw an honesty, a loyalty that could not be ignored. He befriended them, guardians of a hidden paradise, and coveted their lands. He viewed the hills around Khe Sanh and marveled at the rusty-red laterite soil, a sight as beautiful and rich as the earth of Tuscany, he said. It was a region of lavish vegetation, triple-canopy forests rising sixty feet, bamboo thickets, and elephant grass sometimes as tall as a man. Tigers of gigantic size, the *tigre royal d'Annam* (royal tigers of Annam), roamed there; the same tigers that, when squeezed from their homeland, attacked human intruders. In fact, years later, in 1937, Major Howard Stent, then a battalion commander in the "Chinese Marines" (Fourth Marine Regiment) visited Khe Sanh to hunt tiger, such was the notoriety of the striped beasts. And underneath it all was a ubiquitous ruddy clay, fertile in its eagerness to pour forth plant life that triumphed in its exuberance.

In 1922, Poilane returned. It was then that he first cultivated his coffee trees. Chari trees were planted, with nine beans brought from Tonkin. The Chari tree came from Africa, a hardy specimen with fat trunk, long branches, and broad leaves, an ideal plant for the wealthy soil of Khe Sanh. His bride, the teenager Madam Yvonne Bourdeauducq, a Parisienne of high standing, whom he married on a short visit to France in 1925, was his companion. Together they toiled—plant and prune. But it was ten years before red cherrylike fruit, the coffee bean, blossomed. Bru tribesmen plucked the trees and aired the beans to dry, not only from Chari trees but also now from Robusta and Arabica trees, acres and acres. True to his botanical passions, Poilane, recognizing the synergism of climate and soil, introduced a variety of fruit trees in his plantation. Avocado, mango, banana, and persimmon groves dotted the landscape. Madam Bourdeauducq perched in trees and killed roving tigers. Not that she disliked the animals, but the vengeful beasts mauled and ate her peasant workers. Other planters followed, including Benedictine priests from Hue who took over the plantation of Madam Bourdeauducq after she and Papa Poilane divorced. Their breakup sent her just a mile up the road to begin her own coffee plantation. But she did not last. It was as if she had become an alien, or perhaps she sought only a more elegant life in Paris, her land lent as a departing gift to the fathers.

As for Eugene Poilane, he remarried, a woman of the Tay-Nung tribe they said, siring a total of ten children by both wives, five after age sixty. To work his prosperous plantation, Poilane brought in lowland Vietnamese eager to find employment, adding to the montagnard Bru workers. Both tended the coffee beans, thinning trees and turning soil. The Vietnamese would not live with the Bru. There was contempt for them. They considered the Bru to be uncivilized brutes. So each resided in their own villages. The Bru puzzled at the wanton behavior and hatred of their fellow countrymen. Entirely without gile, warm and accepting, the Bru lived apart and in tune with their own customs. Over the years, the populations of Khe Sanh swelled. By the 1960s it was almost two thousand—Bru in one spot, Vietnamese in another. The French built a fort near

Khe Sanh village in the 1940s, later abandoned after their exodus in 1954. Referred to as the Old French Fort, it was used for a time by American special operations troops in the early 1960s. War brutalized Khe Sanh. Eugene Poilane saw his plantation burned by the Japanese in 1945 and by the Viet Minh in 1953. It was so dangerous that he and his clan took refuge in an abandoned (and notorious) French prison at Lao Bao, just inside the Laotian border. But he always returned. Politics, French or Vietnamese, had little interest for him. It was nature, wild and unencumbered, that captivated and held him. Papa Poilane, by then plump and sporting a bushy white beard, was an icon of the region, a true godfather to his families. Yet this did not prevent tragedy. In 1964, he was gunned down by Viet Cong guerrillas who probably mistook him for the Quang Tri district chief they were intent on assassinating.[6]

More settlers arrived around Khe Sanh. John and Carolyn Miller, missionaries and Bible translators, came in 1961. They lived among the Bru, learning their dialect and transcribing the Bible in a language that had no written form. Father Pierre Poncet from the *Société des Missions Étrangers de Paris*—the Foreign Missions Society of Paris—arrived from Paris. He also mingled with the Bru, traveling from house to house on his motor scooter. One of Eugene Poilane's sons, Felix, who was born at Khe Sanh, returned to Vietnam in 1957 accompanied by his French wife, Madeleine. They took over management of his mother's plantation, the one maintained by the Benedictine fathers. Felix Poilane was pleased to return and enjoyed the company of his loyal Bru workers. His wife had a bit more trouble acclimatizing but eventually embraced the lifestyle and the friendship of her montagnards. "You will be a queen here," she recorded one of the Benedictine fathers telling her. Madeleine Poilane renovated the plantation house, a sixteen-room mansion that had been poorly maintained by the Benedictines, and named it Petite Fleur (Little Flower). Production soared. Shortly several tons of arabica, robusta, and Chari shipped to Dong Ha. So productive were the plantations that the South Vietnamese president, Ngo Dinh Diem, paid a visit in 1959.[7] And it was just up the road, between Eugene and Felix Poilane's plantations, that in 1962 American soldiers, with their wrinkled tiger-striped fatigues and stylish green berets, wanted to build an airstrip. It was a plateau—called the Xom Cham Plateau—of about seventy-five acres at an elevation of almost 1600 feet. The French had used it for their aviation. That flattop of red earth would eventually become the Khe Sanh combat base.

23

"Eye" Corps

On March 8, 1965, two battalion landing teams of the US 9th Marine Expeditionary Force splashed ashore on the beaches outside of Da Nang, South Vietnam. Their intended focus was perimeter security around the sprawling Da Nang Air Base. A US presence there began in 1955 but ramped up after attacks—largely exaggerated—by the North Vietnamese on the USS *Maddox* in the Gulf of Tonkin in August 1964. Combat aircraft from the 3rd Tactical Fighter Wing, the 18th Tactical Fighter Wing, and the 27th Tactical Fighter Wing were now crammed into barely finished parkways, wingtip to wingtip, inviting targets for saboteurs. And guerrilla activity had become noticeably more brazen. In the last half of 1964, armed Viet Cong (VC) units struck at outposts and hamlets in South Vietnam. On November 1, 1964, the American airbase at Bien Hoa suffered an audacious mortar attack that killed a number of personnel and destroyed or damaged twenty-two American aircraft. Overcrowded airfields at Tan Son Nhut, Bien Hoa, and Da Nang now lay exposed, with only token Vietnamese security. The Bien Hoa attack infuriated members of the Joint Chiefs of Staff and Defense Secretary Robert McNamara. Immediate retaliation began under the air operation Rolling Thunder. Unfazed, members of the Viet Cong 409th Battalion attacked Camp Holloway near Pleiku the night of February 6, 1965, killing eight US servicemen and injuring 126. "We're going to die. We're all going to die," an American soldier was heard to say.[1] Another brazen Viet Cong raid in the coastal city of Qui

Nhon two days later killed twenty-three Americans and wounded twenty-two at a US Army billet. President Johnson had had enough, and so had his Joint Chiefs. South Vietnam was crumbling. Corruption and intrigue ruled its government. Spotty protection of American assets was inviting retribution from willing Viet Cong rebels. South Vietnam chairman Phan Khac Suu's armed forces were close to incompetent. Americans were at risk. Send in the Marines, was the unanimous decision. But to allay fears of American involvement Marines were to be used only for base security—and for a limited period of time. The first destination was Da Nang, a mere 125 miles from the North Vietnamese border.

And so on that sunny day in March, Marines left their landing craft in full battle dress on the scenic beaches around Da Nang, and pretty Vietnamese girls in pastel áo dài greeted them with smiles and garlands of flowers—not quite the reception their fathers received on Iwo Jima. Hammered home was the directive from the Joint Chiefs of Staff: "[T]he U. S. Marine Force will not, repeat will not, engage in day-to-day actions against the Viet Cong."[2] General William Westmoreland was put in charge of the entire operation, named Military Assistance Command, Vietnam (MACV), perhaps to stress the assistance rather than the intrusion. Throughout the war, MACV was the joint command for US forces in South Vietnam, and it became synonymous with American meddling.

Among those in Washington clamoring for revenge there were few level heads. Maxwell Taylor, the ambassador to South Vietnam, was one of them; he felt the Marines were not armed, trained, or equipped for jungle guerrilla warfare and worried the United States, like France, would fail to adapt to conditions in Vietnam.[3] It was not usual Marine doctrine to occupy and hold territory. They were trained for amphibious operations, to strike swiftly, complete the mission, and withdraw. Occupying troops would then replace them. This had worked exceptionally well in the Pacific Theater during World War II. Indeed, commanders felt, the use of Marines instead of army paratroopers would give the impression of a short stay, just to allow time for adjustments in the South Vietnamese government. But skeptics wondered. Had that also not been the case in Korea, a surprise Inchon landing, liberation of Seoul, stabilization of the battlefield? Yet before long there they were, Marines deep into North Korea, in terrain and tactics and climate distinctly unfamiliar. Now, Vietnam and the broad strip of land separating North and South called the Demilitarized Zone, or DMZ, could prove to be another North Korea. Like elite French paratroopers a decade before, Marine "grunts" would be forced into the ground in bunkers and trenches, turning their offensive elan into a stale, stationary defense, biding their time with endless, seemingly meaningless patrols, waiting for the inevitable assault by a largely unseen enemy.[4]

Those Marines found themselves in a region of South Vietnam referred to as I Corps (pronounced "Eye" Corps in the vernacular) Tactical Zone. The Army of the Republic of Vietnam (ARVN) had divided South Vietnam into four "tactical" zones for political and military oversight. The most northern zone, I Corps, comprised the provinces of Quang Tri, Thua Thien-Hue, Quang Nam, Quang Tin, and Quang Ngai, the closest provinces to the DMZ. The DMZ had been marked out as a corridor roughly six miles wide running east-west, straddling the seventeenth parallel, and generally following the Ben Hai River.[5] The Geneva Accords of 1954 specified that "all military forces, supplies and equipment shall be withdrawn from the demilitarized zone" and that "[n]o person, military or civilian, shall be permitted to cross the provisional military demarcation line unless specifically authorized to do so by the Joint Commission."[6] While the intent was to provide a sort of no-mans land of inactivity, the DMZ was hardly demilitarized, the area crowded with Viet Cong guerrillas and North Vietnamese regulars. It was a strategic fulcrum for Hanoi. To the north, this wilderness sheltered thousands of North Vietnamese troops and was a staging area for incursions into South Vietnam. By 1968, it was estimated that forty thousand of the People's Army waited just on the other side of the DMZ. These so-called demilitarized sanctuaries also housed North Vietnamese cannon, which lobbed high explosives at Marines mired in muck and rain who had silenced their guns in obedience with ridiculous rules of engagement applying only to them. I Corps itself was a hornet's nest of criss-crossing North Vietnamese supply routes heading south into and out of bordering Laos. Honeycombed limestone caves and caverns on the eastern, Laotian, slopes of the Annamites provided natural barriers for detection on the ground or by air. Choking those trails was vital to the security of South Vietnam. For good or evil, Westmoreland needed his troops poised on the border of the DMZ.

I Corps was the bellwether for all of South Vietnam. Americans had been there since 1962. Special Forces A teams—Green Berets—were sent then, twelve-man units practiced in weapons, communication, and health care. Recruitment and training of local villagers was their aim, special militia called Civilian Irregular Defense Groups (CIDG). Mostly these were rustic montagnards with no love lost for lowland Vietnamese. From across the Laotian border they snooped and harassed Pathet Lao rebels, Viet Cong guerrillas, and North Vietnamese regulars. The Green Berets knew well the maze of paths through Laos to South Vietnam, tracks soon to be known collectively as the Ho Chi Minh Trail. Secluded in their fortified camps like frontier cowboys, these Special Forces trusted no one and slipped out unannounced for their clandestine deeds—but also in a paradoxical twist, offering humanitarian aid. The ultimate mission was to "win the hearts and minds."[7]

By May, the Marine presence had mushroomed to an entire division, the 3rd, and the 1st Marine Aircraft Wing, both placed under overall command of the 3rd Marine Amphibious Force (III MAF) with legendary Major General Lewis Walt in command. Within a year, even more Devil Dogs arrived, elements of the 1st Marine Division. I Corps became their singular AO—area of operations.[8] Of course there were ARVN troops as well, and furtive, clandestine activities of Special Forces prowling the back country. The Viet Cong felt their collective American heel as they pared back pestering of local peasants. But an ominous substitute was heavy traffic of North Vietnam regulars. Ho Chi Minh's timetable called for serious efforts at unification. Infiltration of the South shortly began in earnest.

The government of South Vietnam would not improve. From the top down, nepotism, vice, and stark incompetence reigned. A meager defensive ring of US troops around encampments was not going to turn the tide. Within a month, President Johnson countermanded the Joint Chiefs of Staff. By his authorization, at the urging of General Westmoreland, American units commenced offensive operations up to fifty miles from their bases—"search and destroy" were the buzzwords. Body counts. Kill more VC. Yet his concept of "enclaves"—keeping American troops in carefully contained coastal compounds to limit their exposure—was ineffective and short lived. The Viet Cong and, soon, Giap's Peoples' Army roamed the countryside and villages and haunted mountain retreats and sanctuaries, taunting and tormenting GIs hunkered behind their barbed-wire fortifications.

The 3rd Amphibious Force and its Marines had settled in. Tents, prefabs, Quonset huts, watchtowers, and concertina wire signaled sprouting communities in typical American fashion. Patrols roamed, flexing Marine muscle—M-14s locked and loaded—itching for contact with VC. Hand-in-hand with military action came medical support for the ubiquitous health care resources an expeditionary force demanded. Navy Commander Almon Wilson rolled his 3rd Medical Battalion through the earthy, narrow streets of Da Nang in June 1965 in caravans of noisy diesel-belching deuce-and-a-halfs. Wilson's outfit would be configured into four member companies, one deployed for each Marine regiment and one larger division hospital. At first, these were stark tent billets reminiscent of the typical MASH unit of Korean War vintage, laid out in orderly fashion—admission, triage, resuscitation, and two or three operating spaces. The medical staff were mainly young doctors with only a few years at most of experience. "Collect and clear" was the guiding principle. Officially, that meant evaluate, resuscitate, and evacuate—period. Any surgery was to address resuscitation and stabilization only: salvage from life- or limb-threatening injuries.[9] However, actual experience differed. Dr. (Captain) William Mahaffey, an anesthesiologist at 3rd Medical Battalion's C Company, "Charlie Med," divulged that in late 1965 and 1966, "Some people assumed that's all we did—stabilization. No way. We did definitive surgery." This included, apparently, a number of vascular cases.[10]

It was a stark existence in the Vietnam of 1965. Doctors of Charlie Med considered their experience "as a camping trip gone sour." Tents were old, sometimes rotting, hygiene and mess primitive—everyone ate out of cans and crapped in slit trenches. Wooden barracks with tin roofs eventually went up, but showers were still fifty-five gallon drums pouring water into large fruit-juice cans punched with holes—no hot water, of course. Screens were the only ventilation. And it was hot and dusty as only Da Nang's summers could be.

Indeed, the boys of Charlie Med were neophytes. Few had seen combat or, for that matter, much trauma at all. Fortunately, their chief, forty-one-year-old Almon Wilson was an old salt who had served as an ensign in four assault landings in the Pacific during World War II. Korea and rigorous surgical training in Utah gave Almon the credentials for a capable and patient mentor for his men. There would be much to teach—and soon, he reckoned: "We were going through the typical learning curve of young surgeons in a war . . . a new population of surgeons has to learn war surgery . . . in the civilian sector few injuries are true counterparts of combat injuries."[11]

In July 1965, headquarters, C Company, and most of D Company of 3rd Med were located in Da Nang; B Company and a platoon of D Company along with Force Logistic Supply Unit #1 (FLSU #1) at Chu Lai, a coastal town and Marine base about sixty-five miles southeast of Da Nang;[12] and A Company and FLSU #2 put at Phu Bai, an airfield and Marine Corps enclave northwest of Da Nang, close to the Imperial City of Hue. Sharp clashes with small groups of Viet Cong predictably produced a number of victims from automatic gunfire. That fall, Marine skirmishing picked up, and by December, Charie Med had been thoroughly baptized in combat medicine. During Operation Harvest Moon, a three-battalion foray into Viet Cong territory, Marine and ARVN troops battled entrenched guerrillas, rooting out most and driving off the rest, but not without a price. In one twenty-four-hour period, Charlie Med's shock and resuscitation teams worked on ninety-four wounded. "It was obvious from our Harvest Moon experience that we did not have enough ORs to keep up with the heavy casualty load," Wilson wrote to General Lewis Walt.[13] Almost immediately, Third Med in Da Nang, Chu Lai, and Phu Bai got several more Quonset huts, all for surgery and intensive care. Commanders prepared for the worst.

Paul Pitlyk was fresh from neurosurgery training at the Mayo Clinic and new in private practice, but even as a neurosurgeon Pitlyk was bored. That was when he made the radical decision to join the navy, "for the purpose of being assigned to a position with maximum need and excitement." Navy recruiters gladly ushered him in. After a whirlwind orientation he was standing in sweltering heat on the blacktop of Da Nang Air Base. It was late 1965. His bosses had assigned him to the sprawling Naval Support Activity Hospital under construction in Da Nang, to be the crown jewel of Navy medicine in Vietnam. But for Pitlyk that assignment was not to be. Viet Cong sappers, using satchel charges and raining in mortars, had just blown the place up, leveling much of the compound. Instead, he was off in a jeep to Charlie Med some nine miles distant with a nervous driver who couldn't wait to dump him off and get back. Charlie Med was in the boonies then, not entirely a safe neighborhood.[14] Concertina wire and armed guards made that clear. Inside, hardback tents were his billet and work space. It seemed more like a prison than a hospital. But behind its utilitarian design, the compound was remarkably equipped. He toured the shock tent, just off the helipad, the x-ray tent, and then a sandbagged tent with two cramped operating areas separated by a canvas curtain. Last in line was a larger tent containing forty cots for postoperative recovery. Foxholes manned by Marines with automatic weapons dotted the perimeter. Somewhere out there, people wanted to kill him. This was not Rochester, Minnesota. Excitement? Oh, there would be plenty of that. Before Naval Support Hospital Da Nang was finally finished, Charlie Med was *the* go-to hospital. Casualties came right from the battlefield—bloodied and bandaged. Too often the thumping of incoming choppers signaled more arrivals. Pilots loved the place—wide-open spaces for landing. They flocked to Charlie Med. Yes, Dr. Pitlyk, salutations from the tropical paradise of Vietnam.[15]

By 1966, Southern I Corps was a hotbed of activity. The entire 1st Marine Division had arrived in March and set up headquarters at Chu Lai. The place was an Americanized sea of billets and buildings and huts. On March 20, 1966, the 1st Med Battalion landed and shared tent space occupied by B Company, 3rd Med Battalion. And just in time. Between March 20 and 25, the 7th Marines tangled with the Viet Cong in northern Quang Ngai Province in Operation Texas, and brought in over one hundred wounded. The 1st Med was packed, with both operating rooms working, bandages and blood littering the floors. Surgeons got the message. Combat surgery was surge business—dozens at a time. No steady trickle here.[16] Like Commander Wilson before him, Commander Robert Mitchell clamored for more operating rooms, and got two more. He also dispatched a shock and resuscitation team to the Quang Ngai airstrip to sort through casualties fresh from battle. On their first venture in April during Operation Hot Springs, the team handled forty-five, medevacing thirty-eight to other facilities and returning seven to duty. Early interdiction, Mitchell felt, was instrumental in salvaging critical wounded and shortening helicopter transport times.[17] Other campaigns followed. Marines were determined on ousting "Charlies" who had infiltrated southern I Corps. Operations Kansas, Washington, and Colorado all supplied a steady stream of combat wounded to Chu Lai surgeons. The 1st Hospital Company arrived in April 1966 to back up the 1st Med Battalion. Extra doctors and corpsmen could be pulled and used if needed. For the time being, the hospital company itself would locate two miles from 1st Med in hardback buildings. A separate surgical unit was set up in MUST housing with triage, resuscitation, and operating spaces, enough room for upwards of fifty mass casualties.[18]

Back in Da Nang, Dr. Pitlyk's ultimate duty station, the Naval Support Activity (NSA) Hospital finally opened in January 1966. It had been a tortuous process. The hospital was put just outside of town, not too far from a stretch of sand later named "China Beach." Da Nang itself was a bleak little village in 1965, with rows of French-era one- and two-story stucco buildings bordering muddy, sewage-laden streets, without streetlights; it was pitch black after sundown. Throughout wafted the stink of raw sewage, drifting even across the Han River into more modern American dwellings. The Viet Cong rushed the hospital compound, still not complete, in October and used satchel charges to blow up much of what had been built. Intruders were cleared, damage removed, security improved, and building resumed. In mid-January, the place opened, with 120 beds. With expansion through 1968, it became the largest land-based medical facility in all of Vietnam, eventually providing over seven hundred beds for Marine and navy personnel. A vast complex, dozens of Quonset huts, were interconnected by cement walkways covered with wooden planking. The place soon had three receiving and resuscitation areas, four operating rooms, blood banking, and even a naval medical research unit. A chopper pad sat just outside "receiving," the area lined by canvas litters and corpsmen ready to empty arriving Chinooks.[19]

As at army evacuation and station hospitals, a wide scope of specialty care was provided: general, thoracic, plastic, orthopedic, and urologic surgery; neurosurgery; and medical specialties. Most doctors, though, were young GMOs—general medical officers—used primarily for triage—"sorting" would be the word used—and resuscitation. They learned quickly the ramifications of incompetence. There was no margin for error for horribly wounded Marines. In explosive, punishing war trauma—high thigh amputations, degloving groin and rectal injuries, open chest wounds—hemorrhage was colossal, rapid access for fluid and blood infusion imperative. It was quick, decisive business. Balk, freeze up, fumble and someone dies. The mental and physical stress slammed into surgeons' sanity. There was one disaster after another. Letters home told of fatigue, of utter inanition: "This past week . . . we've had quite a few patients. . . . Our census has risen abruptly from around 120 to 125 to 145 . . . and the crew is pretty seriously overtaxed. In particular is . . . our anesthesiologist who's been working around the clock for what must . . . seem like days and days and days."[20]

James Chaffee was a corpsman assigned to the NSA Hospital from 1967 to 1969. His task was to unload the big Chinooks and Sea Knights, bodies sometimes stacked one on top of another. Stretchers were taken right into the receiving areas and put on sawhorses. Weapons were removed, clothes cut off, vital signs taken, and three intravenous lines placed—sometimes with broad slashing cutdowns near the groin to find a large saphenous vein. First blood pressure and pulse were scribbled across chests with black markers. "Seeing chests with 0/0 and 0 was not uncommon," he said. Those were the boys who needed blood, and lots of it. Physicians engaged with laser focus, an intensity few knew before and would never know again. Author and Vietnam combat veteran Tim O'Brien described the attitude: "No time for sorting through options, no thinking at all; you just stuck your hands in and started plugging up holes."[21] It was a veritable ballet of practiced skill and teamwork. As combat doctors know, there is nothing like military triage and resuscitation in wartime. Nothing in civilian practice compares to it.

The daily stress was too much for some. Not uncommon were requests for transfer. They had seen enough—enough shattered boys and blood and raw tissue. And moans and cries and death. Too much for too long. Chaffee never forgot the images, even years later: "Circling above the room in my mind's eye, I can see the concrete floor covered with clotting blood like great mounds of liver, naked young men littering the room on blood-stained green stretchers."[22]

Paul Pitlyk understood that. Over at Charlie Med, the days and weeks after his arrival were filled with "a deluge of battered and broken bodies." Despite reports from the helicopters, one was never sure exactly what would be brought in. A number of casualties were dead on arrival, maybe 5 or 10 percent. They were put in body bags and stacked to the side. Others, he saw, had cataclysmic injuries from which there would be no survival: sheared skulls, holed chests, men with feeble pulses and gasping, agonal respirations. They were given slugs of morphine and also set aside. The rest were fair game. In alive, out alive was the maxim. All too often it just did not happen that way. Those were the heartbreaks. And sometimes doctors were at fault. He was one of those on Commander Wilson's learning curve: "It quickly became apparent that I was in over my head. . . . My fears about a lack of actual operating experience were justified. Mistakes happened. The war happened. I probably killed some kids back in those early days at Charlie Med, killed them through my efforts to save their lives."[23]

Jim Chandler was a fully trained surgeon. As soon as he finished his seven-year residency at Columbia Presbyterian Hospital in New York City, he headed straight for Camp Pendleton, California. After an orientation of three or four weeks, he was off to Da Nang, a newly christened lieutenant commander in the navy. It was February 1966. Charlie Med was his first assignment. Little had changed since Paul Pitlyk's arrival. Personal tents were still canvas, no hardbacks. There was no ventilation, it was hot, and on the perimeter of the hospital grounds there was only a solitary Marine guard standing between him and the great beyond. But he never got to his "hooch," (slang for quarters), not that day. No sooner had he stepped from his jeep than mass casualties came in. Off Chandler went. His first cases were a number of Marines "who had been literally broiled in an armored personnel carrier that got hit and then caught fire. They came in kind of stuck together. It was horrid. . . . So I just went into the operating room and got them apart and resuscitated. I don't think any of them survived."[24]

All his training did absolutely no good that day. It was a different kind of surgery, a different world. Amazing that humans could get so smashed and still live long enough to test the wills of the medical profession, their frames unrecognizable, more dead than alive. Doctors pumped spent physiology with a pretense of hope. It was for those times—those rare times—when one sad case actually came back, soul and body again united. But it was a sorcerer's balm. Fogs of tragedies blanketed even the most miraculous rescues, leaving many lost in a pale of grief.

Meantime, up in northern I Corps, Poilane's little paradise of Khe Sanh lay smack on the route into Laos from coastal Dong Ha and not too far from the DMZ. Americans knew it and so did Hanoi. Through the Col D'Ai Lao they poured, venturing into Khe Sanh, a natural gateway to the south. Even the French had been aware of its strategic value, building a fort in 1950 about one mile east. Up from the village past Poilane's place was the Xom Cham Plateau, a flattened strip of acreage on which the French had leveled a rough landing strip. Sneaky Special Forces types had been rummaging around there for years, first showing up in 1962, sometimes linked with supersnooping CIA operatives intent on nothing admitable. In fact, in December 1965, the Xom Cham compound was made a forward operating base (FOB) for the highly secret MACV-SOG (Military Assistance Command, Vietnam Studies and Observation Group—also known as Special Operations Group), housing all kinds of spies and "fringe" military. Their game was clandestine harassment, political bullying, capture of prisoners, sabotage, and intelli-

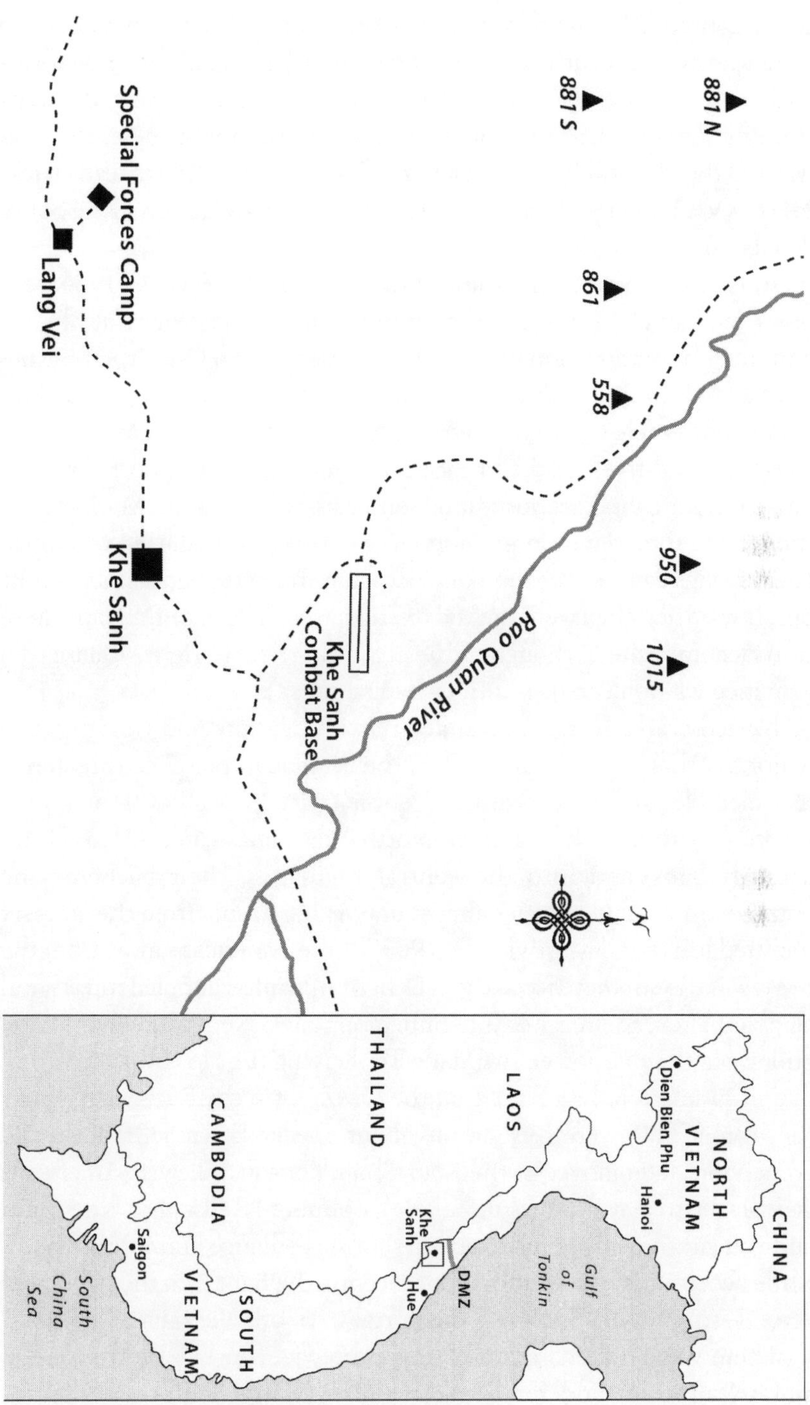

Map 5. Vietnam and the Khe Sanh area, 1968.

gence gathering. It was Special Forces on steroids. Small groups of Green Berets and other sleuths conducted cross-border operations into Laos—and even over the DMZ into North Vietnam—under the code name Shining Brass, feeling out Viet Cong and North Vietnamese, their reports to this day still highly redacted.[25] What did they find? Steady trickles of NVA regulars[26] heading south, filtering in and around Khe Sanh. Trouble was in the making.

In fact Marine reconnaissance units visited Khe Sanh in 1964, sent to spy on Viet Cong in the area after insurgents had systematically blown a number of bridges along Route 9. "Advisory Team One" the Marines were called, in line with official American posture of advisement only. It was a miserable few weeks Gyrenes spent on Tiger Tooth Mountain, a five-thousand-five-hundred foot peak some eight miles north of Xom Cham. Cold canned rations, mud, and rain hounded the Marines, but they found themselves in the middle of constant traffic back and forth, NVA troops came so close on one occasion that a firefight almost broke out. It was then they were yanked off Tiger Tooth back to Da Nang. Mission accomplished, though. Shining Brass had it right. Quang Tri Province was fomenting seditious happenings.

No secret, really. Hanoi was keen on unification, and I Corps was a major marshaling area. After 1965, the American presence threatened its timetable and upset local insurgent activity. A swell of troop movements sent tens of thousands of North Vietnamese around the DMZ, through Laos, and into the central highlands, their backbreaking portage, trucks, and bicycles almost impossible to spot from the air—six hundred tons per day arriving by 1966.[27] Lure Americans away from the coast was the strategy. Force them to fight in triple-canopied forests, tall elephant grass, and rugged Annamite mountains. Neutralize their armor. Hide from their airpower. In Quang Tri, leaving the Ho Chi Minh Trail, over Route 9 from Lao Bao, from the DMZ down the Rao Quan Valley they came. They were very curious about Special Forces FOB at the old French fort, later moved to the Xom Cham Plateau. Likewise Americans were eager to stay. In Westmoreland's opinion, "Relinquish Khe Sanh and you gave up all those advantages [of surveillance and interdiction], while accepting the inevitability of carrying the fight into the populated coastal strip."[28] Khe Sanh was the portal to South Vietnam.

There was no denying, trouble was brewing. In fall 1966, General Lewis Walt, commander of III MAF, shifted Marine units farther north, near the DMZ. Headquarters, 3rd Marine Division, moved from Da

Nnang to Phu Bai. Even farther north, at Dong Ha, a forward command post was placed. The 1st Marine Division headquarters then shifted from Chu Lai to Da Nang. Just below the DMZ, Route 9 was crucial. Keep it open to Americans. Deny the enemy access to deep I Corps and keep them from outflanking and encircling Marines along the DMZ. Westmoreland's Khe Sanh was a choke point. By October 1966, a battalion of Marines landed on the Xom Cham Plateau and set up a perimeter. The combat base was born.

The 3rd Med Battalion shifted north as well, following the anticipated violence. Year's end found A Med still at Phu Bai and B Med having moved to Da Nang and An Hoa. C Med, Charlie Med, remained at Da Nang, and D Med had been sent up to Dong Ha. D Med—Delta Med—was vital, the most northern surgical unit, almost to the DMZ. It had three operating rooms and thirty beds for combat wounded. It was a minifortress of steel barriers, corrugated Quonset huts, covered walkways, and a watchtower stuck in the middle of nowhere. Delta Med saw it all, not just combat wounded. In February 1967, Corpsman Paul Churchill saw one Marine who had been mauled by a tiger just outside Khe Sanh. "It was almost as though a surgeon had removed his biceps. The humerus was lying there perfectly clean and just white as snow. It wasn't even bleeding." Dr. Gustave Hodge, the surgeon on duty that night, remembered the fellow saying a tiger grabbed him by the arm, dragged him from his foxhole, and shook him like a rag doll. He finally punched the animal in the nose and managed to fire off a few rounds. The tiger ran off, and he called for help. The wound was irrigated and dressed and the patient medevaced out to a waiting hospital ship, arm saved.[29]

24

Indian Country

By 1967, intelligence reports had confirmed that areas near the DMZ were critical in Hanoi's efforts to insert regular army troops. In response, General Westmoreland designed the "strong-point obstacle" system, OPLAN 11-67—code name Practice Nine—a series of battalion-sized combat bases just south of the DMZ extending from Dong Ha west in a six-hundred-yard-wide swath through Gio Linh, Con Thien, Cam Lo, and Khe Sanh. Counterinsurgency efforts, Westmoreland called them. It would forever be known as "McNamara's Line" after its strong endorsement by the secretary of defense. Marine commanders were not fond of the concept, tying down their troops in defensive and reactionary roles. One Marine officer described it as "just one more 'happening' in the Defense Department's Alice in Wonderland approach to insurgency."[1] Marines, in the meantime, busied themselves with constructing bunkers, clearing tracks of land for fields of fire, and improving Route 9 between Dong Ha and the Laotian border—and hunkered down to take a pounding. At Khe Sanh, the Marine garrison had been downsized to a single rifle company and a few cannon. The combat base—the Xom Cham Plateau—sitting as it was on the far edge of McNamara's Line, was no longer a priority. There would only be enough Marines to protect the airstrip and send occasional patrols into the countryside. But the North Vietnamese had different ideas. The base represented an unwelcome presence. And General Giap, whatever his thinking, found out how dearly Americans would pay to keep it occupied. Shelling began in earnest in March, and probing efforts against the perimeter put General

Walt on notice that the North Vietnamese were nosey. As a result, another company of Marines was flown in to reinforce.[2]

Three major hills overlooked passages into Khe Sanh from the northwest: Hills 861, 881N (North), and 881 South (S), the latter two separated by a sloping saddle.[3] Together with Dong Tri Mountain, these high points dominated the landscape and commanded a view of the plateau. Yet the strategic hilltops were miles from the combat base itself—Hill 881S was over four miles distant—all through dense underbrush, elephant grass, and jungle. After sharp clashes with enemy troops in those hills, reconnaissance teams surmised there was a growing North Vietnamese presence around Khe Sanh. In fact, the worry was that Hanoi intended to take over the combat base. Hill country was already in its hands. It fell to infantry of the 3rd Marines to drive them off.[4] On April 24, 1967, bloody fights known as the Hill Battles began. Marines roamed up and down impossible terrain, enduring bitter clashes in bush, on near vertical slopes, and facing almost invisible trenchlines. Add downpours and it was miserable going. Lieutenant Jim Lally was the sole medical officer for these assault platoons, and he had ten corpsmen. Frontier medicine it would be. There was lousy weather, hideous terrain, and few options for critical cases except to get them the hell out. That is, if they didn't die on the way. And the dead went anyway. After an ambush on Hill 861, Captain Michael Sayers described the awful ordeal of lugging out his company's casualties: "We were carrying KIAs and WIAs in ponchos [borne by] four men to a litter. The heat deteriorated the bodies rapidly and they bloated fast. Almost impossible to carry in the dark, the mud, and the rain. Many times we stopped our march to retrieve a body that had fallen out of a poncho and rolled down a hill."[5]

The NVA were dug in deep. Bunkers, spider holes, and dugouts covered hilltops. They were literally gutted by artillery and napalm-rich air strikes, balding the crowns of those scarred slopes. But it still took the infantrymen to pry them out one at a time with grenades, rifles, and even knives. Landscape turned into moonscape, brought home by vivid photographs from journalist Cathy Leroy in the pages of *Life* magazine. Stark, stripped woodlands "evoked ghosts of Iwo Jima and Pork Chop Hill," according to *Time* magazine.[6] And, for the first time, the specter of Dien Bien Phu, the French debacle of a decade before, crept in. Would the same fate befall Khe Sanh, the press wondered? The geography of these primitive highlands was eerily similar.[7] Marines had a different name for the place: "Indian Country," no home for the tender hearted. Wild firefights—rattling off clips of M-14s and M-16s—clubbings, stabbings. Back and forth the skirmishes waxed and waned, advance and retreat—and charge again. Fallen Marines were pulled to safety by corpsmen, dragged or carried through thickets to scratched-out landing zones, heaved on choppers, and sent to the combat base and Lally's aid station, or what there was of it: "The now almost forgotten art of chest auscultation and percussion were indispensable in triaging the wounded . . . medical supplies were somewhat limited. . . . Although intravenous fluids and morphine were plentiful, one rarely had whole blood to administer. We had basic surgical instruments, and the few chest tubes that we had we used sparingly."[8]

Corpsmen were heroes; easy targets as they hunched over victims, wrapping wounds, pushing morphine. Michael Gibbs, corpsman for Kilo Company was one of those. Giving first aid to wounded Marines, he was hit in the back; moving to another fallen Marine he was hit in the leg. The next day he was shot again and killed. Six other corpsmen perished in the two weeks on the hills, a sacrilegious, lonely place for brave men to die.

Marines kept whacking the NVA, who kept whacking them, until from sheer attrition and exhaustion, the North Vietnamese gave up and melted away. It all cost the Marines dearly. In two weeks of vicious fighting, 155 had died and 425 were wounded. Smelling trouble, a special clearing platoon of Charlie Med had been sent to the combat base on April 27 (the remainder of Charlie Med moved up to Phu Bai from Da Nang that same month), but most casualties had been flown out. Quick survey and treatment by Lally and gone. D Med at Dong Ha got them, 353 wounded—it was damage-control stuff: stop the bleeding, stabilize, and evacuate—sending a number back to A Med at Phu Bai and the NSA Hospital in Da Nang.[9]

But Hanoi was not done with Khe Sanh, not by a long shot. Through the summer Giap's bo doi (ground troops) slipped back in, silently. Before long, Route 9, the only passable road to the coast, was cut off. Ground traffic was halted; bridges were out, ambushes likely. Any garrison at Khe Sanh would subsist on the air. Navy Seabees extended and reinforced the dirt airstrip at the combat base. Rock crushers were brought in for a heavy gravel foundation; steel matting was laid down. On October 27, twin-engine C-123s and quad C-130s began to make daily appearances.

The North Vietnamese had returned. Enemy sightings proliferated, and a few seen meant many hidden. Operations Crockett and Ardmore

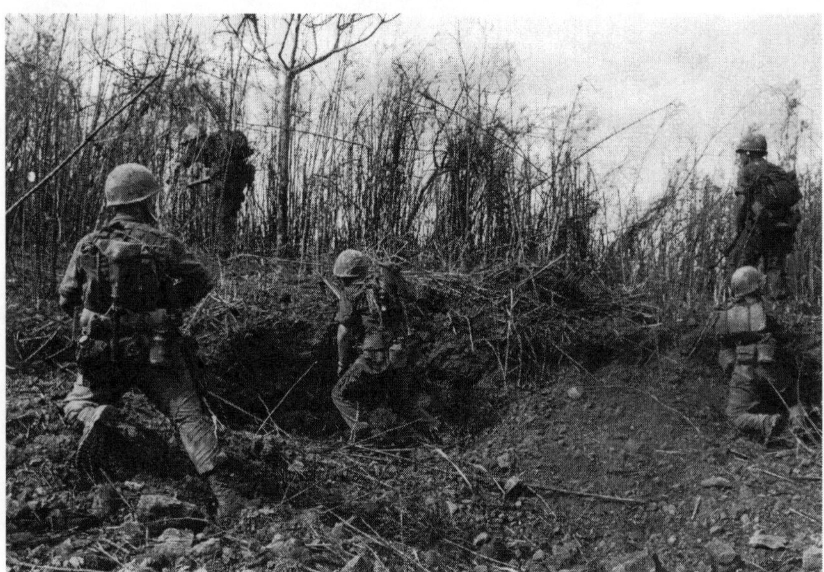

Company G, 2nd Battalion, 3rd Marines assault Hill 881 N, on April 29, 1967. (*National Archives*)

scoured the hills, uncovering nests of North Vietnamese. Sharp exchanges followed. More Marines were pumped in. By fall, a full battalion of the 26th Marines occupied the combat base. Mustachioed Colonel David Lownds, a veteran of Saipan and Iwo Jima and Korea, assumed command in August. Next door, Special Forces of FOB-3 moved in, dug bunkers, and tried to coexist with restless Marines. An uneasy peace prevailed: "The Marines tended to view the Green Berets as an undisciplined rabble, while the Special Forces saw the Jar Heads as a collection of clumsy, overarmed, overheavy units who would never be able to cope with the VC [Viet Cong] and NVA."[10]

No one liked it. One Special Forces trooper had said Khe Sanh "was cold, terrible. For combat operations, it was pitiful; it was terrible. You could not depend on decent weather."[11] With the onset of the monsoon season, that proved only so true. When there were no outright downpours, the steady drizzles, called crachin, seemed to soak everything.[12] Tents, bunkers, supplies never really dried out. More Marines headed for the hills, an entire battalion—outposts on this harsh frontier—bolstering defenses with trenches, bunkers, and endless rows of wire. Cargo planes brought supplies into the airstrip, and they were shuttled to helicopters, then choppered to outpost stations in foggy weather—or sometimes not. Corpsman William Gerrard remembered his time on Hill 881S: "Once or twice we got down to one meal a day. . . . The best we ever had was two meals a day eating C-rations." He came off the hills with seventy days' growth of beard and twenty pounds lighter. "We had been living on less than a canteen of water the whole time we were up there." They were supposed to spend only one day up there, they were told. Somehow, it just didn't work out that way.[13]

Single-file columns of faded green dungarees, pith helmets, rubber sandals, and slung Kalashnikov rifles snaked their way through vegetation thick enough to hide an elephant. On bicycles and backs, bo doi and thousands of dan cong—civilian volunteer porters—lugged provisions and ammunition and guns without a sound, without a whimper. Ducking into caves, creatures of the night, they were barely noticeable even from above. Thousands flocked just as they had to Dien Bien Phu. The glorious revolution moved forward, every fighter, every peasant worker a small cog in a big, grinding wheel. This enemy, a new enemy, would crumble like the last, the hated French. All colonial imperialists would drown in cesspools of their own making. So said the songs on long treks south. By December, at least two North Vietnamese divisions had arrived and were locked in around Khe Sanh.

The Marines sensed their isolation. Their strategic hilltops were laced with dugouts and trenches and concertina wire. Vegetation was cleared one-hundred-fifty-feet out from perimeters. At MACV, inescapable comparisons of Khe Sanh and Dien Bien Phu were topics of conversation. A letter to the editor of the *Washington Post* from historian Arthur Schlesinger Jr. argued that once the North Vietnamese had surrounded the base, "a humane or intelligent leadership would have arranged for the immediate evacuation of the men." "Whatever we do," he went on to say, "we must not reenact Dien Bien Phu."[14] Meanwhile the combat base bristled for an attack. One company commander wryly remarked "I can smell . . . the enemy."[15]

As the New Year broke, a Marine listening post just beyond the main perimeter picked up activity. A squad sent to investigate found six Asians in what appeared to be Marine uniforms loitering about. When they failed to respond to a challenge and one seemed to go for a grenade, Marine sentries cut them down. Five were killed and the sixth man limped away. All the dead proved to be ranking officers of the People's Army. Khe Sanh, the Marines assumed, must be high priority. A third battalion of the 26th Marines was brought in. All the regiment's battalions were now in one location, the first time since Iwo Jima. Security on the hills tightened, making sure all approaches from the northwest were under surveillance. By early January, Colonel Lownds had three battalions of infantry, one battalion of artillery, a Special Forces group, montagnards of FOB-3, and several army 175-mm guns at Camp Carroll and "the Rockpile" were ranged in.[16] There was also a CIDG group of Special Forces and montagnards at their heavily fortified camp near the village of Làng Vei on Route 9, five-and-a-half miles from the combat base and only a mile-and-a-quarter from the Laotian border. A small MACV advisory team, and a Marine Combined Action Company Oscar—the Marine counterpart of the Army's CIDG militia-advisors—were housed in the village of Khe Sanh itself. Strange bedfellows: None of the Special Forces had anything to do with Lownds and would have liked to have had nothing to do with the Marines, unless they needed bailing out. The whole affair was hush-hush. The special ops guys talked in subdued tones and kept buttoned up about their mysterious incursions. They were under different command, all the way to Da Nang and Saigon.

Would it be another Dien Bien Phu? There were uncanny similarities: a comparable American tactical mind-set—establishing enclaves segregated from the native population; an outpost in a remote valley surrounded by hills; long, insecure supply lines; total dependency on aerial resupply; and predictably lousy weather. Inevitably the analogy stuck. Jules Roy's book *The Battle of Dienbienphu* was popular reading at the time. And what was critical, really critical, for the defenders, was that the Marines' water supply lay almost a third of a mile outside the base perimeter. North Vietnamese tampering with that would have disastrous implications for the garrison. By late 1967, President Johnson had taken a personal interest in the situation, reassured, of course, by his commanders that Khe Sanh could be successfully held. In January, the White House came to resemble a military command post. Don Oberdorfer, in his book *Tet*, wrote, "The President and [presidential advisor Walt] Rostow were mentally in the trenches with the boys."[17] Ambassador Maxwell Taylor felt Khe Sanh had "Dien Bien Phu written all over it."[18] Roughly six thousand American troops were surrounded—trapped, some would say—by upward of twenty thousand North Vietnamese regulars and their well-concealed artillery. To some extent it was Giap's call. Would he want to make this another Dien Bien Phu—albeit at an enormous cost—or feint and draw American attention from the rest of his

Phase 2 offensive that was to strike elsewhere in South Vietnam? Some suspected the worst. On the Marine Corps' "birthday," November 10, 1967, Colonel Lownds told his men, "You all will soon be in the American history books."[19]

With abruptness it began. Just after midnight on January 21, Marines occupying Hill 861 were suddenly attacked. The first victim was a corpsman, "Doc" Malcolm Mole, twenty years old. Out for an early morning walk, he was hit by a rocket-propelled grenade and instantly killed. Then the North Vietnamese opened up with volleys of automatic fire. The surprised Marines were almost tossed off the hill, but determined leadership and savage hand-to-hand combat finally drove back the attackers. Several hours later, just before dawn, the 1st Battalion, 26th Marines guarding the combat base perimeter received approximately one hundred mortar rounds and twenty rockets in their sector alone, hitting the main ammunition dump. Almost one thousand five hundred tons of ammunition erupted in a huge fireball, spewing shrapnel and live rounds all over the immediate area. Some shells, glowing red hot, landed in the trenches, and Marines had to gingerly cart them away. Later in the morning, a second blast of stores of the plastic explosive C-4 occurred with such intensity that thick roofing timbers cracked.[20] The People's Army had placed its opening bid on Khe Sanh.

Dr. Edward Feldman was a New Yorker, born in 1941. He grew up in Queens and eventually, after a convoluted path, graduated from the Kansas City College of Osteopathic Medicine in 1966. Shortly afterward, "greetings" by his Selective Service Board labeled him "1A." By hook or by crook, Feldman finagled a spot with the navy, and he was commissioned in August 1967. Even with the usual snafu of military transportation, he was in Da Nang by Christmas. His first assignment was B Med at Phu Bai, but that didn't last long. On January 3, Feldman was scurrying out of a C-130 onto the rusty clay of Khe Sanh. His work station would be the two brown tents of the 1st Battalion aid station, one for storing supplies and the other for sick call and casualty care. Dangling light bulbs provided dim illumination for minor surgery but nothing big, it was stressed. A limited inventory of surgical instruments—scalpels, hemostats, scissors, needle drivers, and small retractors—guaranteed that. Surgery was reserved for boils, ingrown toenails, and thrombosed hemorrhoids. Serious stuff would be sent over to Charlie Med. Feldman was not a watcher, he was a doer. Within five days, he was in the bush, volunteering for a battalion-sized search-and-destroy mission. There was no enemy contact but plenty of physical activity.[21] In fact, in the process of stumbling up and down slopes in stifling humidity, Feldman managed to break his precious IV bottles and lose nine pounds. The NVA was out there, about that he had no doubt. "I don't know how they could not have seen a thousand guys walking through the woods."[22]

But January 21 was different, with detonations of thunder and fire. Feldman remembered every minute of that morning as he scrambled to get dressed: "I was very frightened. And I can underline the word 'very.' I was trying to tie my boots and my hands were shaking. I was in no position to help anyone in this bunker [his personal bunker] by myself."[23]

The rounds sounded like "freight trains" coming in and punched holes "the size of a Volkswagen." Aid station tents had taken a direct hit and were aflame and in tatters. Injured were quickly transferred to the holding bunker. One of the first casualties was a Marine with a belly wound, as it turned out some sort of "pipe" sticking out of his abdomen. All took a step back. Unexploded ordnance was the immediate concern. He was placed in a corner and sandbagged. With some trepidation ("If anything bad happens, just get rid of these personal letters of mine," he told a friend), Feldman removed the canister, pushing tissue off of it, and disposed of it outside. The poor fellow then went into shock and was rushed over to Charlie Med, where a liver laceration was repaired. After that he was off to Phu Bai, alive. Feldman saw sixty more casualties that day, now something of a celebrity. His summary comment about that whole day: "many brave deeds by young men." Ed Feldman's tour was up in February, but he would not leave. Pleadings to Commander Brown, head of the 3rd Med Battalion, to stay were heard and granted. He would be assigned to Charlie Med.[24]

The small group of army advisers (Green Berets), Marines of CAC–Oscar, and a number of Bru warriors inhabited the Huong Hoa District Compound near Khe Sanh village. Their post included an old French fort built in colonial days and an adjacent landing zone. That morning of January 21, mortar rounds fell on them, too. Behind the barrage, in thick morning fog, came North Vietnamese, crawling up to the perimeter undetected. Now they were almost upon the defenders. Medic Jim Perry, always with a Thompson submachine gun and an automatic pistol, jumped from his bunk and joined other Green Berets firing through the mist at approaching shadows. Khe Sanh was under attack. For the next twenty-four hours, Perry's team fought off hundreds of North Vietnamese troops. A relief force flown in of ARVN troops and some American advisers was ambushed at the landing zone by North Vietnamese. It was a massacre. Thirteen American pilots and seventy-four ARVN troops were cut down.[25] Nevertheless, Special Forces, Marines, and Bru tribesmen somehow prevailed, killing many enemy and forcing a withdrawal of the rest. However, under attack and most certainly surrounded, Lownds had his own problems at the combat base. No more could he commit artillery or troops for the district compound. It had to be abandoned. Helicopters descended, loaded wounded and refugees, and sped over to the combat base, medic Perry one of the last out. Green Berets, Marine CAC people, and Bru warriors hit the bush, sneaking past North Vietnamese troops on foot for eight kilometers, heading for the combat base. Lownds opened the doors for them—all except the Bru. Marines distrusted natives, no matter what ethnicity. Too many spies and saboteurs, they figured. The gates shut. Seventy-seven days of siege had begun.

LIEUTENANT COMMANDER JAMES FINNEGAN's father insisted his son serve in the military. A steelworker from Pittsburgh, his dad was kept out of the military during World War II. Hard hats were vital to the effort. Young Jim was an Irish kid from the tough side of the tracks. College was a struggle. A little bit of a rebel, a little restless, he was floundering at the University of Pittsburgh. On advice from high school teachers, he transferred to LaSalle University in Philadelphia. It was a total rebirth. Finnegan excelled and placed among the freshman class at Hahnemann Medical College. A standout in medical school, Finnegan won a spot at the Hospital of the University of Pennsylvania for surgical training. The days were grueling, with rigorous duty under the new surgery chief, Jonathan Rhoads. But what caught Finnegan's eye was the trouble brewing in Vietnam, and his father's words echoed in his head. After three years of residency, Finnegan begged his navy recruiter to be sent overseas. Dr. Rhoads, a longtime supporter of the military, understood. "[Your] place is preserved," he told Finnegan. "So when you're ready, you'll be welcomed back."

Finnegan's navy odyssey took him from Camp Lejeune to San Francisco to Okinawa and finally Da Nang. The Marine Corps—Semper Fi, baby. And they loved their doctors. "Doc, if anything happens to you, it means that every Marine around you is dead," one burly sergeant told him. His military occupational specialty? Surgeon of course, after three years of surgical residency. He went to D Med up at Dong Ha first. Near the DMZ there was no dearth of business. It was immersion. No toe testing—jump in. Tons of casualties. Finnegan kept things simple. His principles: "stop the bleeding, get rid of the bad parts, put the other stuff back together." And then in February, James Finnegan, tough kid from Pittsburgh, was on a Huey gunship into Khe Sanh. Relieve some shell-shocked doctor, they said. His first impression? "What is this? What are we doing here?" Charlie Med was an assembly of canvas tents surrounded by sandbags. Second impression: there were way too many holes in that canvas. Three other doctors met him. Joe Wolf, the anesthesiologist with six weeks of training; the famous Ed Feldman; and former battalion surgeon Don Magilligan. Finnegan was the head surgeon, though. It was he who would get Marines through or not. Under him at Charlie Med, anything was doable. Without him, men would die.[26]

These were young doctors, some barely out of internship. None had seen such violence, and what training they had after medical school was structured, supervised. Not here. No senior members to give careful guidance, to look over their shoulders. They were on their own. For some it was a maturing experience, full of good and bad, successes and failures, and they were grateful for the ones they could save. For others, it was complete destruction. Seeing young boys die from their ineptitude was crushing. At times it was mind-bending. So much damage, so much urgency, so many dead, so many more. Was this their idea of medicine, of healing? Medical training was supposed to be a rational, structured process of progressive competence and autonomy, albeit with careful supervision. That was the sane approach, tried and true. Here? Not the slightest resemblance to structure. Guilt or remorse? That would come, but not right away. Not enough time for that. The next case was waiting. And the next and the next. Navy surgeon Al Levin recalled, "It was mud, screams, and the terrible smell of death." But then, maybe just as bad, he recounted, "[T]he soldiers would look at me like I was God, like I could put this mess back together. But a lot of times, there was nothing I could do. I remember the sense of timelessness. Except for helicopters, I might as well have been in the mud in Gettysburg or Valley Forge—that's how much I could do for those guys."[27]

So here they were now, Jim Finnegan, Joe Wolf, Ed Feldman, and Don Magilligan: the core of Charlie Med, Second Platoon. The outfit first set up in four fifteen- by thirty-foot tents, one for sick call, one for supplies, and two for living quarters. Once the shelling began, sandbags were piled high and tents transformed into triage areas. Too dangerous for sawhorses—no one would stick their head above sandbag level—litters were put on the ground. Doctors treated them there, on hands and knees. Jim Thomas remembered those days. Dr. Thomas had just completed one, and only one, year of internship under Dr. Ben Eiseman, a Vietnam veteran himself, at the University of Kentucky. Thomas was a native of Ashland, Kentucky, an old Appalachian steel mill town. He attended all-black Booker T. Washington High School there, one of the last to graduate before desegregation closed it in 1962. Morehead State University was next and then the new University of Kentucky College of Medicine. Thomas was in one of the first graduating classes. After a surgical internship, he entered the navy as a commissioned officer. By July 1967, he was in Vietnam, a battalion surgeon. His first experiences were horrific. He was in a bomb crater aid station "full of dead and dying." From there it was Phu Bai and the MUST confines of A Med. Now a tested veteran, Thomas helped in triage and even did some minor surgery. Someone noticed. For his skill and cunning, Thomas, too, was ferried to Khe Sanh and Charlie Med. His tiny sunken "hooch" was small comfort. Most of those early days were spent upstairs in the triage area, crawling from casualty to casualty, cutting away pants legs, peeling off bandages, probing wounds, suturing. It was far too hazardous to stand.

There was Thomas that Sunday morning, January 21, bending over a Marine who had lost half his jaw, hit by shrapnel full in the face. There was gurgling, stridor—signs of airway obstruction. A tracheostomy was the only hope, otherwise the kid would asphyxiate. Had Thomas ever done one before? Doubtful he had. With his helmet firmly in place, Thomas made the standard low neck incision—too shallow. Deeper still, he knew. Dig for the trachea. Damn, there's a lot of blood. Found it. Another cut across the windpipe. A gush of air. Shove in a tube. Bag him! Good, breathing easier now. "[T]he operation went very well," he later wisecracked. But one never got too cavalier there, if only because personal safety was so arbitrary. Flying shrapnel was almost a daily occurrence. "You never knew whether or not you were going to get hit . . . guys would bring their wounded buddies in and then walk out and get blown away." The best salve? Keep busy. Care for your patients. Stay occupied. Don't think too much. Thomas was a stoic individual, like many of his friends there. But the surly exterior that he exhibited so well later in life surely belied an acknowledgment of human fragility learned at Khe Sanh. For those who knew him better, it was at the heart of his ready compassion.[28]

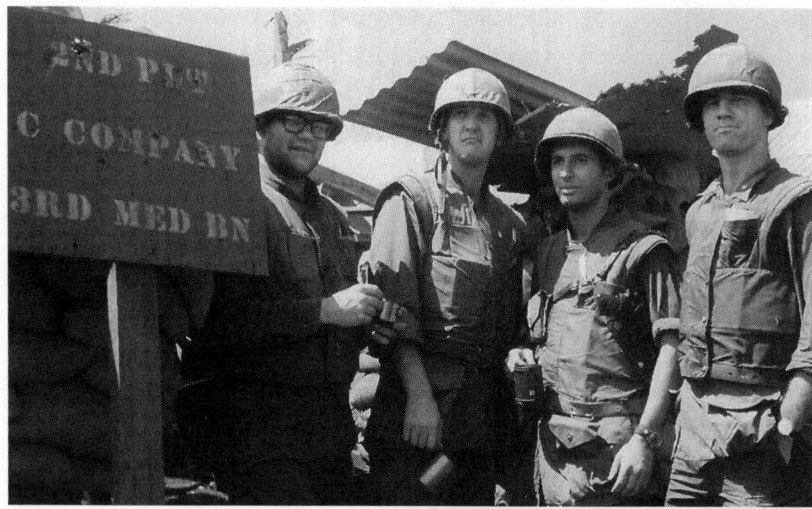

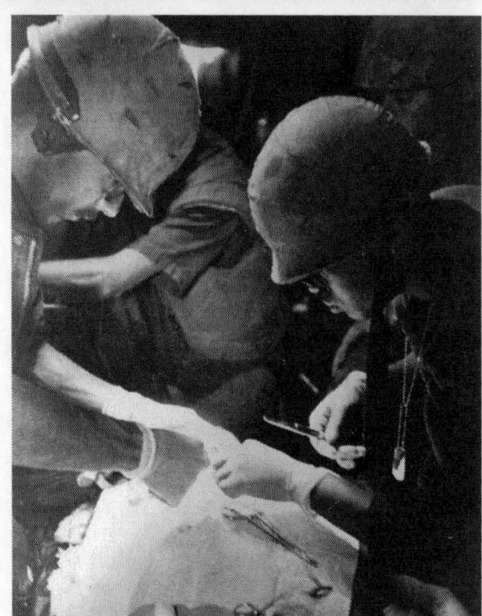

Top: physicians of Charlie Med: from left to right, Lt. Joseph Wolfe, Lt. James Finnegan, Lt. Edward Feldman, and Lt. Donald Magilligan. Right: Dr. James Thomas engaged in an emergency procedure on a fallen Marine at Charlie Med at Khe Sanh. (*Navy Bureau of Medicine and Surgery*)

Those thunderclap explosions of January 21 wiped out almost 98 percent of the base's ammunition—1,422 tons someone calculated.[29] The following day, the 1st Battalion, 9th Marines, hustled aboard helicopters and flew to Khe Sanh. Colonel Lownds now had four infantry battalions and one artillery battalion at his disposal, a grand total of 6,053 officers and enlisted.[30] Lieutenant Colonel John Mitchell's 1st Battalion—the "One-Nine"—was placed outside the perimeter on a couple of low hills and began shoveling out its fortifications. Bunkers were built, fighting holes sunk, and "tactical wire" laid. The airstrip itself, damaged by the barrage of the twenty-first, was hurriedly repaired, but replenishment of ammunition and evacuation of casualties assumed top priority. Too short now for heavy C-130s, the two-thousand-foot airstrip saw steady traffic of lighter C-123s. Twenty sorties delivered 130 tons of ammunition and, along with Marine helicopters, evacuated a number of wounded from Charlie Med.

It became a daily occurrence at the combat base, the distant "pop" of mortars or "thump" of artillery and then the whine and swish of incoming rounds seconds later. Anzio vets had called them screaming meemies and whistling willies. All prepared for a deafening blast that seemed always too damn close. On Monday, January 22, almost ninety rounds of rockets and mortar hit the base, the first coming even before the morning mist dissipated. Four more Marines died. The day after that, one heavy artillery shell killed four Marines in a bunker, obliterating bodies. Colonel Lownds demanded that his Marines dig deeper and pile higher. Many of the prepared positions were constructed for only one battalion of infantry. Now there were what amounted to two to three battalions within the wire, all needing to burrow in. Marines became subterranean denizens, scooping out eight- by eight-foot dugouts with timber pillars for support. Overhead were planks, runway matting, sandbags, loose dirt, and more sandbags. Some men used discarded 105-mm artillery casings and drove them into the bunker tops like nails. The trenchlines, reminiscent of those at Dien Bien Phu, were also sandbagged with partial covering of runway matting. Would it all be thick enough? Could anyone dig deep enough? And what about those huge, armor-piercing shells lobbed from miles away, would *anything* stop them? In all probability, no.[31] But fortunately, like bumpers on a pinball machine, control of the hills afforded an effective stopgap as North Vietnamese artillery bounced off their slopes. Deny them those hills and take away the ability to directly fire onto the base.[32] Giap's long range artillery had to locate farther away and fire indirectly—less accurate and not as spontaneous. Co Roc Mountain, to the west across the Laos border, was one location. "Hill 305" was another, over six miles from Hill 881S. Most rounds, it seemed, came from there. Salvos had to be aimed by forward observers. But North Vietnamese guns were well camouflaged, hard to pinpoint and target.

Yet Marine spotters were on the lookout. Muzzle flash "winks" from as far away as Co Roc were picked up by Marines on Hill 881S; sometimes only a whoosh overhead alerted them. They then radioed and warned the combat base of incoming: "Arty, Arty Co Roc" or "Arty Arty

305." At the base, the radio operator would activate a truck horn wired to a pole, giving everyone maybe ten seconds to find cover.[33] Yet even with indirect fire, shells were giants: 122-mm rockets, 82- and 120-mm mortars, and 130- and 152-mm cannon blew craters in the soil—or anything else they touched. Kill zones ranged out to half a football field, and casualty zones over three-hundred feet. Blasts were deafening—leaving ears ringing—and mind numbing. Concussions were not unusual, with men behaving much like punch-drunk boxers.[34]

The airstrip was a particularly hazardous place. The NVA pounded it mercilessly. As soon as aircraft approached, spotters in the hills called in mortar and artillery. And with planes on the tarmac, salvoes picked up, often bracketing aircraft and killing service personnel who were unable to hear incoming sounds drowned out by engine noise. With trepidation, men scrambled to and from airplanes, always mindful of the inevitable ordnance coming their way. The 3rd Reconnaissance (Recon) Battalion was stationed near there, committed to base protection if the North Vietnamese breached the perimeter. It took a beating. On January 24, a 152-mm shell penetrated a 3rd Recon bunker crowded with twenty-two men. Apparently the round had a delayed fuse. The shell drilled right through the roof and exploded. Four were killed outright, all the rest were wounded. Those who died were found in tiny pieces. It was a repeated occurrence. By mid-February, the 3rd Recon had suffered terrible losses: seventy out of 120 members had been either killed or wounded.[35]

For anyone, any time "on deck" was Russian roulette. Exploding ordnance sent flying fragments everywhere, even the tiniest potentially lethal. At Charlie Med, casualties were stripped naked and searched for small nicks and bruises that could indicate penetration. And as a rule, there were many. Graphic conditions often distracted from more subtle, ominous happenings. On January 27, a Marine private was struck standing outside his bunker. His buddies carried his body over to the aid station and pleaded for the doctors to do a tracheostomy. He was gasping, choking it seemed. The doctors took a look and put him over in a corner; a fragment had embedded in his head, mincing most of his brain. His gurgling respirations were simply agonal death rattles. Three days later, a rocket landed, killing a Marine who had been at Khe Sanh only twenty-four hours; his "utilities" (battle fatigues) were still pressed and green. The same blast took off a finger and punched a kidney hole in a second Marine, standing right next to him—he survived. Minimize time in the open. The "Khe Sanh Shuffle" caught on: no more than fifty meters in one half-slouched running shot; one eye ahead and the other to the side—the nearest trench always in mind—ears pricked for that fateful whoosh and whistle.[36] But there were times necessity ruled. Dr. Finnegan recalled: "Having a bowel movement takes on a whole new meaning when you have to time it between mortar attacks. Try to imaging sitting on a piece of plywood with a hole cut in it that just barely accommodates one butt while wearing a steel helmet and flak jacket."[37]

One lance corporal refused to have a bowel movement the few days he was at the combat base, afraid that going outside to the "shitter" would get him killed. Having a smoke, taking a piss, idling in the sun, all were activities that now could have grave consequences. More than one Marine standing next to his fortified dugout was hit. Of course showers were out of the question. It seemed absurd to be standing naked in the open just to wash off some blood and dirt. And after a few days, everyone smelled the same anyway. But errands above ground were risky despite their necessity and brevity: now and then individual Gyrenes were picked off by those random shots. Seventy-nine wounded were brought to Charlie Med on January 21. The day after, there were forty-nine, then twenty-five, then thirty-seven, and then forty-eight. By the end of January, surgeons had seen 372 patients.[38]

25

Scotland

OFFICIALLY, 3RD MARINE DIVISION OPERATIONS IN WESTERN QUANG Tri Province were known as Operation Scotland, but after January 21, all eyes were centered on the Khe Sanh combat base. To the public and forever more in history, Operation Scotland would be synonymous with the siege of Khe Sanh. Following evacuation of Khe Sanh, few doubted the presence of large numbers of North Vietnamese troops. The place was crawling with them—upwards of twenty thousand enemy soldiers, some estimated; others put the figure at forty thousand. Route 9 was in their hands, the hill country in their sights. The Xom Cham garrison's last major reinforcement, the 37th Ranger Battalion of ARVN forces, arrived January 28. Lownds put them just outside the perimeter at the end of the runway, in an area called the Gray sector. It was around Gray on January 31 that forward observers detected "many NVA [North Vietnamese Army] around . . . carrying baskets and weapons." Sappers were at work, inching their trenches forward, eerily similar to what happened at Dien Bien Phu.[1] One Marine wrote a poem addressed to no one. He stuck it to an envelope with a piece of chewing gum:

At night I hear them digging,
like woodworm in timber,
creeping towards me.
Digging with shovels, inside the earth.[2]

It was at Dien Bien Phu that the Viet Minh burrowed below ground until they were within yards of French strongpoints. Then hell was unleashed. Waves of storming troops rushed over the top so close that defenders were quickly mauled. Lownds was determined not to let that happen on his watch. He was not going to sit behind his wire and fret. They were Marines, after all. Patrol and recon, patrol and recon. The 1st Battalion of the 26th Marines completed six platoon-sized combat patrols and one squad patrol, and set up three night ambushes during February, every now and then a brief firefight but mostly probing for NVA.[3] Where was the enemy? How close were they? Patrols were kept within five hundred meters of the perimeter, close enough to withdraw to safety. Outside that zone, Arc Light B-52 strikes systematically pulverized any moving thing. But inside the wire, it was business as usual. Almost daily shipments of North Vietnamese artillery dropped with unpredictable randomness, some days worse than others.

Giap wanted those hills around the combat base. He hurled his young troops with indiscriminate viciousness. Early in the morning of February 5, the 2nd Battalion, 26th Marines caught it on Hill 861. Tear gas (officially known as "CS") at first nearly panicked defenders, but not for long. Jarheads met the enemy head on. The fight quickly turned into a donnybrook with "knives, bayonets, rifle butts, and fists," according to historian Moyers Shore. Hand grenades were tossed like hot potatoes, sometimes as close as ten meters. If a target had no body armor, the American-issue M26 grenade was highly lethal. Showers of shrapnel felled the enemy in heaps. Marines, on the other hand, had flak-jacket protection. In spots, handguns were pulled and gunfights erupted reminiscent of the OK Corral. "It was pandemonium. . . . It was like watching a World War II movie," said Captain Earle Breeding, head of E Company. The enemy "didn't know how to cope with it . . . we walked all over them."[4] And then as quickly as it all began, it was over. Silence—that breathless realization of survival. Clouds kept cordite heavy in the air. Almost mechanically, Marines collected their casualties: seven killed and seventeen wounded. Those alive were first taken to the 2nd Battalion's aid station on adjacent Hill 558, a large shell hole soon full of sick and wounded. As for the dead, Private Mike DeLaney recalled: "There were bodies everywhere. . . . I had never seen young dead people. . . . I had sat around the day before smoking cigarettes and sharing C-rations with some of the dead young people on that hill. Their skin was gray and rubbery; they didn't look human anymore."

Khe Sanh's ubiquitous fog made helicopter evacuation dangerous. Lance Corporal Bill Maves, of the Tactical Air Control Party, anguished over whether to ask pilots from Da Nang to risk their lives trying to land. He had around thirty-five wounded who needed to be moved out: "This forced upon me the biggest decision of my life. . . . I had emergency medevacs [critical patients] waiting in the landing zone who would not live another hour if I waited. If they [helicopters] couldn't get in, more would die with the longer wait. I looked at the men lying there and told Da Nang to send the birds."

Standing bolt upright in the landing zone, Maves shot a red star cluster in the air when he heard the choppers nearing. The birds landed one at a time, safely, snatched the injured, and lifted off for Da Nang or Dong Ha or Phu Bai. Mission accomplished.[5]

The scruffy tents of Charlie Med came down. Bombardments were going to destroy the place—and everyone in it—Finnegan figured. He pleaded with the command staff for better protection. Shortly afterward, Seabees arrived with a backhoe and dug a hole ten feet deep, buttressed the walls with timber, and covered the roof with Marston matting and sandbags—it was the new triage and treatment room. There was even a ramp entrance so litter bearers would not need to maneuver down stairs. No more slouching on the ground. Now there was a real system. When wounded arrived, corpsmen removed all combat gear and clothing, recorded vital signs, and drew a tube of blood for typing. All areas of the victim's body were searched for fragment entry points; armpits, scalp, buttocks, anus, and scrotum were notorious for concealed skin breaks, "armpits and assholes" as the saying went. Physical examination was imperative. No x-rays were available. The only blood test was blood typing. Tetanus toxoid was given. Any litter patient automatically had an intravenous catheter inserted—large veins were sought, brachial or cephalic were preferred—and fluids started. With patients in shock, saphenous vein was accessed via cutdown in the groin. Sterile intravenous tubing was inserted directly into the vein. For blood transfusions only type-specific blood was given; there was no crossmatching done. And for the worst cases—patients in cardiac—everyone pitched in. Two dozen of the 220 wounded seen at Charlie Med arrived like that, all but one from hemorrhage. There was not enough blood for an empty heart to pump. Thoracotomy—and quickly—was the answer: A generous slash across the chest, just below the nipple line. Right through pectoralis, right through rib space. Cram in rib spreaders, crank open, snip through pericardium. Then cradle the heart: internal cardiac massage—literally squeezing by hand while blood was pumped in. Finnegan's crew claimed success in most cases. Otherwise major surgery was avoided. Patients were stabilized and flown out, except on those rare occasions when the weather turned nasty or the North Vietnamese were particularly busy pummeling the airstrip. Dr. Feldman remembered one of those times. An ARVN soldier came in, obviously bleeding from a belly wound. Nothing was landing. The four physicians huddled and decided there was no other option. "We opened him up from stem to stern, did whatever had to be done."[6] And for departing patients—total anxiety. There was no worse moment than waiting in trenches for medevacs to light. Marines knew it and the North Vietnamese knew it. In came the shells.[7]

At daily briefings, Colonel Lownds began talking "what ifs." Finnegan surmised a North Vietnamese assault was around the corner. What about the doctors, he asked. A "reaction force" would come to their aid, he was assured. And how soon? Well, he was advised, "go back and make sure that your docs and corpsmen all have sidearms, M16s, and grenades, and that you also dig fighting holes." Madness, he thought, pure madness. Of course his team never had a plan for self-defense, no fighting holes, no ready weapons. They were much too busy for all that. That sergeant was right: If he or his men had to use weapons, Finnegan was sure every other Marine around them would be dead—and they shortly would be, too.

Marines were not the only ones catching it. The Special Forces A-101 detachment—that "undisciplined rabble" of lanky, easygoing provocateurs—at Xom Cham, the combat base, had moved its camp west in the vicinity of the village of Lang Vei in 1967 to make room for Marines—and Marines were glad of it (their snoopy SOG team, of course, stayed behind at FOB-3). The CIDG Bru had gone with them. Much too close to Laos, Lang Vei had already been a VC target. That was back in May 1967. Infiltrators had opened the gates and let Viet Cong buddies in who attacked and killed two Americans. They were eventually driven off, but it exposed flimsy camp defenses. The entire compound was moved a kilometer to the west. The new Lang Vei camp was situated just off Highway 9. Reinforced bunkers were sunk, strongpoints fortified, fields of fire cleared, and barbed wire strung. It now was a veritable castle. Twenty-four Green Berets and 463 militia occupied a compound that bristled with automatic weapons, light artillery, and even antitank rockets.[8] Even more Laotian militia and their American advisers were located at the old camp, just down the road. "The 'Greenies' [Green Berets] were not social animals," Tim O'Brien remembered, "Animals . . . but far from social. . . . Secretive and suspicious, loners by nature."[9]

On February 6, just before midnight, Lang Vei GIs were awakened by volumes of artillery fire. It was a prelude to a full-out infantry and tank attack. "Tanks in the wire" was the cry over intercoms. North Vietnamese rolled in from three directions and soon punched through the perimeter. The castle was breeched. Soviet PT-76 tanks pointed their 76-mm guns and fired point blank. The North Vietnamese were everywhere, running through the base, shooting from every direction, pounding on bunkers with grenades and satchel charges. At the same time, over at the combat base, a coordinated artillery barrage started, rounds screaming in at a rate of six per minute. One estimate put the total at 550 rockets and mortar rounds by morning, the heaviest bombardment yet. Marine gunners hunkered down, unable to focus their fire on Lang Vei. Shells also cratered the airstrip, preventing a relief force of Green Berets from Da Nang from landing. American advisers and Laotian troops attempted to rescue the Lang Vei garrison on five attempts, all repulsed by the North Vietnamese. A call went out for Leathernecks to saddle up. That was nixed by Generals Cushman (III MAF), Tompkins (3rd Marine Division), and Westmoreland (MACV). It was a trap, they felt, to lure Marines out only to be ambushed. At daybreak, the Lang Vei garrison was finished; all troops were killed, captured, or scattered. Later in the day, a reaction force of Green Berets helicoptered from FOB-3 and evacuated what wounded they could find. Montagnards—combatants and refugees—fearing for their lives, sifted through to the combat base but were turned away by Lownds; VC were thought likely to be mingled among them.[10] Ten Green Berets were killed or listed as missing, including specialist Les Moreland, a medic who was left behind in the throes of a fatal head injury after attempts to move him were met with delirious agitation. For the safety of the entire group escaping from the command bunker, he was not taken. One other adviser, Sergeant Eugene Ashley, later awarded the Medal of Honor, died after being carried by medic Richard Allen to the old Camp Lang Vei. Shot in the chest, he needed mouth-to-mouth resuscitation all the way but soon succumbed. The brave CIDG militia also lost 209 men. Virtually all the Americans still alive were wounded.[11]

Back at MACV headquarters, worries skyrocketed. Reports were unnervingly close to Viet Minh strategy at Dien Bien Phu. Whittle away at the perimeter, overrun outlying strongpoints, and then move in on the interior. Now Khe Sanh and the CIDG camp at Lang Vei were lost. Americans at the combat base were becoming isolated—and surrounded.[12] Colonel Reamer Argo, the command historian, painted a dismal picture of the embattled garrisons at Khe Sanh. His assessment of encircled forces was pessimistic, based on a review of historical experiences, including the most recent at Dien Bien Phu. Defenders would feel hemmed in and lose the initiative, the ability to maneuver and respond. This sense of helplessness would disable many. A defeatist attitude would surface, with men bracing for a final onslaught, convinced there was no escape, no victory. They would sit in their foxholes and bunkers and trenches and wait and wait. That was not the Marine instinct. They had a distinct loathing for the Khe Sanh Shuffle. Frustration climbed, Jarheads itching for action. Westmoreland railed at Argo's report, convinced that Khe Sanh was different, that air power and artillery support would turn the tide. And his reputation was on the line for taking a stand there. "[W]e are not, repeat not, going to be defeated at Khe Sanh. I will tolerate no talking or even thinking to the contrary," he spit, maybe more to convince himself than anyone else.[13] In Washington, President Johnson, equally obsessed with the Marine's predicament, even contemplated the use of tactical nuclear weapons, a proposal that, of course, was never carried out. Yet, he savagely unleashed Arclight strikes to the extent that the tonnage of conventional bombs dropped on the North Vietnamese around Khe Sanh soared to the destructive power of a small nuclear weapon.

February was a bloody month. The North Vietnamese chipped away at the Marines' perimeter. Stark hilltop outposts dotting the boundaries of the combat base were the juicy targets. A particularly brutal attack occurred on a small rise, Hill 64 (not for sixty-four feet in elevation but sixty-four Marines, as the story goes), about five hundred meters from the wire. It was manned by a platoon of Marines, Alpha Company, 1st Battalion, 9th Marines—Alpha One of the One-Nine, they called themselves. They were the hard-luck boys, the "walking dead," a name given to them after their stunning losses a year earlier at Con Thien, just south of the DMZ. Now at Khe Sanh, One-Nine was suddenly attacked early in the morning of February 8. North Vietnamese troops rushed the wire with grenades, satchel charges, and Bangalore torpedoes. Many Marines were caught in their bunkers, barely awake, explosives chucked in their midst. Defenders were soon fighting for their lives, swinging entrenching

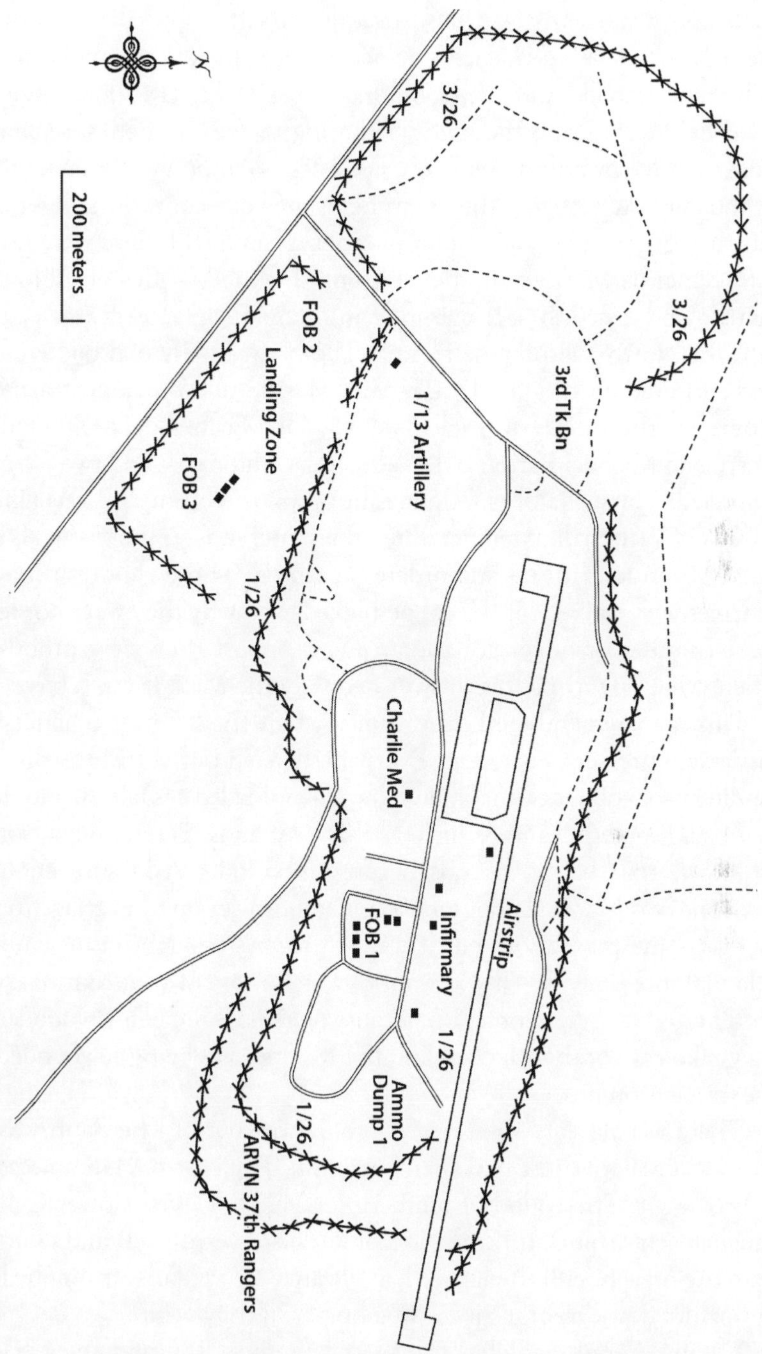

Map 6. Khe Sanh combat base, February 1968. The location of Charlie Med is shown as well as the general defensive positions of the 1st (1/26) and 3rd (3/26) battalions, 26th Marines.

tools and water cans—an obscene orgy of kill or be killed. Another grenade toss developed, each side occupying some of the small summit. When the grenades were gone, Marines threw rocks. The small surviving band held out during the night, squatting in their trenches, separated from their foe by only a number of sandbags—abrupt, vicious encounters in the dark. Where was the damn help, they cursed. At first light, the North Vietnamese organized for another try, and still there were no reinforcements. Marines fired everything they had—rifles on full automatic—and tossed their remaining hand grenades in a stormy melee that sent the North Vietnamese reeling. The NVA finally had had enough and slithered away, gone by the time Marine reinforcements arrived. However, the price was high: twenty-four Marines dead—including Corpsman Michael Barrett of Los Angeles, California—and twenty-nine wounded.[14] First Platoon "Alpha One" took the brunt and was almost wiped out. With rising temperatures, the stench was stifling. Lownds had had enough for Hill 64 and ordered it closed. Those gaunt, unshaven Marines who walked off it were perplexed as to why they were not reinforced sooner or never got the artillery support they were promised. There were no satisfactory answers. For Charlie Med, it was a busy day.

Finnegan remembered those times when the "mortar magnets"—medevac choppers—came in. Everyone headed out with litters to the landing pad—about twenty meters away—unloaded casualties, and shuffled back, sometimes in as little as thirty seconds. Sure enough, somewhere in that ballet, rounds began to explode. And sure enough, someone was hit. A wall of sandbags had been set up from triage to the pad for some protection, but it was not always enough. Finnegan had told Colonel Lownds: "If you want us to take care of your Marines, you better provide some protection because our troops are being wounded as they take care of the Marines and the Marines are being rewounded in the evacuation process."[15]

There was no easy solution. The only way out of Khe Sanh was by air. Yes, air supply, just like Dien Bien Phu. The North Vietnamese delighted in it. The sound of lumbering C-123s or even slower C-130s caught their attention. Enter coordinates, shove in shell and charges, slam the breech, pull the lanyard, and watch misery sail. Or simply drop projectiles down mortar tubes. Whoomp! Off they went.

Marine Aerial Refueler Transport Squadron 152 and the US Air Force 834th Air Division got the call. There was awful weather, short approaches, and the enemy's incessant shelling—never a good day—but

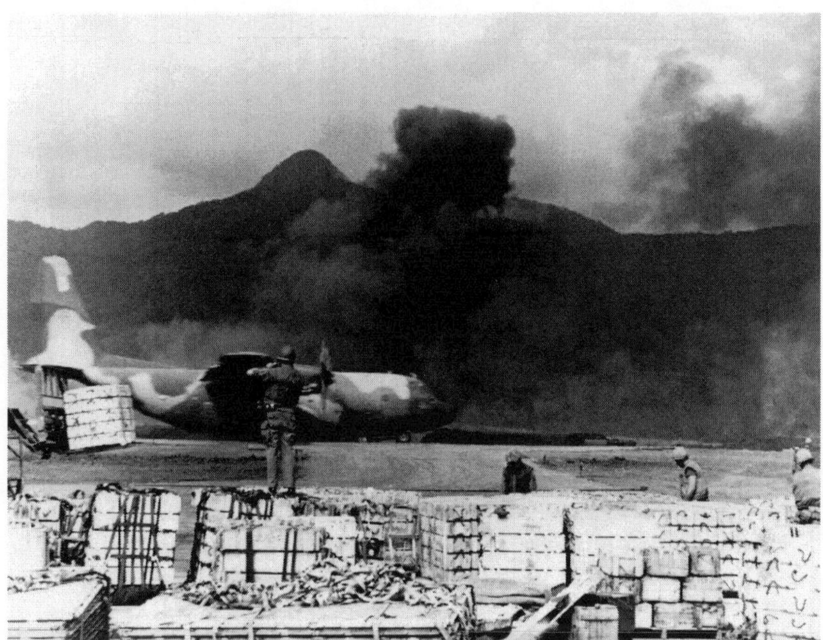

A C-130 Hercules transport plane taking off from the Khe Sanh landing strip in January 1968. (*National Archives*)

they got through. A steep approach from the east, drop three thousand feet per minute, roll out, taxi right to the tarmac, drop off supplies, pick up wounded, turn around, rev engines, and take off—sometimes a blast with jet assist—all within three minutes.[16] In January, the 834th delivered over three thousand six hundred tons of supplies. The Marines and air force combined met target deliveries of 235 tons per day. But there were consequences. Three times in late January, aircraft were struck with .51-caliber rounds on approach, and on one occasion, mortar fire damaged a parked plane. But on February 10, a KC-130, a modified tanker version of the C-130, carrying six full fuel bladders and two pallets of cargo was hit on approach, setting the cargo department ablaze. Right after touchdown a spectacular fireball appeared, and before the plane came to rest, two more explosions occurred. The aircraft was soon a raging inferno. Through efforts of the ground crew, five of the ten aboard survived. Four other crew died in the flames and a fifth later succumbed to pneumonia brought on by extensive burns.[17] The next day two more C-130s were hit. A 122-mm rocket landed just fifteen feet away from one while it was emptying of troops. One Marine was killed outright and another died later at D Med in Dong Ha. Four others were wounded and evacuated.[18]

Slow, plodding C-130s were too inviting for enemy gunners. It was bound to happen again. On February 12, General William Momyer, MACV deputy commander for air operations, suspended Hercules landing operations at the combat base. Crashes on approach and takeoff or fiery spectacles down the runway could kill scores of crew and passengers—all displayed on nightly television. Smaller, more maneuverable C-123s took over resupply missions—for the air force, that is. Marine KC-130s continued to land—and opened up regular shooting galleries. On February 22, one KC-130 took eight rounds of .51-caliber hostile fire on approach, and a second plane was bracketed by mortar and automatic-weapon fire on takeoff.

Pilots seemed fearless. They kept coming despite the weather and gunfire. There were breathtaking approaches, near-vertical takeoffs. The crews knew supply was vital to survival—*the* lifeline. At Charlie Med, doctors were in constant need. In those busy months of January and February, material was consumed fast. Blood, splints, dressings, instruments, chest tubes, endotracheal tubes, and sutures were quickly devoured as wounded rolled in and out. If the weather prohibited landings, parachute drops were used. Containers that could hold almost seventy tons of ammunition, petroleum, and rations were pushed out, hitting the ground within a radius of 150 yards. Starting in February, radar guidance could plant parachute drops within one hundred yards, even in total cloud cover. Over two days that month, 280 tons of material was deposited by radar. To avoid any tarmac down time, the air force employed extraction systems virtually feet from the ground: on approach, C-123s opened their doors, and containers were yanked out by billowing parachutes or hooks snagging cables stretched across the runway.

For arrivees, it was strictly choppers from bases at Dong Ha, Phu Bai, or Da Nang—and a definite "Come to Jesus" moment. Bruce Geiger, an army officer in charge of an Air Defense Artillery battery at Khe Sanh described his first plunge into the combat base: "As we began our descent, we saw tracer rounds streaking past the windows through the thick clouds. The crew chief shouted that we would have less than ten seconds on the deck, and we had better be off the ramp or know how to fly! . . . Incoming mortars and artillery rounds exploded all around. . . . The pilot didn't even land the chopper. The crew chief lowered the tailgate to the

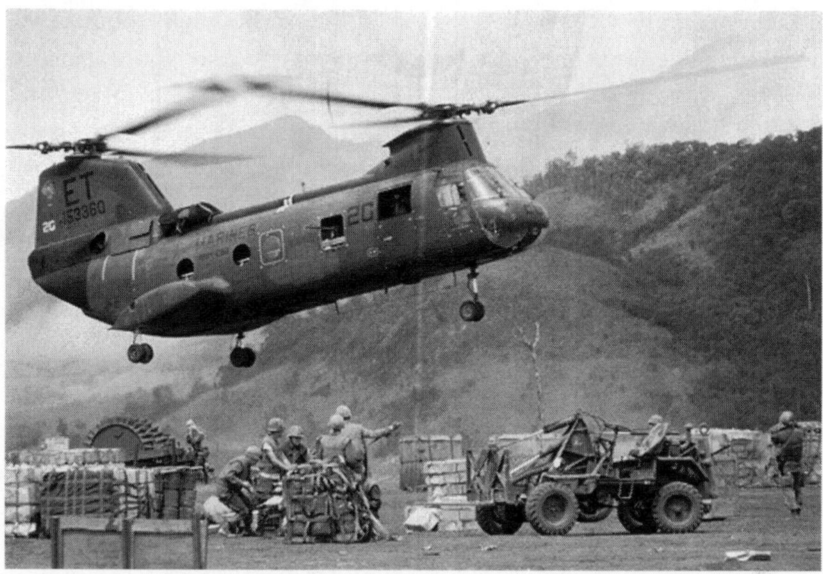

A CH-46 Chinook helicopter resupply at Khe Sanh combat base, February 22, 1968. (*National Archives/US Marines*)

ground as the chopper hovered and we were dumped out like a heap of garbage from the rear of a sanitation truck."[19]

He said they scattered like rats for the nearest trenches, and scared out of their wits, waited for the barrage to end. The air bristled with gunfire and whizzing shell fragments, as if the ghosts of the highland dead were hissing, "Welcome to Khe Sanh!"

It was even worse on the hills where almost half the Marines lived. There were no parachute drops there. Supplies came in by helicopter only, almost daily. At first, UH-34s, those bulbous-looking Sikorskys, and twin-rotored Chinook-type C-46s shuttled material straight from the combat base. But the North Vietnamese caught on to that. Even behind revetments, they zeroed in on helicopters with amazing accuracy. "We were losing aircraft on the ground up there at a rate faster than we could replace them," said Major Arthur Crane, operations officer for VMO-6, the Marine observation squadron.[20] In fact, during February, rocket, artillery, and mortar fire badly damaged thirteen CH-46 aircraft of HMM-262 while sitting on the ground at the combat base, including eight that were supposedly protected by revetments.[21] It all came to a head on February 22. A huge CH-53 Sea Stallion from HMH-463 had unloaded supplies and was waiting to pick up wounded from Charlie Med when incoming rounds fell near the chopper. Rather than taking off immediately, Captain James Riley kept his ship on the ground, blades whirling, hoping to load and scoot. Sure enough, a round came much too close. He aborted, buttoned up, and tried to levitate out just to save crew and passengers. Screeching noises and vibrations were probably the last sensations for him. The chopper slammed back to the ground and the main rotor tilted, slicing through the cockpit. Riley and copilot Cary Smith were killed instantly, one decapitated and the other cut in half. For General Tompkins, that was the last straw. No more helicopters would be stored at the combat base. Missions would fly directly from Dong Ha to the hilltops. For the combat base itself, the routine was as speedy as the cargo planes. Choppers zipped in, unloaded their cargo, piled in medevacs, and zipped out, all in less than a minute. During February alone, crews of HMH-463, as daring as any and flying Sea Stallions, made 544 sorties from Dong Ha to the combat base or hilltops.[22]

To be sure, those were wild trips into Indian Country. Thumping choppers came down the Rao Quan Valley, sometimes in near-zero conditions. Rolling clouds, the bane of Khe Sanh, first covered hilltops, making approaches more than tricky. And with the thwap-thwap of rotor blades, the North Vietnamese would lie on their backs, point guns in the air, and wait for choppers to fly across. Over the landing zone (LZ), mortar fire soon registered and added to the pelting. Within half a minute, choppers were invariably bracketed as they dumped off cargo. Medevac patients had to be ready, litter teams poised. Walking wounded often shouldered the litters, and all piled into chopper bellies in one ignominious leap. Pilots did not dally; they could hear the splat of bullets against their hulls. On at least one occasion, machine-gun fire sawed off the tail rotor of a UH-34 just after takeoff. Hill 881S became a veritable helicopter graveyard. Five wrecks could easily be seen scattered around the hill by the time the siege ended, some thought even more.[23] For newbie Marines arriving, the invective was shouted to get the hell off. Corpsman David Steinberg of India Company on Hill 881S recalled: "Replacements would jump off the helos and supplies would just fall off. . . . Any time we got resupplied was the time for a corpsman to worry. We got three or four mortar rounds in every time a chopper came in. Almost every time, we had casualties. Most of them were new guys who were getting off the chopper."[24]

Those poor rookie Marines had no clue what to do. Shoved out onto a barren hilltop, they stood, gawking, like the first day of school. Few knew right away to bolt for the trenches, few even knew where the trenches were. And then, with uncanny timing, mortar rounds began to fall. There were explosions, fresh Marines toppled—"Corpsman up!" was the call—and the medics went to work. They dreaded these days, struggling to loosen bulky packs on the freshly wounded arrivals, and keeping their heads down as more shells hit.[25]

Single-file columns of fat Sea Stallions and Chinooks—daisy chains, they were called—were easy prey. The enemy was getting expert at hosing their soft underbellies as they flew over. Mortars were already ranged in on the LZs. In February alone for HMM-364—the "Purple Foxes"—eighty-nine sorties were fired on, twenty-four hits scored, and five of their crew killed.[26] In fact, on a single day in mid-February three helicopters were shot down trying to reach hilltop fortifications.[27] Colonel William White, commander of VMO-6, came up with a counter called "Super Gaggle." Helicopters were escorted by A-4 Skyhawks and Huey UH-1E gunships out of Chu Lai. Jets and gunships "prepped" the area with rockets and napalm, then choppers rumbled in, cargo slung low in nets. In less than a minute, while gunships laced surrounding terrain, material was dropped and medevacs picked up. Four Super Gaggles and forty tons could be sent this way each day. The hit rate was reduced in half. "My guess, based on knowledge of Hill 881S casualties both before and after Super Gaggle, is that it saved 150 to 200 casualties and perhaps half a dozen birds," said Captain (now Colonel) Dabney years later.[28]

The weather was still capricious. Those days of "zero-zero" conditions—ceiling and visibility confined to a few feet—were especially tough. There were no medevacs. On one occasion, bad weather kept Corporal Homer Taylor grounded. Struck in the head and shoulders by a mortar round ("three or four good sized holes in his head and a hole through his right lung," an officer wrote), he was losing consciousness—and vital signs. Over the next thirty-six hours his condition worsened, but there was still no evacuation. After forty hours—and no medevac—Corporal Taylor died. "Lack of help" was the official explanation.[29] In hill country, battalion surgeons did as much as they could. Dug-out aid stations provided fluids, bandaging, and morphine but not much else. At least one casualty on Hill 881S died while waiting three days for a medevac helicopter; thick mist, like a shroud, kept anything from landing. Bleeding outpaced the supply of intravenous saline. Even the dead died again—lingering in body bags, stored in a "body bunker," rotting away in the heat. In his memoir, *Khe Sanh and the Mongol Prince*, Reverend Ray Stubbe, the Lutheran chaplain for the 1st Battalion, 26th Marines, included a remark by Captain William Dabney, commander of India Company garrisoning that hill: "Ever watch rats crawling in and out of ponchos holding what's left of [men] hit by a 152 [mm artillery round]? The troops did! They were up there five days. Weather socked in. Ripe. We were told we couldn't bury them. We did anyway. Had to."[30]

The stench of human decay filled their nostrils. And not just any stench, and not just any decay. These were friends, comrades, men who just a while ago laughed and joked and talked of home. For the besieged, death must be put away; seen and removed. Focus on surviving. A keenness is imperative. No distraction of what could happen to them. Dying must be separated from living. In the film *Full Metal Jacket*, the character Animal Mother looks at a crop of dead Marines. His only comment: "Better you than me." Bury and move on. No good living in tombs. The chewing gum poem said as much:

I want to get out of this tomb,
out of this waiting
And if I get out they'll kill me . . .
God, I'm tired . . . [31]

AROUND THE COMBAT BASE, digging continued—over two thousand meters of digging. The North Vietnamese dug at night, the crunch of shovels slightly louder now. Trenches snaked toward the perimeter from southeast and west, from near Poilane's plantations and Route 9 to within thirty meters of the wire. "Some nights you can hear the NVA digging their tunnels, just coming closer and closer to the base perimeter," one Marine told a correspondent. "It's spooky, man."[32] Leathernecks doused the place with rockets and high explosives and napalm, but the Vietnamese kept digging. Snoops had also learned of buildups just over the Laotian border. Sharp probes on the Gray sector, too. Looking for gaps maybe? Something was up.

Hell broke loose on February 21. Almost two hundred rocket, mortar, and artillery rounds fell on the 1st Battalion. There were sixteen casualties for Charlie Med. The next day was worse: 238 rounds came in, someone counted. On February 23, 1,307 more rounds (who was counting?).[33] One hit an ammunition dump, cooking off one thousand six hundred rounds. Marines peered into darkness and morning fog fully expecting a surge of little green men. They hunkered in their trenches and holes and

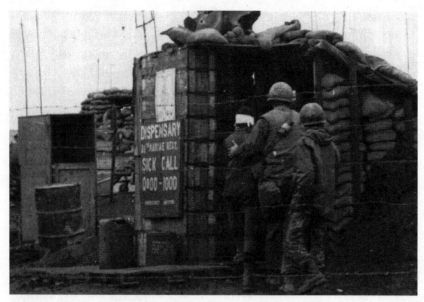

Dispensary (infirmary) of the 26th Marine Regiment at Khe Sanh. (*National Archives*)

took the blasts, one after another. For some it was simply too much. Aid station Corpsman Rod DeMoss recalled: "Two Marines escorted a gunnery sergeant into the regimental aid station. He came in shaking, wouldn't talk, had both hands holding his helmet down on his head, and every time a round hit he would shake. He was, of course, suffering from shell shock."[34]

Sunday, February 25, marked a dark passage in Khe Sanh's saga, as if lifted from the pages of a Euripidean calamity. It was the day of the "Ghost Patrol": 3rd Platoon, Bravo Company, 1st Battalion, with twenty-year-old Second Lieutenant Don Jacques in the lead, forty-six men behind him. Jacques, wonder boy, youngest officer to complete the Basic School—officer candidate school—in eighteen years. A real gung ho Marine. Off they went, heading south outside the wire, looking for the enemy. Jacques was supposed to check in with his commanding officer, Captain Ken Pipes. But the fog was thick. Beyond five hundred meters, maybe six hundred meters or more, they humped. Three North Vietnamese were loitering on Poilane's plantation road—bait. They ran. Jacques wanted action, and here it was. "Let's go get them," he said. It was a classic L-shaped ambush. The platoon caught automatic fire and mortars full face. Men dropped in clumps. "The screaming and shouting was so loud you couldn't hear your own voice," one private said.[35] Maneuver? Impossible—enemy all around. Marines hugged the earth and tried to hide in tall grass. By 9:30 AM it was all over. Survivors said it lasted maybe ten minutes. Corpsman John Cicala, wounded, tried to help other injured, including a buddy shot through the eye. He was still conscious. Cicala crammed a battle dressing in the red hole—there was nothing else to do. The Marine asked for his weapon, that was all. Cicala went to others—there were plenty. He was hit again in the neck and again through his flak jacket into his lung, creating a sucking chest wound. He plugged the hole with cellophane from a cigarette packet and crawled back toward the wire. A few survivors managed to disengage and pulled away, staggering in twos and threes back to the base, many not making it in until sundown.[36]

Don Jacques stood tall, covering his men. Why he stood straight up no one will ever know, but an NVA gunner got him, stitched right across his groin by a lonesome machine gun. Both femoral arteries opened up. Blood poured like geysers. Corporal Gilbert Wall crawled over and tried to stop the bleeding, but it was useless. "All this time he was trying to talk to me but I couldn't understand him . . . shortly I noticed a change in the color of his face. It was turning white."[37] Don Jacques was dead in minutes. What were his last thoughts? Total disbelief? Or did he simply "pass quietly from the stormy shores of time"?[38] Lieutenant Jacques had been close to his parents. He often wrote of Vietnam and his exploits. One of his last letters was written February 8. An invincible Gyrene, he scoffed at the hazards. Youthful immortality and the panache of the Corps ruled: "Well, they haven't gotten me yet. . . . But my men and I will be all right no matter what comes. We are all well and morale is high. . . . But old Don is pretty lucky (knock on wood), and home I'll come, I'm sure . . . I'll close with love in my heart for both of you. Love, Don."[39] Maybe in those final moments, immortality was indeed revealed. Marines carried Jacques's body back, the only confirmed killed in action. Twenty-five men did not return. It was April before they were found.[40]

Yes, it was a black day at Xom Cham. The North Vietnamese had won big. A grim reality settled in of impending doom. Everyone braced for an all-out attack, much like at Dien Bien Phu, with hordes of green-helmeted troops barreling across the wire. David Leitch, a correspondent for the (London) *Times* who had bribed his way into Khe Sanh, put it this way: "It was beyond human endurance. . . . It was like being in one of those medieval sieges where you knew you actually had to lose because you didn't have water, and they were going to get you and cut your throat. Meanwhile, you had a day or two to live, and you had to live like a man."[41]

Live like a man? Reverend Stubbe remembered how men tried. Through February and into March, the bombardments, almost daily now, began to eat away at sanity. Despite their bravado and gallows humor, there was a deep streak of looming calamity, and whenever possible they sought safety, mostly below ground, as if that was somehow their impervious sanctuary: "And I remember how nervous they all were . . . they all seemed like they wanted to be in the bunker all the time. It was like their womb. It was warm. They had a little candle. They were making coffee. I kept telling them that the trench [just outside] out there is safer than the bunker. . . . But anyway they were all in there."[42]

Safer outside? Lieutenant Robert Brett, better known as Father Robert Brett, the Catholic chaplain for the 2nd Battalion, 26th Marines, would say no—if he could talk. Father Brett had been unflagging in shepherding his troops, visiting hill country and saying one service after another for the few Marines who could congregate at any one time. On February 22, as he waited for a helicopter to take him to Hill 558 and crouched in a trench covered with steel plating and two or three layers of sandbags, an armor piercing projectile fell, penetrated all those layers, and exploded, killing the young priest and his clerk instantly.[43] Another chaplain, Reverend Walter Driscoll, would also say no. He was struck in the spine by flying shrapnel and his legs suddenly went flaccid; he was paralyzed below the waist.

Above ground the place, war correspondent Robert Pisor wrote, had turned into "a reeking trash heap," full of the detritus of combat: thousands of shell casings, torn boots, shrapnel pieces, shreds of canvas, and broken timber. Here and there were ripped, bloodied flak jackets, their occupants long gone. "Smoke and the smell of things burning lifted the back of the tongue almost to gagging."[44] In the FOB-3 compound, discarded and opened C-rations containers began to attract rats. These were not the small, coquettish laboratory animals; they were often as large as a cat. During the day, their homes were the sandbagged bunkers, but after dark, dugouts came alive with the scurry of tiny feet, often across the bodies of sleeping troopers. Some were even bitten, and when evacuations were not forthcoming, painful rabies vaccinations were required. Several of the Bru Montagnards caught the creatures, boiled them, skinned them, and dined. It became something of a camp delicacy when C rations, standard fare for the garrisons, turned intolerable.

And what about Charlie Med? Five hundred thirty-one casualties arrived from February 1 through 24, an average of twenty-two per day. Of course, it was that surge phenomenon only combat can bring. Numbers ranged from a low of four to a high of sixty-one, on February 7. Dr. Finnegan remembered: "It soon became difficult to distinguish one day from another. The wounded arrived at all hours, sometimes one or two at a time and at other times one or two dozen. . . . We fought hard to save these boys. . . . We treated each Marine like he was priority one."[45] With all the commotion of resuscitation, that medical bunker was a bizarre scene: it was eerily quiet. On a visit to Charlie Med, Reverend Stubbe recorded in his diary: "The patients that are in C Med are amazingly calm. None scream. A few moan softly. They all look and gaze at their wounds, some very ghastly indeed, but portray no emotional response. They are numb. We are numb."[46]

The wounds could be heartbreaking. There were traumatic amputations, sometimes two on the same person. Head wounds, facial wounds, blindness, charred flesh, exposed bone and tendons. A corpsman commented, "I don't want to look at that, but I have to."[47] Discarded bloody clothes, flak jackets, ponchos, and bamboo poles were strewn about, incriminating evidence of human destruction. Finnegan was truthful: "we knew the joys of saving a man and the gut-wrenching feeling of losing one."[48] Ambulance driver Daniel Sullivan recalled the orderly chaos of Charlie Med and one sad case. He had brought in the only survivor of a huge explosion: "A gun pit crew had taken a direct hit. Three out of four dead with the only one alive possibly losing both legs and his left arm. Two doctors and a corpsman worked feverishly on this Marine until they got him stable. The poor Marine was awake and saying, 'I want to live. I want to live.'"[49] Transferred to D Med at Dong Ha, the stricken Marine lost both legs and an arm, and died anyway.

Evacuations were kept to a minimum. The reasons were apparent to anyone. First, it was probably safer to remain on base and under cover than lying in trenches waiting to be medevaced. Second, manpower was at a premium. Replacements were infrequent, and many units were already undermanned. In February, the 1st Battalion, 26th Marines—the main unit responsible for defense of the combat base itself—had 117 combat wounded, but only thirty-one needed evacuation. In March, 96

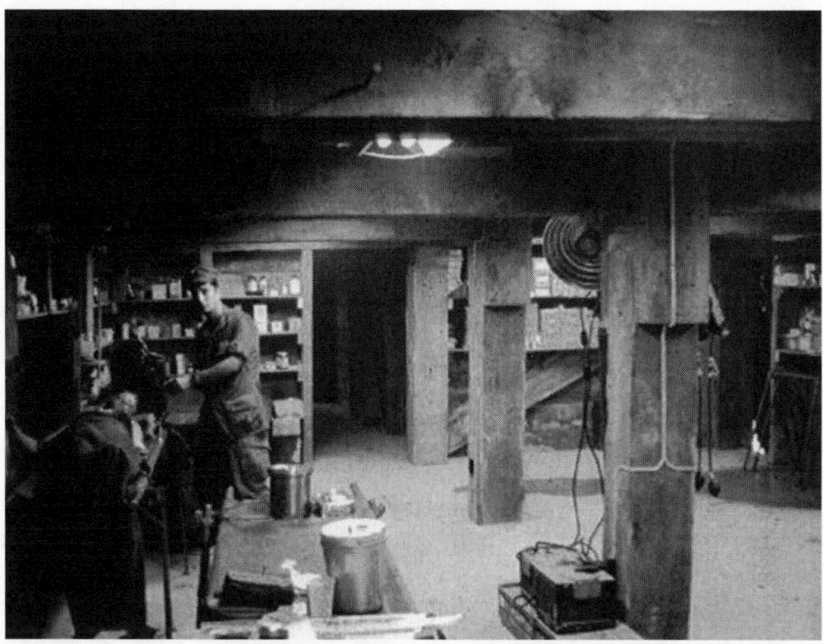

Charlie Med bunker at Khe Sanh. (*Courtesy Ed Feldman*)

of 238 were sent.[50] Most were treated and released from the battalion aid station. Dentist Robert Birtcil and regimental surgeon Casey Firlit could handle minor wounds: cleansing, suturing, dressing. Birtcil himself suffered a minor wound "dogtrotting" (his version of the Khe Sanh Shuffle) across the base during a barrage. The Marine directly in front perished from the same blast.

In truth, the North Vietnamese might have been preparing a major assault. The night of February 29, they attacked the ARVN sector manned by South Vietnamese rangers. Unbeknownst to the North Vietnamese, they had all been picked up by sensors. No sooner had they massed for assault than B-52 Arc Light strikes, artillery from Camp Carroll, and fighter-bomber raids plastered their ranks. A few reached the outer wire but no farther. Scores were later found dead in their trenches, armed with Bangalore torpedoes and satchel charges. Marines were convinced there would be more. To them there was no letup. Small unit probes kept them vigilant, fully expecting another Dien Bien Phu. "I think most of us had already accepted the fact that we were going to die.

No one said that. . . . But . . . we acted that way," recalled Chaplain Stubbe in an interview.[51] War correspondent Michael Herr put their fears this way: "[W]hat if all of those gooks that you think are out there are really out there? What if they really want Khe Sanh. . . . And what if they pass over every barricade we can put in their way . . . and kill every living thing, defending or retreating . . . and take Khe Sanh?"[52]

Giap may have lost his appetite for frontal assaults, but incoming artillery and mortar fire did not let up, averaging 150 rounds a day, peaking to 1,109 rounds on March 23.[53] Each time, one or two or three Marines were caught in the open and felled, particularly if they chose not to wear their flak jackets, which became a problem as the weather warmed. Hanging out above ground was tempting fate, but many did it. There were yo-yo emotions of confidence and dread—and a duality of behavior. Nineteen-year-old Corpsman Robert Topmiller confessed: "Sometimes at Khe Sanh, I performed my duties and took risks that today seem extraordinary. Yet, on other days, I experienced a paralyzing trepidation that rendered me unable to move. I cannot really explain the difference but I believe that every human has a limit and many understand when they begin to approach it."[54]

March 8 was the day Jonathan Spicer got it. It had already been a rough start at Charlie Med. The gun-pit triple amputee had just come in and gone out, barely alive. People were still cleaning up the mess. Then, a number of Marines, maybe as many as twenty, wounded and corpsmen, grouped around a waiting chopper—a bad idea. In came a round, and with freakish accuracy, it exploded in their midst. Two died outright.[55] Spicer, a slender young Marine, dropped. He had refused to take cover, insisting on carrying Marines to the chopper. He was hand-carried right over to Charlie Med. Doctors found him pale, pulseless, and lifeless. Finnegan called it: cardiac tamponade. Thoracotomy. Sure enough, a bulging pericardium full of blood from a heart wound. Slicing into the pericardium Finnegan released the pent-up hemorrhage and found a small hole in the left ventricle. Timing his stitches in rhythm with the barely beating heart, he sutured the hole closed. Almost miraculously, Spicer pinked up, his heart began beating, and life returned. He was closed up, bandaged, and medevaced to Dong Ha.[56] But Spicer, a favorite of the men, selfless, courageous, did not recover. He died at the air force hospital in Tachikawa, Japan, on March 14.[57]

Journalists flew into and out of Khe Sanh with some regularity. Fed by almost nightly television news coverage, the American public developed a voracious appetite for the story. They began to suspect a debacle the magnitude of the siege at Bastogne or the entrapment at the Chosin Reservoir. This was the stuff of legends, but it was pure adventure for correspondents and chock full of danger. Adrenaline junkies took the bait: "Khe Sanh has become a testing place for journalists, proving who has courage and who hasn't, or who's got more and who's got less. It's rather stupid business."[58]

One, photojournalist Robert Ellison, had courage but not luck. He died, along with forty-eight other crew and passengers, in the crash of a C-123 that had to circle Khe Sanh's runway. A light plane had suddenly appeared to make an unannounced landing. On coming around again, the C-123 was shot down by enemy ground fire. All aboard were killed. Then there was freelance photojournalist Jarate Kazickas, nicknamed "Sam" by the Marines. A Chinook brought her in. What a sight, she wrote. "The hills around Khe Sanh were a patchwork of lush greens, so many different shades like emerald and jade." Kazickas was what one Marine described as a "raven haired beauty." So there she was, perched on a bunker, interviewing combat engineer Lieutenant William Gay. One round exploded nearby. Gay knew another would follow. Move, he shouted. Kazickas balked, and Gay literally pushed her into his bunker just as a second shell, some thought a 152 mm, blasted. "I've been hit, I've been hit," her tape recorder caught as she fell forward. Gay remembers saying, "I'm hit! Dammit! I'm hit!" Both he and Kazickas took fragments—a fraction of a second later they would have been killed—and she became Charlie Med's one and only female patient. It was a golden moment. After all the mud and blood, grime and rank, here came a beautiful woman down the ramp. Three doctors—Feldman, Finnegan, and Magilligan—stood gawking, frozen for an instant by the incongruity of such glamor gracing their little chamber of horrors. There was the cursory body check: scratches and bruises, not too bad. Then a corpsman squeaked, "There's blood on the seat of her pants, sir." With that, a careful undress, standard practice. Of course, modesty prevailed, but still "a dozen eyes" peered down, as Sam recalled. Then the peach-pit-sized fragment was found, just superficial to her spine. No internal damage. She moved everything quite well, thank you. She wisecracked, "Is it below my bikini line?" Clean and dress. Goodbye Sam, and off she went to Delta Med at Dong Ha.[59] On they went to Lieutenant Gay, a chunk torn out of his ass. "I put my hand between my legs to determine if my penis and genitals had been blown off and came up with a handful of blood."

But penis and testicles remained pristine. He medevaced out on the same chopper as Kazickas. "I can't tell you how important Charlie Med was to the morale of all of us at Khe Sanh," Gay said much later.[60]

Khe Sanh had to be relieved. This siege, this isolation could not last. Plans had been in the works since late January. On March 2, Westmoreland agreed to an operation code-named Pegasus. Two battalions of Marines (2nd Battalion, 1st Marines and 2nd Battalion, 3rd Marines) and three brigades of the 1st Cavalry Division under General John Tolson attacked from Ca Lu down Route 9 west to Khe Sanh. Of course, Route 9 was a mess. What the VC hadn't done the weather had, with dozens of bridges blown up or washed out. Sky troopers leapfrogged across, inserting at points along the way, and flanking the Marines coming by ground.

Just before Pegasus started, the Marines were eager to strike out, take the offensive, to make sure the world knew they were not rescued. Some thought this rash. Never mind, enough sitting. Marines were saddling up. The immediate objective was south of the combat base, Hill 471 and plantation country—the same area of the Ghost Patrol and its unclaimed dead. Captain Pipes and Bravo Company were given the reigns in a revenge match with the North Vietnamese—but the North Vietnamese were waiting. On March 30, Pipes and his men blew through the wire in full battle gear. Approaching Hill 471, Bravo Marines were clobbered with mortar fire and pinned down. Volleys were so thick Pipes said he could see them fly through the air. After a four-hour fight, Pipes took them back to the base, recovering the bodies of two of the missing from Don Jacques's "Ghost Patrol." But they also took ten of their own dead and one hundred wounded. There was lots of activity at Charlie Med. "The sky was so filled with choppers, it looked like a swarm of mosquitoes or a bee's nest," Ed Feldman remembered.[61] It was another week before Company D, 1st Battalion ventured across Poilane's access road, battled through a North Vietnamese bunker field, and found the remains. Pieces of seventeen Marines were packaged and hauled in. To Pipes fell the grim task of sorting through bones and flesh of his lost Marines.

Operation Scotland ended the same day Pegasus commenced, April Fools' Day. Marines and Air Cav rolled west. Khe Sanh Leathernecks picked away at their perimeter, eventually storming Hill 881N, the last enemy stronghold in hill country. Finally, on April 7, the linkup occurred. The 2nd Battalion, 7th Cav entered the combat base along Papa Poilane's old plantation trail. Operation Pegasus was over.

With army units moving north, nearer the DMZ, hospitals soon followed. Along Highway 1—the French had called it La Rue Sans Joie (Street Without Joy)—came the 22nd Surgical (from Phu Bai), the 95th Evac (Da Nang), and the 18th Surgical (Quang Tri City, just outside Dong Ha).[62] An army medevac helicopter ambulance detachment of six UH-1 Hueys was also stationed at Quang Tri. The Hueys, a favorite of medevac pilots, were considerably more nimble than Marine Corp Sea Knights and Sea Stallions and easier to land on hospital ships.[63]

Giap gave up Khe Sanh. Whether it was ever his intention to overrun the Marines is unclear, but it was not worth the sacrifice. Or it had already served its purpose—diverting attention from his bigger Tet offensives. MACV would also soon give it up. President Johnson had decided to stay out of Laos. Suddenly, Khe Sanh became more a liability than an asset. "[T]he sole remaining reason for holding it, as a base for a drive into Laos, appeared no longer valid," Westmoreland claimed.[64] On June 19, dismantling of the Khe Sanh combat base began—Operation Charlie. Instead, a new Marine base at Ca Lu, directly on Route 9, would be the hub for Quang Tri Province. Operation Charlie called for removing all usable supplies from the base, including the resilient steel runway matting. On July 5, the combat base officially closed, the last convoy leaving down Route 9. At midnight, July 6, Operation Charlie ended. Communist officials in Hanoi proclaimed the withdrawal of US forces from Khe Sanh a victory for the North Vietnamese People's Army. Jim Finnegan was dumbstruck at the news, "as though we were never there—no airstrip, no bunkers, no Marines, no Charlie Med. . . . Not one cross or helmet to remember the dead Marines."[65]

Khe Sanh was no Dien Bien Phu. One hundred thousand rounds of artillery, mortar, and rockets, and some sixty thousand tons of bombs from high-level Arc Light and fighter-bomber strikes helped see to that.[66] Marine and army guns incessantly pounded the hills, and napalm torched the countryside. The North Vietnamese were hard pressed to move. And if they did, sensors picked it up and all those assembly points where green-helmeted men came together to disperse in their trenches were leveled to dust by 750-pound bombs they never heard falling. Within the combat base and even in the hills, Marines held wisely: enough food, enough ammunition, enough medical care. Air power and Super Gaggles and gutsy pilots ran in and out like freight trains. Precision drops and lightning airstrip extractions delivered tons upon tons of material. Winston Churchill may have said it best when he wrote: "Victory is the beautiful, bright-colored flower. Transport [read "logistics"] is the stem without which it could never have blossomed."[67] A vital part of logistics for any army is the ability to evacuate wounded. This wreaked havoc for the French at Dien Bien Phu and had a disastrous effect on morale. But not at Khe Sanh. Special Clearing Platoon #2 of C Medical Company—Charlie Med—processed 2,031 battle casualties from January 14 through April 22, returning 292 valuable Leathernecks to the lines, and flying the rest out. Few festered for long in the C Med bunker.[68] Hill country wounded went straight to Dong Ha (D Med), Phu Bai (A, B, and the rest of C Med), or Da Nang (NSA Hospital). D Med got the most. Its three operating rooms ran at capacity during February, when 1,304 battle casualties were admitted, and March, when the number rose to 1,679. Khe Sanh Marines had a voracious appetite for blood. Third Med poured in one thousand units in February and almost two thousand (1,894) units in March.[69] No, Khe Sanh was never Dien Bien Phu. Some would say it was never really a siege.[70] That, of course, is all in hindsight. It would not be unduly melodramatic to think so, the mind-set of its garrison a function of relentless North Vietnamese probing and a displeasurable proximity to an enemy who refused to hide his presence. Ask Marines who were there. Ask those on the receiving end of ten thousand incoming shells and rockets. The North Vietnamese were just over the horizon, just beyond the wire, thousands of them, waiting. Giap never gave the signal.

And don't forget to ask the families of the 442 soldiers and Marines and air crew who never came back. Official reporting for Operation Scotland, the siege of Khe Sanh, listed 204 Marines killed and 1,622 wounded—hardly the entire story. Chaplain Stubbe put the figure at 442 dead and over 2,000 wounded—Charlie Med's log book told that tale.[71] Operation Pegasus alone resulted in 92 Marines and Air Cav troopers killed and 667 wounded.[72] And then there was Lang Vei and Khe Sanh.[73]

For the injured, speed set the pace. Speed saved lives. At Khe Sanh and in Vietnam in general, a new kind of medicine was borne: air evacuation right from the battlefield. "The speed with which the injured are taken to a forward hospital is the most unique feature of this war," wrote Dr. Ben Eiseman, navy medical consultant and veteran of the Second World War and Korea. In his opinion, the immediacy of care simplified resuscitation, with volumes of blood lost quickly replaced by volumes given. He concluded: "Wounded in the remote jungle or rice paddy of Vietnam, an American citizen has a better chance for quick definitive surgical care by board certified specialists than were he hit on a highway near his hometown in the continental United States."[74]

Was it true? People at NSA Da Nang felt so. From January to June 1968, during the height of I Corps activity around Khe Sanh, 2,021 casualties were admitted. Almost two thousand (1,962) were released alive, a salvage rate of 97 percent. Only 3 percent of wounded died in the hospital—2 percent if one excluded those who never had a chance, the "expectant" cases. Survival from battle wounds was a startling 98 percent. Why? Speed. The time elapsed from wounding to arrival at NSA Hospital was just short of five hours for survivors and 2.8 hours for nonsurvivors. Once brought through the doors, most were in the operating room in under two hours. What happened in the meantime was blood and lots of it, almost six units for those who survived. For those who died, heroic attempts pushed twelve units in before giving up.[75]

One hundred years prior pioneer anesthetist William Morton, after the Battle of the Wilderness in 1864, observed, "It is the most sickening sight of the war, this tide of the wounded flowing back."[76] Indeed little had changed—it was, perhaps, much worse. "I have evolved from a child to a man, and from a neophyte to a surgeon," thought Paul Pitlyk as he departed Vietnam at the conclusion of his tour.[77] Surgeons had done remarkable things, reversing lethal physiology, rearranging disemboweled and dismembered anatomy, but the emotional toll was insurmountable for many—patients and physicians alike. All lost something, inside or out. Pitlyk reflected: "I also wondered how many young men physically lost their dignity while we the surgeons were emotionally losing ours. . . . [W]ith each succeeding devastating injury, the emotional impact on me lessened. . . . The patient simply became curious anatomic abominations from the battlefield."[78]

For surgeon Jim Finnegan, a scene was embossed in his memory: a Marine at Charlie Med whose nearly severed leg was hanging by only the thick sciatic nerve. Insensate, shattered, and ischemic, there was no alternative but to finish the near-amputation before the young man bled to death. As Finnegan cut across the plump cord of nerve, the Marine let out a blood-curdling scream, a scream that haunted him for years to come, and he asked himself again and again, "What have you done?" Years later, he still admitted "there's hardly a week that goes by that there isn't some reminder that I did what I did."[79]

One of the last victims of the Khe Sanh siege was Papa Poilane's son, thirty-seven-year-old Felix. After making innumerable trips to the combat base, ferrying old and sick villagers to safety, he, his wife, and his children locked up the plantation house and were flown to Da Nang. After word reached him on April 9 that Khe Sanh had been liberated, he was eager to get back to his beloved home and coffee trees. He somehow arranged a return flight on April 13 against the protests of his wife, a modern-day Cassandra who spoke of dire premonitions. She even confiscated his passport, all to no avail. The C-130 he was aboard, a plane of the 774th Tactical Airlift Squadron, suffered engine failure just as it was approaching the Khe Sanh airstrip and crashed on landing, spectacularly sliding off the runway and bursting into flames. Despite heroic efforts of an air force rescue detachment, Felix Poilane did not survive. He was the only civilian onboard and the only fatality.[80] Felix Poilane was buried in France, but he will forever be part of Vietnam, nurtured from birth to death in the red clay of Khe Sanh.

Aftermath

A COMMON DENOMINATOR IN ALL THESE CONFLICTS—BATAAN, Anzio, Bastogne, Chosin, Khe Sanh—was the struggle of fortitude against hopelessness. Courage against despair. If not physical depletion, then a spiritual erosion of worth, of future, of salvation. For caregivers, lack of supplies—even the most rudimentary of salves and opiates—caused consternation to all but the most callous of healers. The corporeal privations of food and warmth, and the existence of rampant disease, were as treacherous as battle wounds. A withering of stamina followed—both mental and visceral—so vital to resistance. For America, this was never so apparent as in the Philippines in 1942. Wretched, they all became. General MacArthur wrote in his memoirs about Bataan: "Our troops were now approaching exhaustion. . . . My heart ached as I saw my men slowly wasting away. Their clothes hung on them like tattered rags. Their bare feet stuck out in silent protest. Their long bedraggled hair framed gaunt bloodless faces."[1]

Dr. John Bumgarner was freed from Bibai prisoner of war camp in Japan on August 18, 1945, after three years of captivity at the hands of pitiless Japanese guards and ruthless work in the coal mines. "I was so overwhelmed that I dropped my head, beat the table with my fist, and cried unashamedly." Diets of rice and unsweetened tea, frigid winters, nonexistent sanitation, and cynical overlords had all taken their toll. Back in the wreckage of Manila, he looked for friends from Bataan. Stricken with tuberculosis because of his time in the prison camps, Bumgarner made a slow, agonizing recovery and returned to the practice of medicine for thirty more years. "I suppose I could easily be critical," he wrote later. "I was a victim, like so many others, of the tremendous turmoil and confusion that inevitably accompany a terrible war."[2] Some, like Lieutenant Colonel "Riney" Craig, who had set up General Hospital No. 2, endured unbelievable hardships. Craig's story was one of the most pitiful. After surviving the Allied bombing of a Japanese freighter carrying numbers of American prisoners of war, he died miserably, of starvation and dysentery, before war's end. It happened on another notorious freighter, *Brazil Maru*, trapped in dank holds without food or water. Craig's lifeless form was simply tossed overboard. Al Weinstein lived, but he was haunted by memories of the camps: Fellow physicians mentally broken, to be committed to asylums; bruised and battered inmates, subjects of whimsical Japanese brutality; skeleton frames in rags so weak they could not walk; epidemic diseases—diphtheria, dysentery, tuberculosis—felling prisoner after prisoner with no medical supplies to give. And all the desperate surgery necessary on Bataan as equipment vanished and the Japanese closed in—scenes of despondency and suffering. There was no bravado, no sense of heroism, only survival and a painful reentry to civilized life that seemed so incongruous with the past three years.[3]

And those nurses of Bataan, eventually rounded up with General Wainwright's surrender of Corregidor on May 6, 1942, were imprisoned and not liberated until American troops returned to Luzon in January 1945. "The Angels of Bataan" returned home to a mixed audience. Some were hailed as heroes, others were barely noticed—the "Silent Angels" they then called themselves. Physicians and psychologists preferred to work on male prisoners of war, largely ignoring women who endured almost as much. Diseases of captivity gradually crept in: tuberculosis, fungus infections, intestinal disorders, and dental problems, sometimes lasting decades. And with war's end, they once again became, more or less, part of mainstream America, unpretentious, unobtrusive, and still commited to the care of their patients. They were said to have chased the American dream, but not the dream of possesions, the dream of "'values,' of a richer and fuller life." That they attained, if not for others to see then for themselves, in the knowledge that they had given—and received—above and beyond what they ever hoped. One of the Angels, Mildred "Milly" Dalton, before she died in 2013, told author Elizabeth Norman, "We spent our lives helping people, and we did it with honor and love and never looked back."[4]

The horrors of day-to-day life during those times were mixed with an unbreakable bond with those who endured and remembrances of those who did not. "I said a prayerful farewell to Ellen, Gertrude, Rita, Nick, and thousands of others who had lost their lives on the beachhead," wrote a somber Avis Schorer as she departed Italy. "I never ceased thanking God that I had survived Anzio. . . . Our lives had been permanently altered; people who had stayed at home would never understand us," commented June Wandrey after it was all over, victory declared in Europe.[5] On the way home the troop train was strangely quiet, despite vermin-infested cars "smelling of stale tobacco, sweat, and urine. . . . We stared at others in disbelief . . . people immersed in their own thoughts. . . . Tears spilled down my face."[6] For Lawrence Collins with the 56th Evac, his entire overseas experience centered on his nine weeks at Anzio. "Nothing after compared with it," he wrote, adding: "[I]t was a time of intense pride in our nation . . . and in each other. It was a time of consuming interest in our work and a dedication to it. Such pride and such consuming interest . . . seem to compensate for any and all miseries endured in gaining them."[7]

Major Lamar Soutter continued across Germany with the 4th Auxliary Surgical Group, his quiet demeanor, patient voice, and boyish looks making him an icon among enlisted men. Few were aware of his heroics in Bastogne; indeed, even after the war few heard of it. In passing through, he saw the ruins of a German nation, the horrors of Buchenwald, and the poverty of victimized civilians. VE Day found him in Pfeffenhauen, near Munich, among a collection of people from a dozen countries intermingling with concentration camp survivors in their striped prison garb. Bins of Rhine wine were found in a basement. Soutter's men confiscated scores of bottles, and, lacking a corkscrew, without hesitation, Soutter obliged the thirsty group by knocking the tops off against the side of a truck. All partook. Celebration: the war was over.

For Major Albert Crandall of the 3rd Auxiliary Surgical Group, the war ended with his capture by the Germans just outside of Bastogne on the evening of December 19, 1944. He and other prisoners were loaded in boxcars packed sixty tight, and the doors were shut and locked for the next several days. In that suffocating journey he even survived strafing by American planes that killed a number of men in his car and wounded over one hundred. His efforts to treat the wounded were crude, with medical supplies sorely lacking, and the weather was freezing cold. With numerous transfers and shuttling, Crandall ended up in Poland as the Russians were advancing from the east. Soon, German guards, fearing the immediacy of vindictive Soviet troops, lost interest in their captives.

It was then that Crandall and his medical teams began working on Allied prisoners of war, though the weather was harsher and nourishment meager. But he operated with surprising freedom, aided by the Polish underground. Soon they were surrounded by Red Army troops, who were not much more sympathetic than the Germans, being highly suspicious of the American doctors and loathe to give any meaningful help or material. Finally at war's end, like medical refugees, Crandall and a group of American officers made their way to Odessa in the Ukraine, through the Black Sea, Malta, and finally to Marseilles. From there he caught a ride to Naples and then home to Vermont by way of Washington, DC. He remembered those times in captivity as heartbreaking, caring for the thousands of wounded American soldiers with no food, no clothing, no shelter, and no medical provisions. The ravages of frostbite, malnutrition, and disease went unchecked.

Bastogne was rebuilt, brick by brick. Those old stone buildings leveled by air raids or artillery barrages soon regained a new façade. Beleagured residents who fled with the Nazi surge slowly came back, the war now moving east, across the Rhine. Amid the destruction and loss of life, some degree of normality returned. And soon, after the war's end, plaques were erected honoring men of the 101st and 10th Armored in places like Noville, Foy, Longchamps, Jacques Woods, and the Houffalize road where the 326th Medical Company met its end. A small commemorative shrine, the Enclos des fusilles, was erected in Noville honoring the seven civilians tortured and butchered by the Gestapo on December 21. The sprawling Rolle Chateau cleaned out stale bedding and bloody dressings, and regained its former elegance. Gothic Eglise Saint-Pierre and its dominant sandstone bell tower dating from the fifteenth century were declared miracles of the siege, largely preserved and undamaged except, of course, the magnificent stained-glass windows, which were blown out, and two punched holes in the vault caused by enemy shelling. On the Rue de Neufchateau, rubble from that Christmas Eve tragedy was cleaned up and a new structure built, noticeably different from the bordering nineteenth century domiciles. It was eventually occupied by, of all things, a Chinese restaurant. Only a plaque on an outside wall commemorates the loss of life here, over thirty American soldiers and one Belgian nurse, a plaque far too diminutive to reflect the immense sorrow of that night. Le Petit Seminaire, home to the 501st Parachute Infantry aid station, was heavily damaged in February 1945, one entire wing demolished, and was not completely restored until 1947. It still held a prominent place in the town at the point La Grand'rue intersects the roads leading to Noville and Clerveaux. And passing out of town, north to Foy and Noville, remained Heintz Barracks, a tribute to the steel of American commanders during those uncertain days. Toward the rear of the compound, the dilapidated buildings that lodged so many wounded still stood, vacant reminders of the bleak fortunes awaiting so many—until arrival of the airborne surgeons. Just across the street was the Ancien Cemetiere, where two heroines of the siege were to be placed within yards of one another, Renée Lemaire and Augusta Chiwy. And, over the years, the town recaptured its charming simplicity, the battles and memorials fading from local nostalgia, the visiting veterans gradually tapering off until the events of December 1944 were found only in dusty history books. Only the streetside bar Le Nuts served reminders: miniature GI helmets full of local Belgian beer.

"The imminent arrival of Chinese Red troops in Korea should have been known," said Dr. Robert Shoemaker. "Was it General MacArthur's ego that compelled him to cross the 38th parallel . . . or was it stupidity?" Like the many military surgeons caught in the cauldron of siege, Shoemaker always regretted not being able to do more for the wounded. "There was always the frustration that we couldn't do enough because of the logistical and environmental situation," he wrote, in rather sterile terms. But in Korea, all under his care became "family." "In Korea they were 'brothers.'"[8] Dr. Ken Holloway sipped his one Christmas drink in the small Korean town of Masan, near Pusan, the poverty and deprivations of many Koreans lining the compound fence easily visible. His mood was melancholy, thankful he had survived "a very terrible ordeal," but not given to the celebrations of some of his colleagues. Why did they make it through? A little luck he surmised, a whole lot of training, and Marine esprit de corps. For Dr. James Stewart, evacuation from Hungnam to Pusan meant a brief period in reserves but then back to the front lines and hideously wounded Marines. Finally, his tour was up. In Tokyo, he bathed in lavish parties as if all were trying to forget or would not remember, and then he leapfrogged across the Pacific to Los Angeles. "I felt the welcome of native soil and breathed fresh, clean air. I was home, my war was over."[9] But it would likely never totally be. War never really leaves those who endure it. There is a stain on the soul, an indelible mark, a badge, perhaps, or maybe a curse. For doctors and nurses, those times of damaged forms, pumping blood, splitting chests, rummaging through trashed arms and legs, and plowing into the wanton waste of shredded bowel—of those nameless faces who breathed their last—would be their constant shadow.

"A great many people wanted to know how the Khe Sanh Combat Base could have been the Western Anchor of our Defense one month and a worthless piece of ground the next," mused Michael Herr. The brutalized ground, stripped of all vegetation, sprouted that summer of 1968 "with a violence of energy . . . as though there was an impatience somewhere to conceal all traces of what had been left by the winter."[10] Khe Sanh eventually became a memorial to the sacrifices and victories of the People's Army. The combat base reverted to a flat, scruffy plot of land, the airstrip soon unrecognizable. Only the red clay could still be scratched out and poured into bottles as souvenirs. A few armored vehicles, tanks, and helicopters were placed about as a feeble attempt at a museum, and peddlers abounded, hawking their numerous battlefield artifacts to any curious visitor. The surrounding hills, sites of so much bloodshed, overgrew that blood-stained earth and sandbags and rusted canisters and regained the brilliance of "emerald and jade," a panorama much like it might have been when Eugene Poilane stumbled across it that sweltering day in 1918. But an indescribable spirit of the place, what the North American Lakota called *chawn-oh-tee-lah*, infected each person who was there, so that Khe Sanh never left them but mingled with their memories and dreams and dwelled in their hearts forever.

AT LAST WHAT THEN CAN WE SAY ABOUT THESE HEROES; that they expended their best years in blinding instants of benevolence; that they traded the very essence of vitality for the suddenness of extinction; that they unwittingly submitted not to the charms of longevity but rather to the torments of compassion.

The strain of devotion had shown heavily on the tent cities of Bataan, Hell's Half Acre of Anzio, the beleaguered field hospitals in and around Bastogne, the frozen slopes of North Korea, and the red clay of Khe Sanh. Likely, and sadly, it will show again on the battlefields of the future. That the depth of devotion comes with a price is undeniable. There is a depletion that must be renewed. Perhaps it is in mercy itself. The quality of mercy illuminates giver and taker. To the recipient it is replenishment; to the bestower, let it be renewal.

Notes

CHAPTER 1. AMERICA'S COLONY, LAS ISLAS FELIPINAS

1. Quotes from Homer Lea, *The Valor of Ignorance* (New York: Harper and Brothers, 1901), 194-196, 251-253.
2. *Lapu-lapu* is a name given by Filipinos in Luzon to reef-dwelling grouper fish named after the legendary chieftan from Cebu who was the first to resist Spanish colonial efforts in the sixteenth century.
3. Douglas MacArthur, *Reminiscences* (New York: McGraw-Hill, 1964), 112.
4. Ibid., 118.
5. Ibid., 29.
6. "MacArthur Made Chief in Far East," *New York Times*, July 27, 1941.
7. MacArthur, *Reminiscences*, 109.
8. Samuel Morison, *History of United States Naval Operations in World War II, Volume 3: The Rising Sun in the Pacific, 1931-April 1942* (New York: Little, Brown, 1948); it is likely, also, that the United States embargo on oil, iron, and rubber shipments to Japan in the summer of 1941—in response to Japan's invasion of China—would force the Japanese to either get out of China or look for other regions where the embargo did not extend, i.e., Malaya and the Dutch East Indies, which put the Philippines directly in their sights. See also, Robert MacDougall, *Leaders in Dangerous Times: Douglas MacArthur and Dwight D. Eisenhower* (Bloomington: Trafford, 2013), 73-75.
9. Quote taken from Murat Halstead's *The Story of the Philippines and Our New Possessions, Including the Landrones, Hawaii, Cuba, and Porto Rico, The Eldorado of the Orient* (Chicago: Our Possessions Publishing, 1898), 5.
10. "Worst-Governed People," *New York Times*, July 18, 1892.

CHAPTER 2. A TREMBLING LEAF

1. As far back as 1922 then Governor-General Leonard Wood felt defending the Philippines against Japanese incursion was imperative, and that loss of the islands would fatally damage American prestige in the Far East. How this was to be done, however, was a matter of much debate and, in the end, relied on time—time to mount a sufficient naval and ground force to provide a serious deterrent to invasion. For further reference see Louis Morton, "War Plan Orange: Evolution of a Strategy," *World Politics* 11 (1959): 221-250.
2. Morton, "War Plan Orange," *World Politics*.

3. "Hearings before the Joint Committee on the Investigation of the Pearl Harbor Attack," Seventy-ninth Congress, First Session, United States Government Printing Office, Washington, DC, 1946. Included is a letter from Admiral Harold Stark to Admiral Thomas Hart, December 23, 1940: "how far we should go in maintaining our position in the Philippines. . . ." See also Admiral Hart's frustration with General MacArthur vented to Admiral Stark in James R. Leutze, *A Different Kind of Victory: A Biography of Admiral Thomas C. Hart* (Annapolis: Naval Institute Press, 1981), 218-219.
4. F. Scott Fitzgerald, *The Crack-Up* [ed. Edmund Wilson] (New York: New Directions, 1945, 1993), 122.
5. The Visayan-Mindanao Force, under the command of Brigadier General William Sharp, was distributed on the southern islands of Panay, Cebu, Negros, Leyte-Samar, and Mindanao. Medical personnel were recruited from local physicians and nurses who, when war was declared, were inducted into the service of the United States. Local civilian hospitals were designated for military use. (Wibb Cooper, *Medical Department Activities in the Philippines from 1941 to 6 May 1942, and Including Medical Activities in Japanese Prisoner of War Camps*, 1946, RG 407 [Adjutant General] NARA, College Park, MD, 92-97).
6. Interview with Maj. Richard M. Gordon, Bataan survivor, by John P. Cervone; "Remembering the Bataan Death March," *Military History* 16 (1999): 30-37.
7. "National Affairs: Bingham on Brownskins," *Time*, October 10, 1927.
8. Ralph Emerson Hibbs, *Tell MacArthur to* Wait (Quezon City: Giraffe Books, 1996), 15.
9. "Mestizas" were Filipino women of mixed race (usually of Spanish and indigenous descent).
10. Public Papers of the Presidents of the United States: Dwight D. Eisenhower, 1960-61, "Remarks at a Civic Reception at the Luneta in Manila," June 16, 1960, Office of the Federal Register, U.S. Government Printing Office, 1961, 495-499.
11. *United States Surgeon-General's Office. Report of the Surgeon-General of the Army to the Secretary of War for the Fiscal Year Ending 1921* (Washington, DC: Government Printing Office, 1921), Record Group (RG) 112 (Records of the Office of the Surgeon General [Army]), National Archives and Records Administration (hereafter designated NARA), College Park, MD, 127.
12. Roster of all Medical Department Officers Fort Stotsenburg, P.I., November, 1941, Philippine Archive Collection, RG 407 (Adjutant General), NARA, College Park, MD.
13. Report of the Philippine Commission: *Baguio as Summer Capital*, 1903, Filipinas Heritagy Library, Manila, Philippines.
14. "*We Look Before and After, and Pine for What is Not*": *A History of Pines Hotel and Baguio*. Filipinas Heritage Library, Manila, 2015.
15. Interview with Major Richard M. Gordon, Bataan survivor, by John P. Cervone; "Remembering the Bataan Death March," *Military History* 16 (1999): 30-37.
16. History, Philippine Medical Depot, RG 407, Philippine Archive Collection, NARA, College Park, MD.
17. 12th Medical Battalion, Philippine Division, Daily Reports, 1941-1942, RG 407 (Philippine Archive Collection), NARA, College Park, MD.
18. Russell, P.F., "Malaria in the Philippine Islands." *American Journal of Tropical Medicine*, 13 (1933):167-178.
19. T. Gerow, "Relief of the Philippines," War Department: Memorandum for the

Chief of Staff, January 3, 1942, RG 165 (War Plans Division), NARA, College Park, MD.

20. Message from General MacArthur to all unit commanders, January 15, 1942, RG-2, Records of Headquarters, U.S. Army Forces in the Far East (USAFFE), 1941-1942, MacArthur Memorial Archives and Library, Norfolk, VA.

21. Ruth Straub Diary excerpts published in the *Chicago Sunday Tribune*, September 20, 1942.

22. Henry G. Lee, *Nothing But Praise* (Hollywood: Murray & Gee, 1948), a book compiled by his parents Thomas and Mabel Lee of poems and letters written by Henry during his captivity. The title comes from a remark by Secretary of War Stimson when he announced the fall of Bataan to wire services on April 9, 1942: "We have nothing but praise for the men who have conducted this epic chapter in American history" ("Japs Conquer Bataan," *Hattiesburg* [MS] *American*, April 9, 1942).

23. Charles-Augustin Sainte-Beuve, *Portraits Contemporains*, Vol. III (Paris: Calmann Levy, Editeur, 1882), 48.

24. James Hopper, *Caybigan* (New York: McClure, Phillips, 1906), 128.

CHAPTER 3. INVASION

1. Diary, Captain Robert G. Davis, MC, USN, 8 December 1941—7 September 1945, RG 389, NARA, College Park, MD, and John Glusman: *Conduct Under Fire: Four American Doctors and Their Fight for Life as Prisoners of the Japanese 1941-1945* (London: Penguin Books, 2005), 59.

2. Information on Captain Carey Smith from Karen Ann Takizawa (granddaughter of Carey Smith), *War Stories (2): The Fall of Corregidor (May 6, 1942)*, Japanese Institutional Repositories Online *(JAIRO)* 60 (2013): 1-33. His 118-page memoir was written after his liberation from a prisoner of war camp in 1945 and, according to Karen Takizawa, was submitted to the United States government. She retained about one-third of the manscript in which Carey described his activities up to his capture on Corregidor in May 1942.

3. Morison, *Rising Sun in the Pacific*, 171.

4. Evelyn Monahan and Rosemary Neidel-Greenlee, *All This Hell* (Lexington: University Press of Kentucky, 2000), 21.

5. Interview with Rear Admiral Ferdinand Berley, MC, USN (Ret.), conducted by Jan K. Herman, Historian, Bureau of Medicine and Surgery (BUMED), February, March, and May 1995, Falls Church, VA.

6. John R. Bumgarner, *Parade of the Dead* (Jefferson, NC: McFarland, 1995), 52.

7. Japanese Land Operations, December 8, 1941 to June 8, 1942, Military Intelligence Service, War Department, November 18, 1942, The Command and General Staff School, Fort Leavenworth, KS.

8. Eugene C. Jacobs, *Blood Brothers: A Medic's Sketch Book* (New York: Carlton Press, 1985), 26.

9. *Ascaris lumbricoides*, or roundworm, was a frequent parasite among Filipino—and American—residents of Luzon as well as the other Philippine Islands. The mature worm, found in the intestinal tract, can reach lengths of over one foot. The fertilized eggs are eliminated in human excrement and, where human feces are used as fertilizer, can persist in the soil for years. With poor hygiene and in a rural, agricultural setting, they are ingested and the life cycle repeats.

10. Dorothy Cave, *Beyond Courage, One Regiment Against Japan, 1941-1945* (Las Cruces, NM: Yucca Tree Press, 1992), 74.

11. Alfred Weinstein, *Barbed-Wire Surgeon: A Prisoner of War in Japan*, (Athens: Deeds Publishing, 2014), 23.
12. Carlton B. Vanderboget, *Report of the Medical Department Activities in the Philippines*, Office of the Surgeon General, May 21, 1945, RG 112 (Surgeon General's Office), NARA, College Park, MD.
13. Vanderboget, *Report of the Medical Department*, 1945.
14. William Fairfield's experiences were described in Paul Ashton, *And Somebody Gives a Damn* (Santa Barbara: Ashton Publications, 1990), 31.
15. Ashton, *And Somebody Gives a Damn*, 33.
16. Vanderboget, *Report of the Medical Department*, 1945.
17. Elizabeth Norman, *We Band of Angels* (New York: Pocket Books, 1999), 13.
18. Ibid., 15.
19. Paul Ashton, *Bataan Diary* (Santa Barbara: Paul Ashton [self-published], 1984), 64.
20. Ibid., 67.

CHAPTER 4. INTO BATAAN

1. "General MacArthur's Proclamation," *Manila Bulletin*, December 26, 1941.
2. The SS *Don Estabon* had evacuated General MacArthur, his family, and his headquarters staff from Manila to Corregidor the evening of December 23.
3. Details of the SS *Mactan* and her skipper found in George Korson, *At His Side: The Story of the American Red Cross Overseas in World War 2* (New York: Coward-McCann, 1945), 16-22.
4. Diary entries by Major William A. Fairfield as part of the Philippine Diary Project, http://philippine-defenders.lib.wv.us/pdf/bios/fairfield_william_bio.pdf, accessed September 16, 2015.
5. James W. Duckworth, Official History of General Hospital No. 1, USAFFE, at Camp Limay, Bataan, Little Baguio, Bataan, and Camp O'Donnell, Tarlac, Philippine Islands, Philippine Archive Collection, RG 407, NARA, College Park, MD.
6. J. M. Goodman, *J. M. M.D. P.O.W.: A Firsthand Account of 42 Months of Imprisonment in Japanese Hands* (New York: Exposition Press, 1972), 14.
7. Norman, *We Band of Angels*, 23.
8. Col. Wibb E. Cooper, *Medical Department Activities in the Philippines from 1941 to 6 May 1942*, RG 407 (Adjutant General), NARA, College Park, MD. Cooper mentions twelve operating teams at work.
9. Ibid.
10. Hospital Number "2", Bataan, PI, RG 407, Philippine Archive Collection, NARA, College Park, MD.
11. Eventually animal visitors would vanish; most large enough to eat had been killed.
12. Norman, *We Band of Angels*, 55.
13. The GMC CCKW 2 1/2-ton 6 x 6 U.S. Army cargo truck—also known as "Jimmy" or a "deuce-and-a-half"—was the backbone of the army's ground supply train during World War II. The intrepid Lieutenant Colonel William Draper North was a physician in the Regular Army who was eventually taken captive and survived imprisonment by the Japanese until his liberation in 1945. This colorful personality is mentioned in personal memoirs of the Bataan experience. He is listed by Colonel Eugene Jacobs as one of his ten "Blood Brothers" in *Blood Brothers: A Medic's Sketch Book*. Quote from "Hospital Number '2', Bataan, PI", RG 407 (Adjutant General) Philippine Archives Collection, NARA, College Park, MD.

14. Maj. Gen. James O. Gillespie, USA, Ret., Recollections of the Pacific War and Japanese Prisoner of War Camps 1941-1945, RG 319 (CMH Refiles: *War Against Japan*), NARA, College Park, MD.
15. Maj. Gen. James O. Gillespie, USA, Ret., Recollections of the Pacific War and Japanese Prisoner of War Camps 1941–1945, RG 219 (CMH, Refiles: *War Against Japan*), NARA, College Park, MD.
16. Hospital Number "2", Bataan, PI, RG 407, Philippine Archives, NARA, College Park, MD.
17. Exact numbers vary, but there is no question that many thousands, perhaps as many as twenty-five thousand, made their way to the Bataan Peninsula.
18. Hospital Number "2", Bataan, PI, RG 407, Philippine Archive Collection.
19. Recollections of General Hospital No. 2 from General Gillespie's personal papers, Army Medical Department Historical Division, Fort Sam Houston, Texas.
20. This had been carefully outlined in War Plan Orange-3. Layac Junction was a town located where all the roads into the Bataan Peninsula joined, a key position for any delaying tactics.
21. Hibbs, *Tell MacArthur to Wait*, 44.
22. Quotes from Hibbs, *Tell MacArthur to Wait*, 49-50.
23. L. Morton, *Fall of the Philippines* (Washington, DC: Center of Miliary History, United States Army, 1993), 264.
24. MacArthur, *Reminiscences*, 129.
25. Calvin G. Jackson, *Diary of Col. Calvin G. Jackson, M.D.* (Ada: Ohio Northern University Press, 1992), 33-34.
26. Ibid., 77.
27. Ashton, *Bataan Diary*, 103-104.
28. William Donovan, *P.O.W. in the Pacific, Memoirs of an American Doctor in World War II* (Wilmington, DE: SR Books, 1998), 29.
29. James W. Duckworth, Official History of General Hospital No. 1, USAFFE, at Camp Limay, Bataan, Little Baguio, Bataan, and Camp O'Donnell, Tarlac, Philippine Islands, RG 112 (HUMEDS), NARA, College Park, MD
30. The clinical term "gas gangrene" is thought to encompass a variety of soft tissue necrotizing infections. The most feared of these is infection with *Costridium* species—so called *Clostridium* myositis which, if not aggressively treated by surgery, is almost universally fatal.
31. Sebastian Junger, *Tribe, On Homecoming and Belonging* (New York: Hachette Book Group, 2016), 70.
32. Carey Smith memoirs as described by Karen Takizawa in *War Stories*.

CHAPTER 5. JUNGLES OF DESPAIR

1. Weinstein, *Barbed-Wire Surgeon*, 41.
2. Morton, *Fall of the Philippines*, 290.
3. Report of Operations of South Luzon Force, Bataan Defense Force & II Philippine Corps in the Defense of South Luzon and Bataan from 8 December 1941 to 9 April 1942, Annex V, RG 407 (Adjutant General) NARA, College Park, MD.
4. Cooper, *Medical Department Activities in the Philippines from 1941 to 6 May 1942*.
5. Maj. Louis Besbeck, *The Operations of the 3rd Battalion 45th Infantry (Philippine Scouts) at the Hacienda at Mt. Natib, Luzon, 15-25 January 1942*, The Infantry School, Fort Benning, GA, 1946.
6. E. B. Miller, *Bataan Uncensored* (Long Prairie, MN: Hart Publications, 1949), 156.

7. Cooper, *Medical Department Activities in the Philippines from 1941 to 6 May 1942*, 38.
8. Jackson, *Diary*, 35.
9. Hibbs, *Tell MacArthur to Wait*, 67.
10. Henry Lee, "Abucay Withdrawal," in *Nothing but Praise*, 15.
11. Surgeon of Luzon Force Report II: Medical, Supply and Personnel. Lt. Col. Glattly commanded medical assets on Luzon and was subordinate to Col. Wibb Cooper, USAFFE Surgeon.
12. Between January 6 and April 8 it was estimated that 2,500 to 3,000 carabao were slaughtered in addition to around 250 horses of the 26th Cavalry and 48 pack mules: G-4 report attached to General Edward King's Luzon Force Operations Report, submitted to Washington on January 29, 1946, obtained through Paul Reuter, a Bataan veteran, and included in Morton, *Fall of the Philippines*, 369.
13. USA vs. Masaharu Homma [Public Trial], testimony of Homma, Vol 26, 3062-3064, RG 331 (Records of Allied Operational and Occupational Headquarters, World War II), NARA, College Park, MD.
14. MacArthur, *Reminiscences*, 133.
15. The pioneer Belgian military surgeon Antoine Depage (1862–1925) promoted a thorough cleansing and removal of all contaminated and necrotic flesh, a resurgence and expansion of the then-considered-antiquated process of debridement—a simple incision into damaged tissue—introduced by the eighteenth-century surgeon Pierre Joseph Desault (1744–1795).
16. G. R. Callender and J. F. Coupal, *Pathology of the Acute Respiratory Diseases and of Gas Gangrene Following War Wounds*, The Medical Department of the United States Army in the World War, U.S. Army Surgeon General's Office (Washington, DC: U.S. Government Printing Office, 1929), 408-409.
17. Report of Operations of South Luzon Force, Bataan Defense Force & II Philippine Corps in the Defense of South Luzon and Bataan from 8 December 1941 to 9 April 1942, Annex V, RG 407 (Adjutant General), NARA, College Park, MD.
18. Cooper, *Medical Department Activities in the Philippines from 1941 to 6 May 1942*.
19. Morton, *Fall of the Philippines*, 254-256.
20. When MacArthur departed for Australia, General Wainwright took command of the USAFFE and General King took command of the defense of the Bataan Peninsula.
21. Morton, *Fall of the Philippines*, 369.
22. A *cavane* has a volume of 80 quarts.
23. Men in combat undergo some of the most extreme stresses possible. Sudden, frightful bursts of energy necessary in modern warfare consume a magnitude more calories than day-to-day peacetime activities, even those of manual laborers. In tropical climates, expenditures are further magnified by the effects of heat and humidity. For combat, American troops could be required to heft an extra forty-five pounds for a rifleman, seventy pounds for a machine gunner, and seventy-five pounds for a mortar man. With forced marches and hostile terrain, estimates of four thousand calories consumed per day were not unrealistic. See *The Role of Protein and Amino Acids in Sustaining and Enhancing Performance* (Washington, DC: National Academies Press, 1999) and S. M. Pasaikos, S. J. Montain, A.J. Young, "Protein Supplementation in U.S. Military Personnel," *Journal of Nutrition* 143 (2013): 1815S-1819S.

24. Victor Hugo, *Carnets intimes*, 1870–1871 (Paris: Édition d'Henri Guillemin, Gallimard, 1953), 87.
25. Cave, *Beyond Courage*, 119.
26. Ibid.
27. The great botanist Carl von Linne (1707–1778), better known as Linnaeus, gave the name cinchona to the tree in honor of the Countess of Chinchon after she was allegedly cured of her fevers by the bark.
28. James O. Gillespie, "Malaria and the Defense of Bataan." Army Medical Department, Office of Medical History, Vol VI, Preventative Medicine in World War II (Washington, DC: Government Printing Office, 1963), 506-507.
29. James O. Gillespie, *Recollections of the Pacific War*, 6. In 1944, physiologist Ancel Keys demonstrated the effects of starvation on mental and physical activities of healthy volunteers in what has since been known as the Minnesota Experiment. With a semistarvation diet physical and psychological effects were astounding: weight loss, loss of muscle mass, weakness, apathy, and emotional volatility. See Ancel B. Keys, *The Biology of Human Starvation*, Volumes I and II (Minneapolis: University of Minnesota Press, 1950).

CHAPTER 6. FLICKERING FORLORN HOPE

1. *E. coli*, *Salmonella*, and *Yersinia* were other pathogens, equally tormenting and capable of nefarious consequences: profuse loss of water and electrolytes, even shock and bowel perforation.
2. Glusman, *Conduct Under Fire*, 149.
3. C. R. George, "Blackwater Fever: the Rise and Fall of an Exotic Disease," *Journal of Nephrology*, Supp. 14 (2009): 120-128.
4. Hibbs, *Tell MacArthur to Wait*, 89.
5. Ashton, *Bataan Diary*, 123.
6. Ibid., 122-126.
7. Morton, *Fall of the Philippines*, 420.
8. MacArthur, *Reminiscences*, 139. His close friend and Philippine president, Manuel Quezon, had departed Corregidor by submarine one month earlier. The two men would be reunited in Australia.
9. H.W. Glattly, Memorandum to the Surgeon, U.S. Armed Forces in the Philippine Islands, March 24, 1942, RG 407 (Records of the Adjutant General), NARA, College Park, MD.
10. Norman, *Band of Angels*, 78.
11. Weinstein, *Barbed-Wire Surgeon*, 67-68.
12. Norman, *Band of Angels*, 80.
13. Donald J. Young, *The Fall of the Philippines: The Desperate Struggle Against the Japanese Invasion, 1941–1942* (Jefferson, NC: McFarland, 2015), 109-115. Father William Cummings was a remarkable minister. A missionary of the Maryknoll Order, he was stationed in the Philippines at the onset of the war. He appeared at the American Army headquarters in Manila and insisted on joining the army as a chaplain. His wish was granted, and he was duly commissioned a first lieutenant. He is most remembered for his phrase: "there are no atheists in foxholes." Father Cummings died in captivity as a prisoner of war on January 18, 1945.
14. Weinstein, *Barbed-Wire Surgeon*, 69-71.
15. Hibbs, *Tell MacArthur to Wait*, 70, 90.
16. Figures from Cooper, *Medical Department Activities in the Philippines from 1941 to 6 May 1942*, 36.

17. Report of Operations of South Luzon Force, Bataan Defense Force & II Philippine Corps in the Defense of South Luzon and Bataan from 8 December 1941 to 9 April 1942, Annex XIV (Medical Report), RG 407 (Adjutant General Reports), NARA, College Park, MD.
18. Ashton, *Bataan Diary*, 131.
19. Jackson, *Diary*, 46.
20. Norman, *We Band of Angels*, 81.
21. Hibbs, *Tell MacArthur to Wait*, 103.
22. Figures from Cooper, *Medical Department Activities in the Philippines from 1941 to 6 May 1942*, 59.
23. Cave, *Beyond Courage*, 114.
24. Norman, *We Band of Angels*, 89.
25. Along with the nurses went three hundred survivors of the American 31st Infantry and navy personnel.
26. Hibbs, *Tell MacArthur to Wait*, 110.
27. Vorin E. Whan, ed., *A Soldier Speaks: Public Papers and Speeches of General of the Army Douglas MacArthur* (New York: Frederick A. Praeger, 1965), 126.

CHAPTER 7. FICKLE ANTIUM

1. Daniele Miano, *Fortuna: Deity and Concept in Archaic and Republican Italy* (Oxford: Oxford University Press, 2018), 56-58.
2. The "Latins" were the forefathers of "Roman" ethnicity and culture. Originally, in the first millennium BC they were probably a number of different tribes, and eventually mixed with another major influence in central *Italia*, the Etruscans descending from north of Rome. See Andreas Alfoldi, *Early Rome and the Latins* (Ann Arbor: University of Michigan Press, 1965).
3. The life of Caius Marcius Coriolanus is famously told by Plutarch, *Plutarch's Lives*, [Dryden translation], Vol. 2 (New York: Little, Brown, 1906), 52-100.
4. Marcus Tullius Cicero, *Cicero: Letters to Atticus* [E.O. Winstedt, translator] (New York: Macmillan, 1912), 125.
5. So named in Pindar's Ode, *For Theron of Akragas* (Agrigento in Italian). Pindar (522-443 BC) described Agrigento as the "loveliest of the cities of mortals" in *Pythia 12. The Odes of Pindar* [Richmond Lattimore] (Chicago: University of Chicago Press, 1942), 5, 93.
6. "Soft underbelly" was a favorite expression of Winston Churchill's and he used it on a number of occasions referring to, of course, the Mediterranean coast line of Europe and, perhaps an easier access to the continent and Hitler's *Festung Europa* through Italy.
7. *Carabinieri* were (and are) the domestic military policing force for Italy, as opposed to the *Polizia di Stato* or civilian police.
8. Trident meeting, "*Papers and Minutes of the Meeting* [including Churchill's quote]," Office of the Combined Chiefs of Staff, The White House, May 1943, RG 165 (Allied Military Conferences), NARA, College Park, MD.
9. Albert Kesselring, *The Memoirs of Field-Marshall Kesselring* (New York: Skyhorse Publishing, 2016), 182-189.
10. The Martin Army Community Hospital at Fort Benning, Georgia, was named after him in 2014.
11. The 15th, 93rd, 94th, and 95th (400 beds) and the 8th, 16th, 38th, and 56th (750 beds) Evacuation Hospitals. Information from Charles Maurice Wiltse, *Medical*

Services in the Mediterranean: Salerno to the Gustave Line (Chapter VI) (Washington, DC: U.S. Government Printing Office, 1987), 225.

12. Evacuation hospitals were initially deployed by Americans in World War I as more or less stationary hospitals some distance from the front lines but close to railway or roadway evacuation routes and capable of providing sophisticated surgical care for battlefield wounds. By the start of World War II, evacuation hospitals were considered the third echelon of care (first echelon: battalion aid stations; second echelon: division clearing companies or field hospitals). In the tangled algorithm of Army-speak, they were considered part of the Army Corps as opposed to divisions or battalions. They remained cumbersome to move (although it could be done) but maintained a distinct surgical orientation, staffed by fully trained surgeons. See D. P. Jones, "The Role of the Evacuation Hospital in the Care of the Wounded" *Ann Surg* 68 (1918): 127-132 and W. F. MacFee, "Plan for Setting up a 750-Bed Evacuation Hospital" *Bull U.S. Army Med Depart* 83 (1945): 61-63.

13. Mark W. Clark, *Fifth Army History: Part 1: From Activation to the Fall of Naples*, Headquarters, Fifth Army, Italy, 1944, Combined Arms Research Library, Fort Leavenworth, KS, 32.

14. USS *Frederick Funston* (APA 89): Report on Operation Avalanche, RG 38 (Action Reports), NARA, College Park, MD.

15. Edward D. Churchill, *Surgeon to Soldiers* (Philadelphia: J.B. Lippincott, 1972), 257.

16. War Diary/Action Reports USS *Joseph T. Dickman* (APA 13), Avalanche, September 1943, and USS *Lyon*, Report of Operations in the Gulf of Salerno, Italy, 9 September and 10 September 1943, all in RG 38 (War Diaries), NARA, College Park, MD.

17. Wiltse, *Medical Services in the Mediterranean: Salerno to the Gustave Line* (Chapter VI), 231.

18. Zachary Friedenberg, *Hospital at War: The 95th Evacuation Hospital in World War II* (College Station: Texas A&M University Press, 2004), 58.

19. Othelia's Story, Operation Avalanche, Part III, Distant Innocence, https://ussbb62.blogspot.com/2015/03/iv-othelias-story-95th-evac-salerno-to.html, accessed April 14, 2017.

20. Martin Blumenson, *United States Army in World War 2, Mediterranean Theater of Operations, Salerno to Cassino*, Center of Military History, United States Army (Washinton, DC: Government Printing Office, 1993), 99.

21. Henry M. Winans, World War II Essays, Special Collections Libraries, University of Texas, Arlington, TX.

22. Kesselring, *Memoirs*, 186.

23. Bill Adler and Tracy Quinn McLennan: *Letters Home: World War II Letters* (New York: St. Martin Press, 2002), 12.

24. Henry Beyle Stendhal, *Rome, Naples et Florence, En 1817*, Œuvres Completes de Stendhal (Paris: Folio Gallimard, 1817), 325-326; translation mine.

25. Clark, *Fifth Army History*: Part 1, 47.

26. Friedenberg, *Hospital at War*, 68.

27. "Christmas in captivity" was the phrase used in 1943. "When will they get here?" was the often asked question. Churchill, for one, had pined for its liberation in 1943. As much as General Clark wanted Rome, he was under no illusions that the Germans would willingly give it away. For further reading see: Robert Katz, *The Battle for Rome: the Germans, the Allies, the Partisans, and the Pope* (New York: Simon and

Schuster, 2003), 138-139, and Jon B. Mikolashek, *General Mark Clark: Commander of U.S. Fifth Army and Liberator of Rome* (Philadelphia: Casemate, 2013), 66-70.
28. Clark, *Fifth Army History, Part II: Across the Volturno to the Winter Line*, 1944, Combined Arms Research Library, Fort Leavenworth, KS, 56.
29. Wiltse, *Medical Services in the Mediterranean: Salerno to the Gustave Line* (Chapter VI), 241.
30. Winans, World War II Essays, 1943.
31. Schorer, *A Half Acre of Hell*, 95.
32. Bill Mauldin, *Mud, Mules, and Mountain: Cartoons of the AEF in Italy* (self-published, 1944).
33. Lawrence D. Collins, *The 56th Evac Hospital: Letters of a WWII Army Doctor*, (Denton: University of North Texas Press, 1995), 121.
34. Warren F. Kimball, *Churchill and Roosevelt: The Complete Correspondence: Volume 2, Alliance Forged November 1942 – February 1944* (Princeton: Princeton University Press, 2015), 563.
35. Clark, *Fifth Army History, Part III: The Winter Line*, 1944, Combined Arms Research Library, Fort Leavenworth, KS, 59, 93-94.
36. Schorer, *A Half Acre of Hell*, 104-105.
37. Paul A. Kennedy, *Battlefield Surgeon: Life and Death on the Front Lines of World War II* (Lexington: University Press of Kentucky, 2016), 79.
38. Ibid., 80
39. Sextant Conference: *Minutes of the Third Plenary Meeting, Held at the Villa Kirk, on Saturday, 4 December 1943 at 1100*, RG 165 (Allied Military Conferences), NARA, College Park, MD.
40. Winston S. Churchill, *Closing the Ring* (Boston: Houghton Mifflin, 1951), 330.

CHAPTER 8. CODENAME SHINGLE

1. The Army's G-3 section was the "operations section," tasked with developing battle plans, including logistics.
2. Carlo D'Este, *Eisenhower: A Soldier's Life* (New York: Henry Holt, 2002), 470.
3. Churchill, *Closing the Ring*, 441.
4. Churchill, *Closing the Ring*, 447-449, including the statements by Roosevelt.
5. John P. Lucas, "The Lucas Diary," entry of January 12, 1944, Archives, U.S. Army Military History Institute, Carlisle Barracks, PA.
6. A *combat command* was a combined arms element peculiar to armored divisions—armor, infantry, field artillery, tank destroyers, and the like—of a regiment or brigade size. It was a flexible organization, a hodgepodge of various battalions and detachments that was mission specific as opposed to a Regimental Combat Team, which was a reinforced regiment of standard infantry battalions.
7. Outline Plan Operation Shingle: Hdqtrs Fifth Army, Copy 47, 12 January 1944, Combined Arms Research Library, Fort Leavenworth, KS.
8. Jarrett Huddleston transcripts courtesy of the Norman Lee Baldwin Collection at the Hoover Institute Archives, Stanford University, Stanford, CA.
9. For further discussion, see Mark Harrison, *Medicine and Victory: British Military Medicine in the Second World War* (Oxford: Oxford University Press, 2004).
10. E. D. Churchill, "The Surgical Management of the Wounded in the Mediterranean Theater at the Time of the Fall of Rome," *Annals of Surgery* 120 (1944): 268-283.
11. Army Medical Bulletin, No. 22, *Tables of Organization, Medical Department*, 1928, 45. *Groupe complémentaire de chirurgie* was an outgrowth of the mobile (auto-

mobile-based) surgical teams called *ambulance chirurgicale automobile* (automobile surgical ambulance, or *auto-chir*, for short) developed in response to the atrocious evacuation and treatment of French wounded during the opening months of World War I. With the *auto-chir*, teams of experienced surgeons could rush closer to the front lines to provide early care to the critically wounded. For a detailed account of their beneficial service, see Alfred Mignon, *Le Service de Santé Pendant la Guerre 1914-1918* (Paris: Masson & Cie, 1926).

12. Medical History, Annual Report, 1944, 2nd Auxiliary Surgical Group, 71, Office of Medical History, U.S. Army Medical Department (AMEDD), Fort Sam Houston, TX.

13. Headquarters Fifth Army: Outline Plan Operation Shingle, 12 January 1944, Combined Arms Research Library, Fort Leavenworth, KS. Estimates for D-Day casualties alone were given at 10 percent of assault troops: Wiltse, *Medical Services in the Mediterranean: Anzio Beachhead* (Chapter VII), 268.

14. *Anzio Beachhead*, 22 January–25 May 1944, Historical Division, War Department, Washington, DC, 1948, 9.

15. Wiltse, *Medical Services in the Mediterranean: Anzio Beachhead* (Chapter VII), 270.

16. Operational Journal for Amphibious Operation "Shingle," 52nd Med Battalion, January-February, 1944, RG 112 (HUMEDS), NARA, College Park, MD.

17. Shock teams were groups of physicians and nurses assigned to begin resuscitation on the critically wounded who, when they arrived, were found to be in shock, i.e., low blood pressure, rapid bleeding, *in extremis* appearance.

18. Headquarters, 52nd Medical Battalion: Annual Report, 52nd Medical Battalion for 1944, 20 January 1945, RG 112 (Records of the Office of the Surgeon General), NARA, College Park, MD.

19. Oral History Collection: Floyd Taylor, MD, recorded June 26, 1998, University of North Texas, Denton, TX.

20. Reports on HMHS *St. David* from Commander Task Group 81.8 and Commanding Officer U.S.S. *Brooklyn*: Action Report—Establishment of Beachhead at Anzio, Italy by combined U.S.-British Amphibious Force—Period 21 January–8 February 1944, RG 38 (Action Reports), NARA, College Park, MD; Commander Task Force Eighty-one: Action Report—Operation Shingle, 22 February 1944, RG 38 (Action Reports), NARA, College Park, MD; Evelyn Monahan and Rosemary Neidel-Greenlee, *And if I Perish: Frontline U.S. Army Nurses in World War II* (New York: Anchor Books, 2003), 242-245.

21. T/O & E stands for "Table of Organization and Equipment." This table itemizes the staffing and equipment in minute detail to be assigned to individual units, such as evacuation and field hospitals.

22. Schorer, *A Half Acre of Hell*, 123-124.

23. Grantley Taylor quotes from *The Massachusetts General Hospital Surgical Society Newsletter*, Robb Rutledge, author, Volume 8, Spring 2007, 1.

24. Friedenberg, *Hospital at War*, 81.

25. Excerpts from a war diary published by Dr. Arthur deGrandpre and donated to the WW2 US Medical Research Center, www.med-dept.com, accessed December 8, 2015.

26. Genevieve Rosales and Eunice Cooke, *Valiantly Done, Lieutenant: 56th Evacuation Hospital, 1944*, RG 407 (Adjutant General), NARA, College Park, MD.

27. Schorer, *A Half Acre of Hell*, 128.

28. Headquarters 56th Evacuation Hospital, RG 407 (Adjutant General), NARA, College Park, MD.
29. The site of the Second Casualty Clearing Station is now "Beachhead Cemetery" containing 2,313 graves of fallen United Kingdom soldiers who fought at Anzio.
30. Headquarters, 120th Medical Battalion, 45th Infantry Division: A History of the Battalion in the Italian Campaign January 1944; RG 112 (HUMEDS), NARA, College Park, MD.
31. This "Order of the Day" or *Führerbefehl* was issued by Adolf Hitler on January 28, 1944, to Kesselring, and is found in a number of sources, including Carlo D'Este, *Fatal Decision: Anzio and the Battle for Rome* (New York: HarperCollins, 1991), 183.
32. *The German Operation at Anzio: A Study of the German Operations at Anzio Beachhead from 22 Jan 44 to 31 May 44*, German Military Document Section, RG 242 (Collection of Foreign Records Seized), NARA, College Park, MD.
33. Quote from Peter Verney, *Anzio 1944: An Unexpected Fury* (London: David and Charles, 1980), 142.
34. Desmond Fitzgerald, *A History of the Irish Guards in the Second World War* (London: Gale and Polden, 1949), 237.
35. Ernest Harmon and Milton MacKaye, "Our Bitter Days at Anzio, Part 1," *Saturday Evening Post*, September 18, 1948.
36. "Surgical Unit with Armored Division," *Bulletin U.S. Army Medical Department* 4 (1945):225.
37. Hollis D. Stabler, *No One Ever Asked Me: The World War II Memoirs of an Omaha Indian Soldier* (Lincoln: University of Nebraska Press, 2005), 84.
38. William O. Darby, *Darby's Rangers: We Led the Way* (New York: Presidio Press, 1993), 204.
39. Milton Lehman, "The Rangers Fought Ahead of Everybody," *Saturday Evening Post*, June 15, 1946.
40. It was rumored that a soldier in the 39th Combat Engineers was actually a German spy and had tipped off the enemy about Lucas's plans with the Rangers.
41. Headquarters, Third Medical Battalion (Journal) 1944, RG 407 (Adjutant General), NARA, College Park, MD.
42. deGrandpre, war diary, accessed December 9, 2015.

CHAPTER 9. HELL'S HALF ACRE

1. Friedenberg, *Hospital at War*, 85-86.
2. Barbara Tomblin, *G.I. Nightingales: The Army Nurse Corps in World War II* (Lexington: University Press of Kentucky, 1996), 105.
3. Ibid., 87.
4. deGrandpre, war diary, accessed January 31, 2017.
5. Medical History (Annual Report 1944) 2nd Auxiliary Surgical Group, AMEDD, Fort Sam Houston, TX.
6. Statistics from the 95th Evacuation Hospital Historical Record and Annual Report 1944, RG 407 (Unit Reports), NARA, College Park, MD. The statistics are at odds with those reported by Dr. Friedenberg in "Hospital at War" who wrote that 1,207 operations had been performed. He may have included minor operations not requiring general anesthesia.
7. Monahan, *And If I Perish*, 261.
8. Ibid., 274.
9. 15th Evac Hospital, RG 112 (HUMEDS), NARA, College Park, MD.
10. deGrandpre, war diary, accessed December 9, 2015.

11. Ibid., 142-144.
12. R. L. Bauchspies, "The Courageous Medics of Anzio, II," *Military Medicine* 122 (1958): 119-128.
13. Headquarters 33rd Field Hospital: Annual Historical Review, 1944, RG 407 (Adjutant General), NARA, College Park, MD, and Excerpts from Evelyn Monahan and Rosemary Neidel-Greenlee, "Anzio Nurses," *Purple Heart Magazine*, May-June 1992, 17.
14. R. Y. White, "At Anzio Beachhead," *American Journal of Nursing* 44(1944): 370-371.
15. Headquarters 33rd Field Hospital APO #464: Annual Historical Review, 1944; Oral History Collection: Floyd Taylor, MD; and Monahan, *And If I Perish*, 269-271.
16. Tomblin, *G.I. Nightingales*, 107.
17. Headquarters Third Medical Battalion APO #3: Unit Report of Operations for Period 1st to Febr 20th, 1944, RG 407 (Adjutant General), NARA, College Park, MD.
18. Collins, *The 56th Evac*, 174.
19. A description of Ellen Ainsworth and her endearment to members of the 56th Evacuation Hospital is lovingly told, quotes included, by her friend and fellow nurse, Avis Schorer, in her memoir *A Half Acre of Hell*, 146-151.
20. Clark, *Fifth Army History, Part IV: Cassino and Anzio*, Chapter VIII, Holding the Beachhead, 129-146.
21. Flint Whitlock, *The Rock of Anzio: From Sicily To Dachau, A History Of The U.S. 45th Infantry Division* (Boulder, CO: Westview Press, 1998), 200.
22. Headquarters, 120th Medical Battalion, RG 112 (HUMEDS), NARA, College Park, MD.
23. Major Lawson's quotes from Headquarters 120th Medical Battalion: A History of the Battalion in the Italian Campaign, February 1944, RG 112 (Records of the Office of the Surgeon General), NARA.
24. Major Lawson's quotes from: Headquarters, 120th Medical Battalion, RG 112 (HUMEDS), NARA, College Park, MD.
25. Statistics from Clark, *Fifth Army History, Part IV: Cassino and Anzio*, 146; the statistics do not include British losses which were prodigious, some units suffering two hundred casualties per day.
26. Collins, *The 56th Evac*, 202.
27. Third Infantry Division Medical Report 1944, RG 112 (HUMEDS), NARA, College Park, MD.
28. R. L. Bauchspies, "The Courageous Medics of Anzio, III," *Military Medicine* 122 (1958): 197-207. Bauchspies put the German losses at more than 5,000 dead, wounded, and missing.
29. Ernie Pyle, *Brave Men* (Lincoln: University of Nebraska Press, 2001), 249-251.
30. Wadis (an Arabic term for watercourses in North Africa) were deep ravines and gullies cut into the soft earth by the action of centuries of draining rainwater. Some were up to fifty feet deep. They were concentrated around the Moletta River Valley in the northwest (British) sector.
31. William Woodruff, *Vessel of Sadness* (London: Abacus, 1969), 152.
32. Pyle, *Brave Men*, 267.
33. Richard Tregaskis, *Invasion Diary* (New York: Random House, 1944), 208.
34. Anecdote found on *The History of the 45th Infantry Division*, http://www.45thdivision.org/history.htm, accessed December 23, 2015.

35. O. C. Leigh, "A Report on Trench Foot and Cold Injuries in the European Theater of Operations," *Annals of Surgery* 124 (1946): 303-313.
36. Peyton, *A Surgeon's Diary*, 147-148.
37. Harrison, *Medicine and Victory*, 164-165; see also M. C. Bricknell, "The Evolution of Casualty Evacuation in the British Army in the 20th Century" (Part 2), *Journal of the Royal Army Medical Corps* 148 (2002): 314-322.
38. Siegfried Sassoon, unfinished and unpublished verse, dated August 10, 1918, in Patrick Campbell, *Siegfried Sassoon: A Study of the War Poetry* (Jefferson, NC: McFarland, 2007), 217.
39. J. A. Ross, "Memoirs of an Army Surgeon," *Journal of the Royal Army Medical Corps* 125 (1979): 32-38.
40. Henry K. Beecher, *Surgery in World War II*, Part I, Chapter 3: "Anesthesia for Men Wounded in Battle," Medical Department, United States Army in World War II [John Boyd Coates, Jr, MC, Editor-in-Chief], Office of the Surgeon General, Department of the Army, Government Printing Office, Washington, DC, 1955, 53.
41. Ross, "Memoirs of an Army Surgeon."
42. H. K. Beecher, "Pain in Men Wounded in Battle," *Annals of Surgery* 123 (1946): 96-105; what to tell men wounded in battle is also discussed by Beecher, a Harvard-trained surgeon and anesthesiologist, in "Preparation of Battle Casualties for Surgery," *Annals of Surgery* 121 (1945): 769-792.
43. Pyle, *Brave Men*, 58.
44. Ross, "Memoirs of an Army Surgeon."
45. Winans, World War II Essays.
46. deGrandpre, war diary, accessed December 9, 2015.
47. Doctor Paul Milligan's story at Anzio in *Legacy of Heroes* [Craig Fisher, Editor] (Rosemont: American Academy of Orthopaedic Surgeons, 2004), 70-71.
48. Peyton, *A Surgeon's Diary*, 153.
49. Ibid., 146-147, 151.
50. "Axis Sally" was a nickname given to Mildred Gillars and Rita Zucca who were employed by the Third Reich to spread propaganda among Allied troops in Italy and Europe. This quote is taken from Rick Atkinson, *The Guns at Last Light: The War in Western Europe, 1944-1945* (New York: Henry Holt, 2013), 417.
51. Wiltse, *Medical Services in the Mediterranean: Anzio Beachhead* (Chapter VII), 284; Headquarters 56th Evacuation Hospital, Office of the Commanding Officer: Essential Technical Medical Data, 14 March 1944, RG 407 (Adjutant General), NARA, College Park, MD.
52. Major sources for the 33rd Field Hospital were: 33rd Field Hospital Annual Historical Review, 1944, RG 407 (Adjutant General), NARA, College Park, MD, and Essential Medical Technical Data Report, 33rd Field Hospital, 1943-1945, RG 407 (Adjutant General), NARA, College Park, MD.
53. Headquarters 56th Evacuation Hospital, RG 407 (Adjutant General), NARA, College Park, MD.
54. Collins, *The 56th Evac*, 166-167.
55. D'Estes, *Fatal Decision*, 308.
56. Memorandum, Fifth Army Advanced Command Post to Colonel Tate, dated February 29, 1944, in David D. Dworak, "Victory's Foundation: U.S. Logistical Support of the Allied Mediterranean Campaign 1942-1945," dissertation, Syracuse University, 2011, 340.

CHAPTER 10. STALEMATE

1. David Nichols, ed., *Ernie's War: The Best of Ernie Pyle's World War II Dispatches* (New York: Random House, 1986), 238.
2. Churchill, *Closing the Ring*, 492-493.
3. Kesselring, *Memoirs*, 195.
4. 82d Airborne Division in Sicily and Italy, After Action Report 504th Parachute Infantry, Combined Arms Research Library, Fort Leavenworth, KS.
5. After Action Report, 701st Tank Destroyer Bn, March, 1944, Combined Arms Research Library, Fort Leavenworth, KS.
6. Pyle, *Brave Men*, 250.
7. Headquarters 56th Evacuation Hospital, RG 407 (Adjutant General), NARA, College Park, MD.
8. Essential Medical Technical Data Report, 33rd Field Hospital, 1943-1945, RG 407 (Adjutant General), NARA, College Park, MD; for processing of the wounded, see Beecher, "Preparation of Battle Casualties for Surgery."
9. Diary of Richard V. Hauver, MD, excerpts February–June 1944, courtesy of the U.S. Army War College, Institute of Military History, Ridgway Hall, Carlisle, PA.
10. R. L. Bauchspies, "The Courageous Medics of Anzio, V," *Military Medicine* 122 (1958):338-359.
11. Peyton, *A Surgeon's Diary*, 159-161. While the Germans had arrayed a wide variety of artillery around Anzio, the *Flak* 8.8 cm gun (88s) was probably the most familiar to support troops and, therefore, the most feared.
12. Wiltse, *Medical Services in the Mediterranean*, 277.
13. Oral History Collection: Floyd Taylor, MD.
14. Memoir of First Lieutenant Ramona T. McCormick with the 94th Evac Hospital, Anzio Beachhead Veterans of World War II, http://anziobeachheadveterans.com/member-memoirs-index/men-of-the-landing, accessed January 7, 2016.
15. Schorer, *Half Acre of Hell*, 160.
16. Diary of Richard V. Hauver, MD, excerpts February– June 1944.
17. Baseball games were not uncommon, folded t-shirts used for bases and slit trenches for dugouts. Volleyball games also sprang up (Monahan, *And If I Perish*, 299); Rick Atkinson, *The Day of Battle: The War in Sicily and Italy, 1943-1944* (New York: Henry Holt, 2007), 488). Exchange of bands between the British and American sectors in the rear areas was frequently done as impromptu "pop" concerts and entertainment for the troops. Scottish highlanders were particularly noted for their bagpipe parades, kilts and all, for hospital personnel; see Harvey Ferguson, *The Last Cavalryman: The Life of General Lucian K. Truscott, Jr.* (Norman: University of Oklahoma Press, 2015), 242; and Fred Sheehan, *Anzio: Epic of Bravery* (Norman: University of Oklahoma Press, 1994), 173.
18. "GI alcohol" was a concoction some attributed to teams of the Second Auxiliary Surgical Group and consisted of a mixture of 95 percent ethyl alcohol (readily available for its use as a sterilizer), chlorinated water, lemon powder, and sugar (Paul A. Kennedy, *Battlefield Surgeon*, 112-113). Some made a form of gin from stills fashioned out of scavenged copper tubing from downed German aircraft, a potent liquor known as "raisin-jack" (Sheehan, *Anzio*, 170). Wine was abundant in the cellars of Anzio and Nettuno as well.
19. Story relayed by Dr. Gurnee's son, Quinby "Skip" Gurnee who kindly communicated with me about his distinguished father.
20. Mark W. Clark, *Calculated Risk* (New York: Harper and Brothers, 1950), 10.

21. Collins, *The 56th Evac*, 204.
22. Annual Report, Surgeon, Fifth Army, 1944. Fifth Army History, pt. IV, 164, lists ninety-two killed, maybe a more accurate figure.
23. Annual Report, 15th Evacuation Hospital, Semimobile, 1 January 1944–31 December 1944, RG 112 (HUMEDS), NARA, College Park, MD.
24. Clark, *Fifth Army History 16 January 1944–31 March 1944. Part IV: Cassino and Anzio*, 168-170.
25. "Via Anziate" refers to the contested Anzio-Albano road leading due north right out of the port town to Campoleone and Route 6.
26. Pyle, *Brave Men*, 298.
27. History 94th Evacuation Hospital (SM) 1943-1944-1945, RG 112 (HUMEDS), NARA, College Park, MD.
28. Memoir of First Lieutenant Ramona T. McCormick with the 94th Evac Hospital, Anzio Beachhead Veterans of World War II, http://anziobeachheadveterans.com/member-memoirs-index/men-of-the-landing, accessed January 7, 2016.
29. Diary, 94th Evacuation Hospital 1944, RG 112 (HUMEDS), NARA, College Park, MD.
30. George W. Tipton, "Surgery Under Stress: World War II, Anzio Beachhead" *Bulletin of the American College of Surgeons* 91(2006): 44-48.
31. Peyton, *A Surgeon's Diary*, 170.
32. Schorer, *A Half Acre of Hell*, 165.
33. Diary of Richard V. Hauver, MD, excerpts February–June 1944.
34. June Wandrey, *Bedpan Commando: The Story of a Combat Nurse During World War II* (Elmore: Elmore Publishing, 1989), 111.
35. Peyton, *A Surgeon's Diary*, 170.
36. The "Anzio walk" was described by Pyle in *Brave Men*, 302.
37. Bauchspies, "The Courageous Medics of Anzio, V": 338-359.
38. "Purple Heart Highway" was the road leading to the docks at Anzio used by ambulances to evacuate the wounded from the beachhead.
39. Collins, *The 56th Evac*, 197-198.
40. LeGette Blythe, *38th Evac: The Story of the Men and Women Who Served in World War II with the 38th Evacution Hospital in North Africa and Italy* (Charlotte: Self-published, 1966), 177.
41. Ibid., 179-180.
42. Ibid., 180.
43. Ibid., 182.
44. Mary T. Samecky, *A History of the U.S. Army Nurse Corps* (Philadelphia: University of Pennsylvania Press, 1999), 225.
45. R. L. Bauchspies, "The Courageous Medics of Anzio, VI," *Military Medicine* 122(1958): 429-448.
46. Headquarters, 38th Evacuation Hospital, Annual Report 1944, RG 112 (HUMEDS), NARA, College Park, MD.
47. H. Snowden, "Latina Province 1944-1950," *Journal of Contemporary History* 43 (2008): 509-526; see also the classic work by Angelo Celli, *The History of Malaria in the Roman Campagna from Ancient Times* (London: John Bale, Sons, and Danielsson, 1933).
48. Worries, largely unfounded, that Atabrine led to impotency abounded. What was real were unpleasant gastrointestinal symptoms at the beginning of therapy, sometimes disabling.
49. Clark, *Fifth Army History*, 167.

CHAPTER 11. BREAKOUT

1. 93rd Evacuation Hospital unit history, RG 112 (HUMEDS), NARA, College Park, MD.
2. Annual Report of the Eleventh Evacuation Hospital Semimobile, 1944, RG 112 (HUMEDS), NARA, College Park, MD.
3. Diary of Richard V. Hauver, MD, courtesy of the U.S. Army War College, Ridgway Hall, Carlisle, PA.
4. Luther Wolff, *Forward Surgeon: The Diary of Luther H. Wolff, M.D., Mediterranean Theater, World War II, 1943-45* (New York: Vantage Press), 89.
5. Wolff, *Forward Surgeon*, 94.
6. Churchill, *Closing the Ring*, 599.
7. Bauchspies, "The Courageous Medics of Anzio, VI," 429-448
8. Headquarters Third Medical Battalion, History of Unit Operations 1 to 31 May 1944, Company D (Clearing Station), RG 407 (Adjutant General); Headquarters 120th Medical Battalion, 45th Infantry Division: A History of the Battalion in the Italian Campaign, May 1944, RG 112 (HUMEDS), all NARA, College Park, MD.
9. Wolff, *Forward Surgeon*, 96.
10. 33rd Field Hospital Annual Historical Review, 1944, RG 407 (Records of the Adjutant General's Office), NARA, College Park, MD.
11. Essential Medical Technical Data Report, 33rd Field Hospital, 1943-1945, RG 407 (Records of the Adjutant General's Office), NARA, College Park, MD.
12. Diary, 94th Evacuation Hospital June 1941 – April 1945, RG 112 (HUMEDS), NARA, College Park, MD.
13. Diary of Richard V. Hauver.
14. History of the 15th Evacuation Hospital, 1944, RG 112 (HUMEDS), NARA, College Park, MD.
15. Peyton, *A Surgeon's Diary*, 181.
16. Wolff, *Forward Surgeon*, 97.
17. Bauchspies, "Those Courageous Medics of Anzio, VI," 429-448.
18. Wandrey, *Bedpan Commando*, 107-108.
19. Figures from Wiltse, *Medical Services*, 268.
20. Bauchspies, "Those Courageous Medics of Anzio, VI," 429-448.
21. Churchill, *Closing the Ring*, 494.
22. Wolff, *Forward Surgeon*, 188.
23. Comment by Col. Joseph I. Martin to the *Clare Sentinel* (Clare County, MI), August 25, 1944.
24. Rudyard Kipling, *Rudyard Kipling's Verse, Inclusive Edition* (Garden City: Doubleday, Page, 1922), "Recessional" (1897), 377.

CHAPTER 12. ARDUENNAM SILVAM

1. First United States Army, Report of Operations, 1 August 1944–22 February 1945. Volumes 1-4, Government Printing Office, Washington, DC, 1945; U.S. Army Operations in the ETO from January 1942 to V-E Day, Control Division and Historical Section, Headquarters Communications Zone ETOUSA, RG 498, NARA, College Park, MD; After Action Report: Third US Army, 1 August 1944–9 May 1945, Vol I, 1945, Combined Arms Research Library, Fort Leavenworth, KS.
2. Von Rundstedt's quotes in Thomas W. Dworschak, *Hitler's "Watch on the Rhine": The Battle of the Bulge*, The Land Warfare Papers, The Institute of Land Warfare, Association of the United States Army, Arlington, VA, 1992.
3. *Herbstnebel* was a less ambitious plan developed by General Walter Model to

counter Hitler's overly optimistic scheme to access Antwerp. It was rejected out of hand by Hitler, but the operational name *Herbstnebel* for some reason stuck.
4. Source for German planning for Operation *Herbstnebel*: Percy Ernst Schramm, *The Preparations for the German Offensive in the Ardennes (Sep – 16 Dec 44)*, A-862, 1954, RG 338 (Foreign Military Studies), NARA, College Park, MD.
5. Julius Caesar: *Commentaria De Bello Gallico*, Book VI, in Caesar, *The Gallic Wars* [H.J. Edwards translator] (Cambridge: Harvard University Press, 1917), 29.
6. *Hohe Venn* (High Venn) specifies an arched plateau on the German-Belgian border; *Schnee Eifel* refers to that part of the upland Ardennes that is thickly wooded, presenting almost a completely arboreal barrier to traffic.
7. Anonymous author, *The Traveller's Guide Through Belgium* (Brussels: AD. Wahlen, Printer to the Court, 1833), 213.
8. Reference of Guichardini to Bastogne as the "*Paris en Ardenne*" (Paris of the Ardennes) was found in Camille Lemonnier, *La Belgique* (G. Van Oest: Brussels, 1903), 730; Dudley Costello, *A Tour Through the Valley of the Meuse* (London: Chapman and Hall, 1846), 313-314.
9. The Antonine Itinerary was ascribed to the Roman emperor Titus Aurelius Antoninus (Antoninus Pius) who reigned from AD 138-161. It has been said that under his wise and benevolent rule a registry of Roman roads throughout the empire was developed, although the exact author of this registry remains obscure.
10. C-SPAN interview with Kurt Vonnegut and Joseph Heller, moderated by Steven Ambrose, sponsored by the University of New Orleans, May 7, 1995, https://www.c-span.org/video/?65129-1/battle-bulge-day&start=0 , accessed April 15, 2017.
11. "Checkerboard" refers to their distinctive shoulder patch.
12. John C. McManus: *Alamo in the Ardennes: The Untold Story of the American Soldiers Who Made the Defense of Bastogne Possible* (Hoboken: John Wiley and Sons, 2007), 15.
13. Samecky, *Nurse Corps*, 240; Headquarters, 102nd Evacuation Hospital (SM) 31 December 1944, Annual Report of Medical Department Activities, RG 112 (HUMEDS), NARA, College Park, MD.
14. John T. Greenwood, PhD: Medical Order of Battle, VIII Corps, as of 15 December 1944, Office of Medical History, Office of the Surgeon General, U.S. Army.
15. Anthony Beevor, *Ardennes 1944: Hitler's Last Gamble* (Falkirk, NY: Viking Penguin Viking, 2015), 129-130.
16. Eisenhower, *Crusade in Europe*, 340.
17. Hugh M. Cole, *The Ardennes: Battle of the Bulge*, Center of Military History, United States Army (Washington DC: U.S. Government Printing Office, 1993), 59-61.
18. "*Ein Letzter Versuch*" (A Last Attempt) containing the phrase *Es geht ums Ganze* is in the John S. Minary Psychological Warfare Collection, ZG 98, George C. Marshall Library, Lexington, VA. The phrase *Es geht um das Ganze* was mentioned in Rick Atkinson's *The Guns at Last Light: The War in Western Europe, 1944-1945* (New York: Henry Holt, 2013), 421. The intercept by the 99th Infantry Division G-2 (Intelligence) files, can be found at the U.S. Army Military History Institute, Carlisle, PA.
19. Brendan Phibbs: *The Other Side of Time: A Combat Surgeon in World War II* (Boston: Little, Brown, 1987), 114.
20. Phibbs, *The Other Side of Time*, 114. Biographer Steven Bach recorded that Marlene Dietrich contracted "the GIs" (dysentery) in the Ardennes, washed her face

and hair and underclothes with melted snow in her helmet, and drank Calvados with the boys. "I'm not afraid of dying," she told the officers (but, being of German heritage, she was afraid of capture). Steven Bach, *Marlene Dietrich: Life and Legend* (Minneapolis: University of Minnesota Press, 2011), 298.
21. The Story of the 107th Evacuation Hospital (SM), RG 407 (Records of the U.S. Army Adjutant General), NARA, College Park, MD, 31.
22. The Henry Swan Papers, National Library of Medicine, Washington, DC.
23. Gellhorn: *Face of War*, 145.

CHAPTER 13. BLITZKRIEG IN THE ARDENNES

1. A German *Kampfgruppe* was a combined arms combat formation. In this particular case, it was commanded by former Himmler staff member, the ruthless Waffen-SS Lieutenant Colonel Joachim Peiper.
2. Information provided by Captain Midderling's Battle History Company "A," 331st Medical Battalion, December 1944. RG 112 (Records of the U.S. Army Surgeon General), NARA, College Park, MD.
3. Clifford Lewis Graves, *Front line Surgeons: A History of the Third Auxiliary Surgical Group* (San Diego: Frye and Smith, 1950), 212.
4. Graves, *Front Line Surgeons*, 253-254.
5. Beevor, *Ardennes 1944*, 143.
6. Comments by Ronald S. Gibbs and William Droegemueller in a memorial for Dr. Taylor published by the American Gynecological and Obstetrical Society, 2015.
7. Headquarters, 331st Medical Battalion, 24 March 1945, RG 112 (Records of the U.S. Army Surgeon General), NARA, College Park, MD.
8. "Bugging out" was a term often used in narratives of the battle. It signified complete detachment from the fight, either running away in fright or, in total dejection, dropping weapons and skulking toward the rear.
9. Headquarters, 331st Medical Battalion, 12 December–31 December 1944, RG 112 (Surgeon General), NARA, College Park, MD.
10. R. M. Citino, "First Blood on the Ghost Front," *World War II Magazine* 29 (2014): 39-45.
11. R. Ernest Dupuy, *St. Vith: Lion in the Way: The 106th Infantry Division in World War II* (Washington, DC: Infantry Journal Press, 1949), 121, 343-344. Interview with George Descheneaux by John Toland and related in his book, *Battle: The Story of the Bulge* (Lincoln: University of Nebraska Press, 1959), 131.
12. Paul Fussell, *The Boys' Crusade: The American Infantry in Northwestern Europe, 1944-1945* (New York: Random House, 2003), 131-132.
13. Cole, *Battle of the Bulge*, 99.
14. Surgeon Report, Headquarters 99th Infantry Division, 8 January 1945, RG 112 (HUMEDS), NARA, College Park, MD.
15. Office of the Surgeon, Headquarters Second Infantry Division Medical Bulletin December 1944, RG 112 (HUMEDS), NARA, College Park, MD.
16. Ibid., 245
17. Report of Operations, Surgeon, First U.S. Army, 1 Aug 44–2 Feb 45, Annex 11, Part C, p. 140, RG 112 (Surgeon General), NARA, College Park, MD; and *The Shield of Phi Kappa Psi*, 65 (March 1945): 115-116.
18. Some details of this evacuation contained in Monahan, *And If I Perish*, 413-415.
19. Annual Report, 67th Evacuation Hospital, Semimobile, 1944, 15 March 1945, RG 112 (Records of the U.S. Army Surgeon General), NARA, College Park, MD.

20. The 28th Infantry Division is the oldest division-size unit in the United States Army. "Keystone" refers to the state of Pennsylvania, the Keystone State, as it was formed from elements of the Pennsylvania National Guard.
21. "Incoming" and "outgoing" "mail" was a GI term used to denote incoming (enemy) or outgoing (friendly) artillery rounds.
22. History of the 110th Infantry Regiment: The Ardennes Breakthrough 16 December 1944 – 15 January 1945, RG 407 (Adjutant General), NARA, College Park, MD.
23. Phibbs, *The Other Side of Time*, 220.
24. Unit Report, 103rd Medical Battalion, 2 January 1945, RG 407 (Adjutant General), NARA, College Park, MD.
25. Military medical parlance ascribes patients as "non-transportable," those too ill or injured to safely move, and "transportable," those patients who are stable enough to transport some distance.
26. Graves, *Front Line Surgeons*, 259-261.
27. After Action Report, 2nd Medical Battalion, Armored, 9th Armored Division, 31 December 44, RG 407 (Records of the U.S. Army Adjutant General, World War II), NARA, College Park, MD, and Division Surgeon Report, Headquarters, 9th Armored Division, 1944, 20 January 1945, RG 112 (Surgeon General), NARA, College Park, MD.
28. The Story of the 107th Evacuation Hospital (SM), RG 407 (Adjutant General), NARA, College Park, MD, 31-32.
29. Ibid., 32-33.
30. Tenant McWilliams: *The Chaplain's Conflict: Good and Evil in a War Hospital, 1943-1945* (College Station: Texas A&M University Press, 2012), 85.
31. History of the 102nd Evacuation Hospital (Semi-Mobile), RG 407 (Adjutant General), NARA, College Park, MD.
32. John S. D. Eisenhower: *The Bitter Woods: The Battle of the Bulge* (New York: G.P. Putnam's Sons, 1969), 8.

CHAPTER 14. SCREAMING EAGLES

1. James M. Gavin, *On to Berlin* (New York: Bantam, 1985), 92.
2. Auxiliary Surgical Team No. 19, supporting the 82nd Airborne Division, did not fare as well in the Normandy landings. Coming in also by glider, one group crash landed, killing the pilot and spilling the men like matchsticks. Another of their gliders was hit by artillery, crash landed and incinerated, the surgeons lucky to get out alive, but all their equipment was lost in the inferno.
3. Leonard Rapport and Arthur Norwood, *Rendezvous with Destiny: History of The 101st Airborne Division* (Saybrook: Konecky and Konecky, 1948), 3.
4. Graves, *Front Line Surgeons*, 278.
5. C. S. Phalen, "Medical Service at Bastogne," *Military Surgery* 100 (1947):37-42.
6. Jerome Corsi, *No Greater Valor: The Siege of Bastogne and the Miracle That Sealed Allied Victory* (Nashville: Nelson Books, 2014), 28.
7. Jack T. Prior, "The Night Before Christmas—Bastogne, 1944," *Bulletin of the Onondaga County Medical Society* (New York), December, 1972. Prior lent a personal recollection of those days at Bastogne.
8. Koskimaki, *Battered Bastards*, 93.
9. Peter Schrijvers, *Those Who Hold Bastogne: The True Story of the Soldiers and Civilians Who Fought in the Biggest Battle of the Bulge* (New Haven: Yale University Press, 2014), 51.

10. McManus, *Alamo in the Ardennes*, 236-237.
11. Ibid., 245-246.
12. Ibid., 250.
13. Prior, "The Night Before Christmas."
14. Charles B. MacDonald, *A Time for Trumpets: The Untold Story of the Battle of the Bulge* (New York: Quill, 1985), 500.
15. Admission and Disposition Report B Company, 80th Armored Medical Battalion, Army Medical Department, Fort Sam Houston, TX, and my personal communication with Sanders Marble, PhD, Office of Medical History, Army Medical Department, Fort Sam Houston, TX.
16. Peter Caddick-Adams, *Snow and Steel: The Battle of the Bulge, 1944-45* (Oxford: Oxford University Press, 2015), 482.
17. Prior, "The Night Before Christmas."
18. Interview with Albert J. Crandall, Major, M.C., 8 June 1945, RG 112 (Records of the U.S. Army Surgeon General, World War II), NARA, College Park, MD.
19. Graves, *Front Line Surgeons*, 277.
20. Phalen, "Medical Service at Bastogne," 37-42.
21. Koskimaki, *Battered Bastards*, 113.
22. Surgeon, 101st Airborne Division, Annual Report, 1944, filed 31 January 1945, RG 112 (Surgeon General), NARA, College Park, MD.
23. Tom Brokaw, *The Greatest Generation* (New York: Random House, 1998), 29-30.
24. Sergeant Natalle and Major Crandall's quotes from Graves, *Front Line Surgeons*, 278.
25. Letter to a Mr. Orton from Dr. Gordon Block, May 19, 1945, contained in Koskimaki, *Battered Bastards*, 115.
26. After Action Report: 326th Airborne Medical Company, 101st Airborne Division in the Battle of the Bulge, RG 407 (Adjutant General), NARA, College Park, MD.
27. Story relayed on http://www.battledetective.com/326th_Monument_Dedication.html, accessed March 11, 2016. While gruesome—and such atrocities certainly occurred during the Ardennes offensive—this discovery is not contained in any official records.
28. Middleton to McAuliffe in Corsi, *No Greater Valor*, 178-179; U.S. elements now trapped in Bastogne included the 101st Airborne Division, Combat Command B of the 10th Armored Division, the 705th Tank Destroyer Battalion, various artillery and engineer units, and fourteen tanks of the 9th Armored Division.
29. Phalen, "Medical Service at Bastogne," 37-42.
30. Schrijvers, *Those Who Hold Bastogne*, 103, 111.
31. "Expectant" is a triage term used for those who are unlikely to survive and thus not ones to consume limited medical personnel, resources, and time. They are made as comfortable as possible.
32. Prior, "The Night Before Christmas." Lt. Col. David Gold, the Division Surgeon, had been captured when the 326th Medical Company was overrun. Major Davidson had been regimental surgeon for the 502nd Parachute Infantry.
33. Prior, "The Night Before Christmas."
34. Jack Prior 1994 interview on FOX uploaded on YouTube by Martin King, https://www.youtube.com/watch?v=XF8N-AqV4ks, accessed 5/17/2016

35. Second echelon medical care in the army of World War II was usually clearing stations, smaller field-type hospitals where patients from the battalion aid stations (echelon I) were taken for further treatment and triage. These were division-level facilities where some surgery could be done if necessary for life-threatening injuries. Such facilities were essentially non-existent in the chaos of Bastogne.
36. Koskimaki, *Battered Bastards*, 279-280.
37. Louis Simpson, "The Way It Was In the Bulge," *New York Times*, December 6, 1964.
38. Fussell, *The Boys' Crusade*, 131.
39. Beevor, *Ardennes*, 189-227.
40. Koskimaki, *Battered Bastards*, 240.
41. Ian Gardner, *No Victory in Valhalla: The Untold Story of Third Battalion 506 Parachute Infantry Regiment from Bastogne to Berchtesgaden* (Oxford: Osprey Press, 2014), 113-114.
42. Actually, the message was more than just the word "NUTS." McAuliffe went on to say that "We continue to hold Bastogne. By holding Bastogne we assure the success of the Allied armies. . . . We are . . . truly making ourselves a Merry Christmas." Merry Christmas message to the troops from General A.C. McAuliffe, RG 407 (Adjutant General), NARA, College Park, MD.
43. S. L. A. Marshall, *Bastogne: The First Eight Days* (Washington, DC: Center of Military History, United States Army, 1946), 134.
44. Figures from H. Rex Shama, *Pulse and Repulse: Troop Carrier and Airborne Teams in Europe During World War II* (Austin: Eakin Press, 1995), 147-291.
45. Surgeon, 101st Airborne Division, Annual Report, 1944, filed 31 January 1945, RG 112 (Records of the U.S. Army Surgeon General, World War II), NARA, College Park, MD.
46. Marshall, *Bastogne*, 139.
47. "K-rations" were individually packaged meals for GIs during World War II that comprised a breakfast, lunch, and dinner serving of canned entrees, usually totaling 8,000 calories and adequate protein per day. See Franz A. Koehler, *Special Rations for the Armed Forces* (Washington, DC: QMC Historical Studies, Historical Branch, Office of the Quartermaster General, 1953), 24-26.
48. Shama, *Pulse and Repulse*, 147-291.
49. United States Army Air Forces, *DZ Europe: The Story of the 440th Troop Carrier Group* (Indianapolis: Hollenbeck Press, 1946), 81-82.
50. General McAuliffe letter to Major General P. L. Williams, 25 January 1945, National WWII Glider Pilots Association, accessed at https://www.ww2gp.org/ardenneslastdrop.php, September 25, 2017.
51. Appendix 3: Daily Casualty Figures, Annual Report, 101st Airborne Division, 1944, Office of the Surgeon, RG 112 (HUMEDS), NARA, College Park, MD.
52. Anecdote from Stevan Dedijer, My *Life of Curiosity and Insights: A Chronicle of the 20th Century* (Lund: Nordic Academic Press, 2009), 140.
53. Major Davidson later claimed that "only about 5 men died of wounds who might have been saved had they been given medical care." Graham A. Cosmas and Albert E. Cowdrey, *The Medical Department: Medical Service in the European Theater of Operations* (Washington, DC: Center of Military History, 1992), 419. It is not clear how he arrived at that figure. The official total by the Division Surgeon, Major Barfield, issued on January 31 of those who died under treatment in medical facilities of the 101st Airborne from December 18 to 31 was 33. Annual Report, Medical

Department, 101st Airborne Division, 31 January 1945, RG 112 (Surgeon General), NARA, College Park, MD. Taking account of all those remote locations where wounded were collected, the figure is almost certainly higher.
54. After the war, for some reason, the name was changed to *Rolley*.
55. Koskimaki, *Battered Bastards*, 326-327.
56. Marshall, *Bastogne*, 165-169.
57. Events in the lives of Augusta Chiwy and Renée Lemaire are taken from Martin King's *L'infirmiere Oubliee: L'histoire inconnue d'Augusta Chiwy, héroïne de la bataille des Ardennes* (Brussels: Racine, 2011), Charles B. MacDonald's *A Time for Trumpets: The Untold Story of the Battle of the Bulge* (New York: HarperCollins, 2002)—which included interviews with Renée's two sisters, Maggie and Giselle—Michael Collins and Martin King, *Voices of the Bulge: Untold Stories from Veterans of the Battle of the Bulge* (Minneapolis: Zenith Press, 2011), Jack Prior's *The Night Before Christmas*; Martin King's *Searching for Augusta: The Forgotten Angel of Bastogne* (Guilford: Globe Pequot, 2017); and FOX news interviews with Dr. Jack Prior and Augusta Chiwy in 1994.
58. Events as described by King, *Searching for Augusta*, 65-67, "besotted," 103.
59. Anecdote reported by Steven Beardsley in *Stars and Stripes*, December 21, 2011.
60. Koskimaki, *Battered Bastards*, 291.
61. William Kerby excerpt from an article published in *The Tigers' Tale*, 10th Armored Division Newspaper, and reprinted in Don Addor's *Noville Outpost of Bastogne – My Last Battle* (Bloomington: Trafford Publishing, 2004), 187-189.
62. From eye-witness testimony it is more likely that Renée was crushed by falling beams rather than, as Martin King speculates, she might have been killed in the initial blast. King, *Searching for Augusta*, 104.
63. Ruth Padawer, "Going Silent: Augusta Chiwy," *New York Times Magazine*, December 27, 2015.
64. "U.S. Honors Belgian Nurse for Valor in World War II," *New York Times*, December 13, 2011, A15.
65. Padawer, "Going Silent: Augusta Chiwy."

CHAPTER 15. AIRBORNE SURGEONS

1. C. S. Phalen, "Medical Service at Bastogne," *Military Surgeon*, 100 (1947): 37-42.
2. Written personal recollections of Major Howard Serrell in diary form kindly supplied to the author by his son, Howard "Chip" Serrell, Jr.
3. The SS *Naushon* was a converted American coastal steamer, handed over to the British in 1942 as part of Lend-Lease and reconfigured as a hospital ship that could hold three hundred patients. It was on loan back to the US Navy for Operation Overlord.
4. Details of the flight were given by Lieutenant Taflinger to Captain Dello Dayton at XII Corps Headquarters in Luxembourg City on January 29, 1945. Lieutenant Taflinger was later awarded the Silver Star for this mission.
5. Serrell, diary.
6. Flight officer was a rank peculiar to World War II. It no longer exists in the US Air Force.
7. Diary 12th Evacuation Hospital October–December 1944, RG 407 (Adjutant General), NARA, College Park, MD.
8. Whipple's philosophy of surgical education is outlined in his 1957 paper "The Training of a Surgeon," *Journal of the National Medical Association* 49 (1957): 295-304.

9. Allen O. Whipple papers, Columbia University College of Physicians and Surgeons, Department of Surgery, compiled by Gael Evans for the Soutter Exhibit at the Lamar Soutter Library, University of Massachusetts Medical School, Worchester, MA.
10. Historical Record 12th Evacuation Hospital, 7 February 1945, RG 407 (Adjutant Genral), NARA, College Park, MD.
11. Almost 40 percent of the 1,283 casualties suffered by the 101st Airborne at Bastogne were due to frostbite and its close cousin, trench foot. Surgeon, 101st Airborne Division, Annual Report, 1944, filed 31 January 1945, RG 112 (Surgeon General), NARA, College Park, MD.
12. Corsi, *No Greater Valor*, 288.
13. Phalen, "Medical Service at Bastogne," 37-42.
14. After Action Report, Headquarters, Third U.S. Army, Part 17: Medical, RG 112 (Surgeon General), NARA, College Park, MD.
15. Doctor Soutter's career is comprehensively told by Ellen S. More: *A History of the University of Massachusetts Medical School: Integrating Primary Care and Biomedical Research* (Worcester: Lamar Soutter Library, 2012). Quotes are from her publication, 45-46.
16. After Action Report, Headquarters, Third U.S. Army, Part 17: Medical, RG 112 (Surgeon General), NARA, College Park, MD.
17. Annual Report 1944, Surgeon, 101st Airborne Division, 31 January 1945, RG 112 (Surgeon General, World War II), NARA, College Park, MD.
18. Each of the medical officers and surgical technicians received a Silver Star for gallantry in action, exemplifying "the highest traditions of the military service of the United States," Soutter, RG 112, NARA, College Park, MD, and Sanders Marble, *Skilled and Resolute: A History of the 12th Evacuation Hospital and the 212th MASH, 1917-2006* (Washington, DC: Government Printing Office, 2013), 39.

CHAPTER 16. RELIEF

1. Martin Blumenson, *The Patton Papers* (Boston: Da Capo Press, 1996), 606.
2. Ibid., 607.
3. Ibid., 608.
4. Koskimaki, *Battered Bastards*, 374.
5. Annual Report, 1944, Headquarters 240th Medical Battalion, RG 112 (Surgeon General), NARA, College Park, MD.
6. Rapport and Norwood, *Rendezvous with Destiny*, 597.
7. The Story of the 107th Evacuation Hospital (SM), RG 407 (Adjutant General), NARA, College Park, MD.
8. 39th Evacuation Hospital messages December 1944 and Daily Log 1944, part 2, RG 407 (Adjutant General), NARA, College Park, MD.
9. History, First Platoon, 60th Field Hospital, RG 112 (HUMEDS), NARA, College Park, MD.
10. Records, 92nd Medical Gas Treatment Battalion, RG 112 (HUMEDS), NARA, College Park, MD.
11. Gellhorn, *The Face of War*, 147.
12. Surgeon, 101st Airborne Division, Annual Report, 1944, filed 31 January 1945, RG 112 (Records of the U.S. Army Surgeon General, World War II), NARA, College Park, MD.
13. Louis Simpson, *Selected Prose* (New York: Paragon House, 1989), 117.
14. Beevor, *Ardennes*, 351.

15. Rapport and Norwood, *Rendezvous with Destiny*, 624.
16. Gardner, *No Victory*, 176.
17. Ibid., 180.
18. Ibid., 182.
19. Koskimaki, *Battered Bastards*, 459.
20. Ibid., 456.
21. Rapport and Norwood, *Rendezvous with Destiny*, 661.
22. Beevor, *Ardennes*, 348.
23. History of the 102nd Evacuation Hospital, RG 407 (Adjutant General), NARA, College Park, MD.
24. McWilliams, *The Chaplain's Conflict*, 87.
25. All from Samecky, *Army Nurse Corps*, 242.
26. Ernest O. Hauser, "Shock Nurse," *Saturday Evening Post*, March 10, 1945.
27. Monahan, *And If I Perish*, 421.
28. Capt. Harry Fisher's comments in Graves, *Front Line Surgeons*, 265-269.
29. Koskimaki, *Battered Bastards*, 513.
30. Gardner, *No Victory*, 215.
31. Rapport and Norwood, *Rendezvous with Destiny*, 822.
32. Ibid., 651.
33. General Middleton's VIII Corps was absorbed into Patton's Third Army in late December.
34. After Action Report, Headquarters, Third U.S. Army, Part 17: Medical, RG 112 (Surgeon General), NARA, College Park, MD.
35. West Point Association of Graduates: "Be Thou At Peace," Jarrett M. Huddleston, Jr. USMA Class 1943, http://apps.westpointaog.org/Memorials/Article/13885/, accessed May 8, 2016.

CHAPTER 17. THE HERMIT KINGDOM

1. William Elliot Griffis, *Corea: The Hermit Nation* (New York: Charles Scribner's Sons, 1894), 7.
2. David Halberstam, *The Coldest Winter: America and the Korean War* (New York: Hyperion, 2007), 63.
3. Redvers Opie, *The Search for Peace Settlements* (Washington, DC: Brookings Institute, 1951), 311.
4. Harry S. Truman, *Memoirs, Volume Two: Years of Trial and Hope* (Garden City: Doubleday, 1956), 333.
5. Gary R. Hess, *Presidential Decisions for War: Korea, Vietnam, the Persian Gulf, and Iraq* (Baltimore: Johns Hopkins University Press, 2009), 9.
6. MacArthur, *Reminiscences*, 334.
7. Truman, *Memoirs*, 343, and Clay Blair, *The Forgotten War: America in Korea 1950-1953* (New York: Random House, 1987), 85.
8. Russell A. Gugeler, *Combat Actions in Korea* (Washington, DC : Center of Military History, 1987), 3.
9. Francis W. Pruitt, "General Aspects of Medicine in Korea and Japan 1950-53," Medical Science Publication No. 4, Recent Advances in Medicine and Surgery (1954), Volume II, U.S. Army Medical Service Graduate School, Walter Reed Army Medical Center, Washington, DC.
10. Armstrong and Bethea quotes from Albert E. Cowdry, *The Medics' War* (Honolulu: University Press of the Pacific, 2005), 66-67.

11. "Korean War Wounded are Quickly Treated," *Spokane Daily Chronicle*, September 20, 1950, 19.
12. Chowdry, *The Medics' War*, 70.

CHAPTER 18. THE ASCENT

1. For a commentary on the Pusan defense, see Bill Sloan, *The Darkest Summer: Pusan and Inchon 1950* (New York: Simon & Schuster, 2009).
2. CINCFE to Joint Chiefs of Staff, Washington, DC, 4 November 1950, Harry S. Truman Library, Independence, MO.
3. The Japanese renamed the Korean "Changjin" to "Chosin" during their occupation.
4. From WWII Japanese air target analysis, 1942-1945, Publication M1653, NARA, College Park, MD.
5. Headquarters X Corps Command Report: Special Report on Chosin Reservoir, 27 Nov to 10 Dec 50, Adjutant General's Office, Washington DC, 1960, Combined Arms Research Library, Fort Leavenworth, KS.
6. Information on Marine operational deployment gathered from the Korean War Project: Special Action Report: Wonsan-Hamhung-Chosin First Marine Division, FMF, Folder 1, Volume 2, and Annex PETER, Special Action Report, 1st Marine Division, FMF, 7 Oct to 15 Dec 1950, NARA, College Park, MD.
7. Information for the First Medical Battalion from Annex HH to the 1st Marine Division Special Action Report for period 8 October–15 December 1950, 9 January 1951, Korean War Project, NARA, College Park, MD.
8. Information for the 1st Medical Battalion gleaned from Annex HH to the 1st Marine Division Special Action Report for period 8 October–15 December 1950, 9 January 1951, NARA.
9. C. K. Holloway, "The Military Aspects of the Chosin Reservoir Withdrawal," *Western Journal of Surgery, Obstetrics, and Gynecology*, 63 (1955):308-311.
10. Mobile Army Surgical Hospitals (MASH) played a prominent role in casualty care in the Korean War. Their proximity to the front lines provided urgent surgical care for life-threatening injuries. For a capsulized account see, Woodard, S. C. "The Story of the Mobile Army Surgical Hospital," *Military Medicine* 168 (2003): 503-513.
11. Salary support for internship and residency was atrocious, hardly meeting minimum wage. Of course doctors were expected to spend most their time in the hospital, marriage and family discouraged.
12. James H. Stewart, MD, "Notes of a Korean War Surgeon," *Space Coast Area Mensa Bulletin* 27, Nos. 6-11 (2009).
13. Oral History with Mr. William Davis conducted by Jan K. Herman, Navy Bureau of Medicine and Surgery (BUMED) Historian, 17 April 2001, Office of Medical History, BUMED, Washington DC.
14. Stewart, "Notes of a Korean War Surgeon."
15. Lynn Montross and Nicholas Canzona, ed., *U.S. Marine Operations in Korea, Volume III: The Chosin Reservoir Campaign* (Washington DC: Historical Branch, G-3, Headquarters, U.S. Marine Corps, 1957), 121.
16. George A. Rasula, ed., *Changjin Journal*, No. 11, http://libraryautomation.com/nymas/changjinjournalTOC.html, accessed 7/12/2016.
17. Morton Silver, DDS, USNR, interview with Jan K. Herman, Historian, BUMED, 12 October 2000, US Navy Medical Department Oral History Program.

18. Company "D" First Medical Battalion, Annex HH to the 1st Marine Division Special Action Report for period 8 October–15 December 1950, 9 January 1951, Korean War Project, NARA, College Park, MD.
19. Charles K. Holloway, *Escape from Hell: A Navy Surgeon Remembers Pusan, Inchon, and Chosin Korea, 1950* (La Jolla: Unpublished, 1997), 100.
20. Robert C. Shoemaker, *A Surgeon Remembers Korea 1950-1951 And The Marines* (Victoria: Trafford Publishing, 2005), 47.

CHAPTER 19. THE DESCENT

1. Annex RR (Appendix 4, Medical), 7th Marines, 1st Marine Division FMF Special Action Report 8 October to 15 December, 1950, NARA.
2. Montross, *U.S. Marine Operations*, 192.
3. Morton Silver interview.
4. Shoemaker, *A Surgeon Remembers*, 56-57.
5. Eric Hammel, *Chosin: Heroic Ordeal of the Korean War* (Pacifica: Pacifica Miltary History, 1981), 123.
6. Reminiscences of Lt. Robert J. Fleischaker, MC, USN, Office of Medical History, Navy Bureau of Medicine and Surgery (BUMED), Falls Church, Virginia.
7. Holloway, *Escape from Hell*, 101-102.
8. "C" Co. 1st Medical Battalion, 8 Oct 1950 to 15 Dec 1950, Annex HH to the 1st Marine Division Special Action Report for period 8 October–15 December 1950, 9 January 1951, Korean War Project, NARA, College Park, MD.
9. Litvin, H. "Frozen in Memory: Recalling the Chosin Reservoir," *Navy Medicine* 91 (2000): 16-21.
10. Ibid.
11. Morton Silver interview.
12. Information and statistics taken from: Special Action Report, VMO-6, 8 October 1950 to 15 December 1950, Annex WW to 1st Marine Division Special Action Report, 5 January 1951, NARA, College Park, MD; and Charles R. Smith [Ed.], *U.S. Marines in the Korean War* (Washington DC: History Division, United States Marine Corps, 2007), 283.
13. For an in-depth review of Marine helicopter activity near the Chosin Reservoir see Ronald J. Brown, *Whirlybirds: U.S. Marine Helicopters in Korea* (Washington DC: U.S. Marine Corps Historical Center, 2003), 28-33.
14. Ordinarily, cold body temperatures—hypothermia—have a distinctly adverse effect on hemorrhaging men. Blood coagulation worsens and bleeding is compounded. It is known as the lethal triad of shock, and often ends in death. However, the air temperature for the Marines at Chosin was so low that, when exposed, blood simply froze.
15. C. K. Holloway, "The Military Surgical Aspects of the Chosin Reservoir Withdrawal," *Western Journal of Surgery, Obstetrics, and Gynecology*, 63 (1955):308-311.
16. Brown, *Whirlybirds*, 32.
17. Jan K. Herman, *Frozen in Memory: U. S. Navy Medicine in the Korean War* (Bangor: Booklocker, 2006), 54.
18. "They Come From Far and Near," *The Harvard Crimson*, March 1, 1935.
19. Information on Peter Arioli Jr. in part obtained from *Journal of the American Medical Association* 145 (March 17, 1951): 836.
20. Annex HH (1st Medical Battalion) to the 1st Marine Division Special Action Report for period 8 October–15 December 1950, 9 January 1951, NARA, College Park, MD.

21. 1st Marine Division Action Report, 3 October–15 December 1950, Appendix 9 to Annex UU, 38–39, NARA. These numbers are at odds with those quoted by Montross and Canzona, who report that 914 patients were flown out on December 2 and "more than 700" on December 3. *U.S. Marine Operations in Korea*, 382.
22. Martin Russ, *Breakout: The Chosin Reservoir Campaign, Korea 1950* (New York: Penguin Books, 1999), 324.
23. Story by Jonathan Bor, "The Cold Is Still an Enemy for Some Frostbitten Korean War Veterans," *Baltimore Sun*, May 26, 1996.
24. Herman, *Frozen in Memory*, 54-55.
25. Russ, *Breakout*, 327.
26. Edward L. Daily, *MacArthur's X Corps in Korea: Inchon to the Yalu, 1950* (Paducah: Turner Publishing, 1999), 72.
27. Montross, *U.S. Marine Operations*, 278.
28. Wolf, S. I., "The Chosin Reservoir: Medical Care in Subfreezing Weather," *Leatherneck* 95 (2012): 18-20.
29. Holloway, *Escape from Hell*, 107.
30. Stewart, "Notes of a Korean War Surgeon."
31. Dylan Bowyer, "Doctor of Chosin Few Recounts Story," July 26, 2013, http://www.hqmc.marines.mil/, accessed July 14, 2016.
32. Preceding quotes from Marguerite Higgins, *War in Korea: The Report of a Woman Combat Correspondent* (New York: Doubleday, 1951), 181-182.
33. Herman, *Frozen in Memory*, 55.
34. Figures from John P. Condon, *U.S. Marine Corps Aviation*, Volume 5, Deputy Chief of Naval Operations, Government Printing Office, Washington, DC, 1987, 28; X Corps report puts the total at 4,526 (Headquarters X Corps Command Report: Special Report on Chosin Reservoir).
35. Headquarters X Corps Command Report: Special Report on Chosin Reservoir.
36. Russ, *Breakout*, 338.
37. Headquarters X Corps Command Report: Special Report on Chosin Reservoir
38. These casualty figures are from Headquarters, U.S. Marine Corps, "Information of Marine action in northeastern Korea," 13 Dec 1950, NARA, College Park, MD. They differ from other "official" sources such as Annex E, Appendix II, First Marine Division Special Action Report, which lists 1,140 total battle casualties and 1,194 total non-battle casualties for the period November 30 through December 4, 1950.
39. Joseph Lister (1827-1912) is generally regarded as the "Father of Antisepsis." His introduction of carbolic acid as an antiseptic agent dramatically affected the rate of post-surgical infections and markedly reduced death and need for amputation in extremity wounds. See Lindsey Fitzharris, *The Butchering Art: Joseph Lister's Quest to Transform the Grisly World of Victorian Medicine* (New York: Scientific American/Farrar, 2017).
40. Holloway, "The Military Surgical Aspects of the Chosin Reservoir Withdrawal," 308-311
41. There are few jobs in the Marine Corps that do not involve proximity to weapons. Fortunately, even service troops—truck drivers, cooks, corpsmen, clerks—were competent infantrymen.
42. Stewart, "Notes of a Korean War Surgeon."
43. Herman, *Frozen in Memory*, 21.
44. Ibid., 57.
45. H. Litvin, "Frozen in Memory: Recalling the Chosin Reservoir," *Navy Medicine*, 91 (2000):16-21.

46. Statistics from First Marine Division Special Action Report, Division Adjutant, Annex E, Appendix 2 and Montross, *U.S. Marine Operations*, 303.
47. Ibid.
48. Shoemaker, *A Surgeon Remembers*, 74.
49. Special Action Report, VMO-6, 8 October 1950 to 15 December 1950, Annex WW to 1st Marine Division Special Action Report, 5 January 1951, NARA.
50. Special Action Report, VMO-6, 8 October 1950 to 15 December 1950, Annex WW to 1st Marine Division Special Action Report, 5 January 1951, NARA, College Park, MD.
51. One C-47 got through on December 8 and took out nineteen, all in almost zero visibility.
52. Headquarters X Corps Command Report: Special Report on Chosin Reservoir.
53. Holloway, *Escape from Hell*, 122.
54. "Devil Dog" was another nickname for a Marine. It was said that Germans, fighting Marines during World War I, used the term *Teufel Hunden*, or Devil Dogs. It stuck.
55. Stewart, "Notes of a Korean War Surgeon."
56. Higgins, *War in Korea*, 195-196.
57. Annex HH (1st Medical Battalion) to the 1st Marine Division Special Action Report for period 8 October – 15 December 1950, 9 January 1951, NARA, College Park, MD.
58. "War: Retreat of the 20,000," *Time*, December 18, 1950, 18-19.
59. Shoemaker, *A Surgeon Remembers*, 80.
60. Litvin, "Frozen in Memory: Recalling the Chosin Reservoir," 16-21.
61. Holloway, *Escape from Hell*, 128-129.

CHAPTER 20. MASSACRE TO THE EAST

1. Roy E. Appleman, *South to the Naktong, North to the Yalu* (Washington DC: Center of Military History, 1992), 736.
2. Seventh Medical Battalion, X Corps: The Loss of Major Oren C. Atchley, Medical Service Corps, Commanding Officer, 7th Medical Battalion, 7th Infantry Division, 24 November 1950, RG 407 (Adjutant General), NARA, College Park, MD.
3. Navarre, letter to Samuel Milner, The Historical Unit, AMEDD, February 19, 1967, courtesy of Sanders Marble, PhD, Fort Sam Houston, TX, 13.
4. Navarre letter, 14.
5. According to Appleman, Captain Drake, Commander of the 31st Tank Company, had urged "the medical company's commander" not to go any farther north that night but to stay at the command center at Hudong-ni (Appleman, *East of Chosin*, 86).
6. Rasula, Galloway: "Medical Company Ambush Hill 1221," *Changjin Journal* 03.25.02, http://bobrowen.com/nymas/Changjinjournal020325.html , accessd July 16, 2016.
7. Jim Blohm's description can be found in Patrick C. Roe, "Destruction of the 31st Infantry: A Tragedy of the Chosin Campaign," Part III, *Chosin Reservoir Korea: November–December 1950*, http://www.chosinreservoir.com/, accessed July 24, 2016
8. Headquarters X Corps Command Report, The Commanding General's Diary for November 28, 1950; Richard W. Stewart, *Staff Operations: The X Corps in Korea, December 1950* (Ft. Leavenworth: Combat Studies Institute, 1991), 4. This infamous

remark by the controversial Almond has been widely quoted as an example of the gross underestimation of the quantity and quality of Chinese troops in North Korea in December, 1950.

9. Memoirs of Colonel John E. Gray (ret), published as "The Chosin Reservoir Campaign" in *RECALL: The North Carolina Military History Society*, 9 (2005): 1-16.

10. Rasula, *Changjin Journal*, 11.27.05, http://bobrowen.com/nymas/Changjinjournal051127.html.

11. Donald Knox, *The Korean War: Pusan to Chosin: An Oral History* (Orlando: Harcourt Brace Jovanovich, 1985), 551.

12. NR: C69953, 28 Nov 50, from CINCFE TOKYO JAPAN SGD MacArthur to: JCS WASH, DC INFO: DEPT AR WASH CD CM, 28 Nov 1950, in *Pertinent Papers on Korean Situation*, Vol. II, 345, Harry S. Truman Library, Independence, MO

13. Report of Major Wesley Curtis, in Rasula, *Changjin Journal*, 09.25.05 http://bobrowen.com/nymas/Changjinjournal050925.html.

14. Navarre letter, 35.

15. Ibid., 46.

16. Ibid., 37-38.

17. Rasula, *Changjin Journal*, 03.25.02, http://bobrowen.com/nymas/Changjinjournal020325.html.

18. Roy E. Appleman, *East of Chosin: Entrapment and Breakout in Korea, 1950* (College Station: Texas A&M University Press, 1987), 212.

19. Knox, *An Oral History*, 553.

20. Steve Vogel, "50 Years Later, an Army Force Gets Its Due", *Washington Post*, December 11, 2000.

21. Rasula, Hugh Robbins: *Breakout*, *Changjin Journal* 02.28.04, http://bobrowen.com/nymas/Changjinjournal040228.html.

22. Knox, *An Oral History*, 554.

23. Ibid., 555.

24. Interview Dr. Yong Kak Lee by Dr. Birney Dibble, *Veterans' Memoirs*, Korean War Educator, http://www.koreanwar-educator.org/memoirs/dibble_birney/index.htm#addendumWritings , accessed August 11, 2016.

25. Navarre letter, 57.

26. Interview with Betty Gregorio Baker, Navy nurse aboard the USS *Consolation* (AH-15), during the Korean War. Conducted by Mr. Jan Herman, Historian, Bureau of Medicine and Surgery, 9 May 2001.

27. Interview with Dr. Yong Kak Lee by Dr. Birney Dibble.

28. Rasula, *Changjin Journal*, 03.25.02.

29. Information from Captain John McGuire in John G. Westover, *Combat Support in Korea* (Washington, DC: Center of Military History, 1955), 115-116.

30. Dwain Lair, "Korean War Nurse Talks of M.A.S.H.", *Bolivar* [MO] *Herald-Free Press*, November 10, 2003.

31. Witt, *A Defense Weapon*, 193.

32. Appleman, *East of Chosin*, 317.

33. Appleman: *Escaping the Trap*, 340.

CHAPTER 21. INDOCHINE

1. Bernard Fall, *The Two Vietnams: A Political And Military Analysis* (New York: Frederick A. Praeger, 1965), 3.

2. Marguerite Duras, *L'Amant* (Paris: Les Éditions de Minuit, 1984), 30.

3. A proclamation found in 1890 in a refuge in the Yen The district of Tonkin, from

Albert de Pouvourville, *Études Coloniales: III: La Politique Indo-chinoise, 1892-1893* (Paris: Albert Savine [Éditeur], 1894), 207.
4. Joseph Buttinger, *Vietnam: A Dragon Embattled* (New York: Praeger, 1967), 453.
5. Report of the Office of the Secretary of Defense Vietnam Task Force (to be referred to as "The Pentagon Papers"): *Vietnam and the United States, 1940-1950*, A-3, RG 330, NARA, College Park, MD.
6. Giap, under Ho Chi Minh's influence, was an educated and brilliant strategist and tactician. His understanding of war is well outlined in Vo Nguyen Giap, *People's War, People's Army* (Hanoi: Foreign Languages Publishing House, 1961).
7. Stanley Karnow, *Vietnam: A History* (New York: Viking Press, 1983), 181. Vietnamese tradition had always pitched a numerically inferior force against apparent superior invaders. It was the art of maneuver, opportunity, and determination that drove the grasshopper to disembowel the elephant.

CHAPTER 22. KHE SANH VILLAGE

1. Thomas Preston, *The President and His Inner Circle: Leadership Style and the Advisory Process in Foreign Policy Making* (New York: Columbia University Press, 2001), 171.
2. Information on the Poilanes from Marie-Laure Tardieu-Blot, "Eugene Poilane (1888-1964)," *Adansonia* 4 (1964): 351-354; John Prados and Ray W. Stubbe, *Valley of Decision: The Siege of Khe Sanh* (Annapolis: Naval Institute Press, 1991), 25-26; "Memories of Vietnam, 1951-1968" (the memoirs of Madame Poilane), Khe Sanh Veterans Association, Inc., Fall 2001, http://www.geocities.ws/ksvredclay/issue-51-memoirs.htm, accessed March 3, 2019; Ray W. Stubbe, *Pebbles in My Boots*, Vol. 3 (Wauwatosa: Self-published, 2014), 20-24.
3. Eugene Poilane was a respected botanist who published a number of scientific botanical papers on Indochinese plants. After his death a three-part installment authored by Poilane was published on fruit trees of Indochina (E. Poilane, "Les Arbres Fruitiers d'Indochine," *J d'Agriculture Tropicale et de Botanique Appliquee* 12 (1965): 235-252; 438-453; 527-549.
4. Tad Bartimus et al., *War Torn: Stories of War from the Women Reporters Who Covered Vietnam* (New York: Random House, 2004), 129.
5. Montagnards were diverse ethnic and cultural minorities, composed of any number of migrant Asian tribes seeking to live in the highland regions of central and northern Vietnam. While thought of as primitive and backward, they developed over time a complex social and economic relationship with lowland Kinh. The Bru tribe inhabited areas of Quang Tri Province. They probably migrated from Cambodia and Laos and settled in the central highlands of Vietnam. See Jean Michaud, ed., *Turbulent Times and Enduring People: Mountain Minorities in the South-East Asian Massif* (London: Routledge, 2000). Bru themselves preferred to be called *Tai So*, as "Bru" was associated with backwardness. Jan Ovesen, "Indigenous Peoples and Development in Laos: Ideologies and Ironies", *Moussons* 6 (2002): 69-97.
6. Viet Cong stood for *Mat tran Dan toc Giai phong mien Nam Viet Nam* (National Liberation Front of South Vietnam). They were also called "Charlie" or "Victor Charlie" by American troops. North Vietnamese regulars were sometimes lumped in with that epithet or simply called "NVA" for North Vietnamese Army. Sometimes no one knew who they were fighting until those captured were interrogated or the dead were inspected for papers. Generically, all enemy could also be lumped under the term "Viets."
7. Excerpts from Madam Poilane's memoirs, fn 787.

CHAPTER 23. "EYE" CORPS

1. Karnow, *Vietnam: A History*, 412.
2. Jack Shulimson, *U.S. Marines in Vietnam: The Landing and the Buildup* (Washington, DC: History and Museums Division, Headquarters, U.S. Marine Corps, 1978), 16.
3. The Pentagon Papers, 22 Feb 1965, Part IV C.4., *Evolution of War*, RG 330, NARA, College Park, MD.
4. The analogy, of course, was Dien Bien Phu where elite French and French colonial paratrooper units burrowed in under relentless Viet Minh artillery barrages, unable to mount much in the way of offensive action. See Bernard Fall, *Hell in a Very Small Place: The Siege of Dien Bien Phu* (Cambridge: Da Capo Press, 1966).
5. Partitioning of Indochina at the 16th Parallel occurred at the Berlin Conference in 1945. The southern part remained in the Southeast Asia Command, the northern section in the Chinese Theater, then under Chiang Kai-shek. The Demilitarized Zone was established at the 17th Parallel by the Geneva Conference agreements (Geneva Accords) of July 21, 1954, spelling the end of the First Indochina War and separating North from South Vietnam.
6. The Pentagon Papers, Part III: *The Geneva Accords* 1954, Articles 5 and 6.
7. Winning the "hearts and minds" of the Vietnamese was a favorite and frequently used line by President Lyndon Johnson, stressing pacification rather than conquest. See Richard A. Hunt, *Pacification: the American Struggle for Vietnam's Hearts and Minds* (Boulder: Westview Press, 1995), particularly 70-71.
8. That is, until mid-1968 when Army elements arrived to bolster MACV capabilities around the DMZ.
9. Leon P. Eisman, *Brief History of 1st Hospital Company, 1st Medical Battalion, 3rd Medical Battalion in Republic of Vietnam* (Falls Church: Navy BUMED, 1973).
10. Jan K. Herman, Oral History with Capt. (ret.) William Mahaffey, MC, USN, 17 December 2003, courtesy Bureau of Medicine and Surgery (BUMED), Falls Church, VA. Procedures on arteries are usually considered quite complex requiring additional surgical expertise.
11. Jan K. Herman, *Navy Medicine: Oral Histories from Dien Bien Phu to the Fall of Saigon* (Jefferson. NC: McFarland, 2009), 68-73.
12. "Chu Lai" was an American settlement, not named geographically but was the Chinese name of Lieutenant General Victor Krulak, Commander of the Fleet Marine Force, Pacific. See Shulimson, *U.S. Marines in Vietnam: The Landing and the Buildup*, 30.
13. Herman, *Navy Medicine in Vietnam*, 72.
14. "Boonies" slang for boondocks, outback, rural.
15. Paul J. Pitlyk, *Blood on China Beach: My Story as a Brain Surgeon in Vietnam* (Bloomington: Universe, 2012).
16. Command Chronology: Headquarters, 1st Medical Battalion, 1st Marine Division, FMF, 19 April 1966, US Marine Corps History Division, The Vietnam Center and Archive, Texas Tech University, Lubbock, TX.
17. Ibid., 4 May 1966.
18. MUST stood for "Medical Unit, Self-contained, Transportable." These were inflatable shelters for ward space and expandable shelters for operating rooms and support sections. They were used throughout Vietnam for fixed medical facilities. Neel Spurgeon, *Medical Support of the U.S. Army in Vietnam 1965-1970*, Chapter IV (Washington DC: Department of the Army, 1991), 65.

19. The Boeing CH-47 Chinook was a workhorse of the army during the Vietnam War. Among other functions each could accommodate up to twenty-four litter patients. The Marine version was called the CH-46 Sea Knight, basically identical in functionality. For a comprehensive review of Marine helicopters in Vietnam see William R. Fails, *Marines and Helicopters 1962-1973* (Washington, DC: History and Museums Division, Headquarters, U.S. Marine Corps, 1978).
20. Captain Bruce Canaga, Transcript of IBM Magnabelt Received from Naval Station Hospital, Danang, 31 March 1966, BUMED History Office, Falls Church, VA.
21. Tim O'Brien, *The Things They Carried* (Boston: Houghton Mifflin Harcourt, 1990), 88.
22. James Chaffee, "NSA Station Hospital, Da Nang: A Personal History," *Navy Medicine* 93 (2002): 9-15.
23. Pitlyk, *Blood on China Beach*, 52.
24. Jan K. Herman, Oral History with Dr. James Chandler, 14 July 2005, courtesy BUMEDS.
25. Military Assistance Command, Vietnam, Special Operations Group (MACV-SOG), Annex N, 1965, 2 June 1966, RG 472, NARA, College Park, MD. Operations by MACV-SOG included maritime, air, and ground surveillance. The SOG team at Khe Sanh was designated FOB-3 (Forward Operating Base-3).
26. NVA were North Vietnamese Army members, sometimes called "The People's Army."
27. Stubbe, *Pebbles in My Boots*, Vol. 3, 8.
28. Westmoreland, *A Soldier Reports*, 336.
29. Jan K. Herman, Oral History with HM2 (ret.) Paul Churchill, USN, 4 January 2006, and Dr. G. Gustave Hodge, 14 February 2004 (San Diego, CA), BUMED.

CHAPTER 24. INDIAN COUNTRY

1. William R. Corson, *The Betrayal* (New York: W.W. Norton, 1968), 78; Lieutenant Colonel Corson was a Marine intelligence officer who became highly critical of the State Department and South Vietnamese government, prompting a reprimand from his beloved Marine Corps. He died in 2000. J.Y. Smith, "William R. Corson," *Washington Post*, July 19, 2000.
2. For an in depth discussion of the barrier project (OPLAN 11-67), see Gary L. Telfer, Lane Rogers, and V. Keith Fleming, Jr., *U.S. Marines in Vietnam: Fighting the North Vietnamese, 1967* (Washington DC: History and Museum Division, Headquarters, U.S. Marine Corps, 1984), 86-94.
3. Actually there were two hills under "861"; Hill 861 and 861A were separated by a similar saddle.
4. A numerical designation of a Marine or army unit, such as "3rd Marines" or 26th Marines, indicates a Marine regiment. If a division-size unit, the number will be followed by the indicator "division."
5. Telfer, *Fighting the North Vietnamese*, 39.
6. "Gnat of Hill 881," *Time*, May 12, 1967, 42, referring to the gruesome barren wasteland of the 1945 World War II Pacific island battlefield (Iwo Jima) during which so many Marines were lost, and the 980-foot denuded hill (Pork Chop Hill) of the Korean conflict repeatedly fought over by American and Chinese infantry in 1953.
7. Dien Bien Phu, like Khe Sanh, was surrounded by hills, but hills held by the Viet Minh, not the French.

8. J. Lally, "The Hill Battles of Khe Sanh: a Marine Corps Doctor Remembers," *Del Medical Journal* 86 (2014):377-397.
9. Command Chronology: Headquarters, 3rd Medical Battalion, 3rd Marine Division, FMF, 10 June 1967, US Marine Corps History Division, The Vietnam Center and Archive, Texas Tech University, Lubbock, TX.
10. Prados, *Valley of Decision*, 55.
11. Stubbe, *Pebbles*, Vol. 2, 24.
12. *Crachin* is French slang for "spit."
13. Herman, *Navy Medicine in Vietnam*, 233.
14. Westmoreland, *A Soldier Reports*, 335; and Bernard C. Nalty, *Air Power and the Fight for Khe Sanh* (Washington DC: Office of Air Force History, 1986), 39.
15. Moyers S. Shore II, *The Battle for Khe Sanh* (Washington DC: History and Museum Division, Headquarters, U.S. Marine Corps, 1969), 27.
16. Camp Carroll was one of nine artillery bases constructed along McNamara's barrier line. It was located south of Route 9 and over a dozen miles from Khe Sanh but easily within range for its 175 mm artillery pieces. "The Rockpile" was a toothpick type 800-foot mountain sprouting from out of nowhere just off Route 9, ten miles from the DMZ and a few miles northeast of the combat base.
17. Don Oberdorfer, *Tet!: The Turning Point in the Vietnam War* (Baltimore: Johns Hopkins University Press, 1971), 110.
18. "A Study of the Strategic Lessons Learned in Vietnam," Volume IV, The BDM Corporation, McLean, VA, 1980, 3-100.
19. Bruce B.G. Clarke: *Expendable Warriors: The Battle of Khe Sanh and the Vietnam War* (Mechanicsburg, PA: Stackpole, 2007), 45.
20. Command Chronology, Headquarters, 1st Battalion, 26th Marines, 3rd Marine Division, 10 February 1968, US Marine Corps History Division, The Vietnam Center and Archive, Texas Tech University.
21. "Humping the boonies" was a favorite term used by U.S. infantry to convey the seemingly endless ritual of searching for enemy troops in the wilds ("boonies" or boondocks) of Vietnam.
22. Jan K. Herman, Oral History with Lt. (ret.) Edward Feldman, MC, USN, 14-15 February 2004, San Diego, CA, Office of Medical History, BUMED.
23. Ibid., Feldman interview.
24. Ibid., Feldman interview.
25. Figures from Prados, *Valley of Decision*, 263.
26. Information and quotes on James Finnegan from Jan K. Herman: Oral History with LCDR (ret.) James O. Finnegan, MC, USN, 9 September 2004, Office of Medical History, Bureau of Medicine and Surgery, Washington, DC.
27. Matthew Naythons, *The Face of Mercy: A Photographic History of Medicine at War* (New York: Random House, 1993), 239.
28. Doctor Thomas's experience is well chronicled by Jan Herman in *Navy Medicine in Vietnam*, 239-241.
29. Command Chronology, III MAF, January 1968, US Marine Corps History Division, The Vietnam Center and Archive, Texas Tech University.
30. Pisor, *End of the Line*, 132.
31. Descriptions from Shore, *The Battle for Khe Sanh*, 56-57.
32. As opposed to Dien Bien Phu where Viet Minh artillery in the hills could aim directly at French fortifications in the valley with devastating effect.
33. Shore, *The Battle for Khe Sanh*, 59.

34. Repeated concussive events almost certainly contribute to a form of traumatic brain injury that may have long-standing consequences. Some clinicians also consider these events a factor in post-traumatic stress disorders.
35. Ray W. Stubbe, *Pebbles in My Boots*, vol. 3 (2014), 63-71.
36. Hammel: *Siege in the Clouds*, 220.
37. James O. Finnegan, *In the Company of Marines: A Surgeon Remembers Vietnam* (Philadelphia: Self-published, 2009), 122.
38. Figures were provided by Rev. Ray W. Stubbe, recorded from his diary of numbers listed in Charlie Med's "green log book" and relayed to the author by written communication. According to Rev. Stubbe, the log book itself has been lost and was probably destroyed some years afterwards.

CHAPTER 25. SCOTLAND

1. Op File: Operation Scotland, 31 October 1967 to 3 April 1968, Marine Corps History Division, US Marine Corps History Division, Vietnam War Documents Collection, The Vietnam Center and Archive, Texas Tech University.
2. Oriana Fallaci, *Nothing And So Be It* (Garden City: Doubleday, 1972), 177.
3. Command Chronology: Headquarters, 1st Battalion, 26th Marines, 3rd Marine Division (Rein), FMF, 1 March 1968, US Marine Corps History Division, The Vietnam Center and Archive, Texas Tech University.
4. Shore, *The Battle for Khe Sanh*, 65.
5. DeLaney and Maves's quotes from Eric Hammel "Khe Sanh: Attack on Hill 861A," *Marine Corps Gazette*, 73 (1989): 40-49. There is obvious discrepancy in the numbers of wounded estimated by Maves (35) and that recorded in the official record. Numbers of bodies are deceiving. Subjective impressions are usually overestimates.
6. Jan K. Herman, Oral History with Lt. (ret.) Edward Feldman, MC, USN, 14-15 February 2004, San Diego, CA, Office of Medical History, BUMED.
7. J. O. Finnegan, "Triage at Khe Sanh," *Surgery, Gynecology, and Obstetrics* 135 (1972): 108-110.
8. Combat After Action Report—Battle of Land Vei, 5th Special Forces Group (Airborne), 1st Special Forces, Period 24 January–7 February 1968, 12 August 1968, OACSFOR, DA, Washington DC, 22 February 1968.
9. O'Brien, *The Things They Carried*, 88.
10. Refusal to admit montagnards was described in Prados, *Valley of Decision*, 326.
11. Combat After Action Report—Battle of Land Vei, 1968.
12. The saving grace was the Marines' control of the high ground, occupying and holding all the hill positions that oversaw approaches to the combat base and direct artillery targeting.
13. Westmoreland, *A Soldier Reports*, 338.
14. Casualty figures from Command Chronology: Headquarters, 1st Battalion, 9th Marines, 3rd Marine Division, 8 March 1968, U.S. Marine Corps History Division, The Vietnam Center and Archive, Texas Tech University. Shore put the number of killed in action at 21 on Hill 64 and five at the combat base. Shore, *The Battle for Khe Sanh*, 71.
15. Herman, Oral history interview with Lt. (ret.) Edward Feldman.
16. Nalty, *Air Power and the Fight for Khe Sanh*, 46.
17. Command Chronology: Marine Aerial Refueler Transport Squadron 152, Marine Aircraft Group 15, 9th Marine Amphibious Brigade, FMF, 8 March 1968, US

Marine Corps History Division, The Vietnam Center and Archive, Texas Tech University.
18. Jack Shulimson, *U.S. Marines in Vietnam: The Defining Year, 1968* (Washington DC: History and Museums Division, Headquarters, U.S. Marine Corps, 1997), 480.
19. Bruce Geiger, "Dusters at Khe Sanh", 1997, http://www.ndqsa.com/khesanh.html, accessed November 22, 2016.
20. Prados, *Valley of Decision*, 381.
21. Command Chronology period 1 February to 29 February 1968: Marine Medium Helicopter Squadron 262, Marine Aircraft Group 36, 1st Marine Aircraft Wing, FMF, 4 March 1968, US Marine Corps History Division, The Vietnam Center and Archive, Texas Tech University
22. Command Chronology, Marine Heavy Helicopter Squadron 463, Marine Aircraft Group 16, 1st Marine Aircraft Wing, FMF, 7 March 1968, U.S. Marine Corps History Division, The Vietnam Center and Archive, Texas Tech University.
23. Shore, *The Battle for Khe Sanh*, 83.
24. Hammel, *Siege in the Clouds*, 209.
25. Studies later showed that the mean number of days a Marine was in combat before he was wounded was five.
26. Command Chronology: Marine Medium Helicopter Squadron 364, Marine Aircraft Group 36, 1st Marine Aircraft Wing, 5 March 1968, US Marine Corps History Division, The Vietnam Center and Archive, Texas Tech University.
27. Shulimson, *The Defining Year*, 483.
28. Dabney, W.H. "Hill 881S and the Super Gaggle," *Marine Corps Gazette* 89 (2005): 69-72.
29. Ray W. Stubbe, *Battalion of Kings: A Tribute to Our Fallen Brothers who Died Because of the Battlefield of Khe Sanh, Vietnam* (Wauwatosa: Khe Sanh Veterans, 2008), 198.
30. Ray Stubbe, *Khe Sanh and the Mongol Prince* (Wauwatosa: Self-published, 2002), 3.
31. Fallaci, *Nothing And So Be It*, 177.
32. Bartimus, *War Torn*, 144.
33. Command Chronology and After Action Report: Headquarters, 1st Battalion, 26th Marines, 3rd Marine Division, FMF, 1 March 1968, US Marine Corps History Division, The Vietnam Center and Archive, Texas Tech University.
34. Hammel, *Siege in the Clouds*, 343.
35. Prados, *Valley of Decision*, 403.
36. The North Vietnamese had a well-planned ambush. Most Marines fell at almost point-blank range (twenty yards according to North Vietnamese sources). The ones who made it into the Viet trenches could not maneuver. "The American Marines were big and tall and they were carrying all kinds of things on their backs and around their waist . . . it was difficult for them to turn or move [in the trenches]." Immobilized, they were slaughtered where they stood. Stubbe, *Pebbles in My Boots*, Vol. 4, 70-71.
37. Descriptions of Don Jacques's death contained in Stubbe, *Pebbles in My Boots*, Vol 4, 53, 56.
38. "Pass quietly from the stormy shores of time," from W. T. G. Morton, "The First Use of Ether As An Anesthetic at the Battle of the Wilderness in the Civil War", reprinted in *JAMA* 42 (1904): 1068-1074.
39. Bernard Edelman, *Dear America: Letters Home from Vietnam* (New York: W.W. Norton, 1985), 83.

40. Information based on USMC Field Historical Interviews, Captain Ken Pipes, Commander, Bravo Company, 1/26; Command Chronology and After Action Report: Headquarters, 1st Battalion, 26th Marines, 3rd Marine Division, FMF, 1 March 1968, US Marine Corps History Division, The Vietnam Center and Archive, Texas Tech University; and an article retrieved from *U.S. Militaria Forum*, http://www.usmilitariaforum.com/forums/index.php?/topic/136751-khe-sanh-february-25-1968-3rd-platoon-bravo-company-1st-battalion-26th-marines/, accessed November 22, 2016.
41. Stubbe, *Khe Sanh and the Mongol Prince*, 3. Lietch made this comment some years after the battle; Leitch wrote an insightful and gritty account of the Khe Sanh siege entitled "Khe Sanh is Quite Takeable," published in the *Washington Post*, February 25, 1968, in which it was quite clear that most Marines on the base felt they would eventually be overrun by the North Vietnamese.
42. Ray Stubbe, Wisconsin Veterans Museum Research Center, Oral History Interview by Jim Kurtz, 2005-2006, transcribed 2008, 59.
43. Herbert L. Bergsma, *Chaplains with Marines in Vietnam, 1962-1971* (Washington, DC : History and Museums Division, Headquarters, U.S. Marine Corps, 1985), 162-163.
44. Pisor, *End of the Line*, 203.
45. Finnegan, *In the Company of Marines*, 83.
46. Ray Stubbe diary, personal communication, November 10, 2016.
47. Ibid.
48. Finnegan, *In the Company of Marines*, 83-89.
49. This was probably twenty-year-old Sergeant Donald Ray Chamblin; the story was told by Lance Corporal Daniel Sullivan in Together We Served, https://marines.togetherweserved.com/usmc/servlet/tws, accessed March 18, 2019. Sergeant Chamblin had only five days left before his tour of duty was up.
50. Command Chronology: Headquarters, 1st Battalion, 26th Marines, 3rd Marine Division, FMF, 1 March and 1 April 1968, US Marine Corps History Division, The Vietnam Center and Archive, Texas Tech University.
51. Stubbe, Oral History Interview, 2008, 59.
52. Herr, *Dispatches*, 113-114.
53. Shore, *The Battle for Khe Sanh*, 127.
54. Robert J. Topmiller, *Binding Their Wounds: America's Assault on Its Veterans* (Abingdon-on-Thames: Routledge, 2015), 4.
55. This was the same incident that wounded Catholic chaplain Reverend Walter Driscoll.
56. Finnegan, *In the Company of Marines*, 97-101. Common practice for lifeless individuals hemorrhaging to death was a quick thoracotomy and internal cardiac massage while blood and fluids were rushed in. Anything less was sure to fail (Edward Feldman, personal communication).
57. Jonathan Spicer refused to be a "shooter" but insisted on being in combat to care for his fellow Marines. He was a tireless litter bearer, risking his life on a number of occasions. He received the Navy Cross for his bravery that day in March 1968.
58. Fallaci, *Nothing And So Be It*, 178.
59. Bartimus, *War Torn*, 129-146; young Jonathan Spicer led the four-man litter crew carrying her to her chopper only hours before his tragic wounding.
60. Herman, *Navy Medicine in Vietnam*, 237-238.
61. Ibid., 237.

62. The stretch of Highway 1 from Hue to Quang Tri was heavily fortified by Viet Minh during the first Indochina War. Ambushes were frequent, the highway being the main thoroughfare from southern to northern Vietnam.
63. Letter, Colonel John A. Sheedy, 67th Medical Group, to Colonel Charles J. Simpson, AHBMED, 28 December 1971, RG 112 (Surgeon General), NARA, College Park, MD.
64. Westmoreland, *A Soldier Reports*, 348.
65. Finnegan, *In the Company of Marines*, 179.
66. Statistics vary on amounts of ordnance used around Khe Sanh. These figures are taken from Shulimson, *The Defining Year*, 283, and Nalty, *Air Power*, 88.
67. Winston Spencer Churchill, *The River War* (London: Longmans, Green, 1900), 276. For tribulations of French wounded at Dien Bien Phu see Fall, *Hell in a Very Small Place*.
68. Brown, 1968.
69. Command Chronologies: Headquarters, 3rd Medical Battalion, 3rd Marine Division, FMF, 8 March 1968 and 4 April 1968 (activities for the months of February and March), US Marine Corps History Division, The Vietnam Center and Archive, Texas Tech University.
70. There are reasons for this position. One can argue that Khe Sanh was never really under siege in the textbook definition: the garrison continued to be supplied by air and was not completely cut off. Others contend that Giap and his NVA were half-hearted in their attempt to overrun the base. In fact one could argue "who was besieging whom?" Perhaps it was more of a distraction for MACV than a true offensive, considering the other ramifications of Tet. For a concise discussion see Shore, *The Battle for Khe Sanh*, 145-151.
71. Ray Stubbe, personal communication with the author.
72. Figures from Shulimson, *The Defining Year*, 724.
73. Combat After Action Report, Battle of Lang Vei, 5th Special Forces Group (Airborne), 1st Special Forces, Period 24 January–7 February 1968, Department of the Army, Washington, DC, 12 August 1968.
74. B. Eiseman, "Combat casualty management in Vietnam," *Journal of Trauma* 7 (1967):53-63. Of course, not all care was provided by "board certified specialists." Many surgeons had not yet completed training but, as far as trauma surgery went, were already some of the best.
75. B. G. McCaughey, J. Garrick, L. C. Carey, J. B. Kelley, Naval Support Activity Hospital Da Nang: Combat Casualty Deaths January to June 1968, Naval Health Research Center, San Diego, CA, and the Naval Medical Research and Development Command, Bethesda, MD, 1986. This material was later published by the same authors as "Naval Support Activity Hospital, Da Nang, Combat Casualty Study" in *Military Medicine* 153 (1988):109-114.
76. Morton, "The First Use of Ether," 1068-1074.
77. Pitlyk, *Blood on China Beach*, 237.
78. Ibid., 127.
79. From Herman, *Navy Medicine in Vietnam*, 234-241, and Herman interview with Lieutenant Commander (ret.) James O. Finnegan, 9 September 2004.
80. Nalty: *Air Power*, 101.

AFTERMATH

1. MacArthur, *Reminiscences*, 135.
2. Bumgarner, *Parade of the Dead*, 175 and 192.
3. Weinstein, *Barbed-Wire Surgeon*; for Craig: Bumgarner, *Parade of the Dead*, 184-185.
4. Taken from a moving tribute in Norman, *Band of Angels*, 243-272; quotes 243, 272.
5. Schorer, *A Half Acre of Hell*, 170.
6. Wandrey, *Bedpan Commando*, 234.
7. Collins, *56th Evac*, 278.
8. Shoemaker, *A Surgeon Remembers*, 134-140.
9. Stewart, *Notes of a Korean War Surgeon*, 44.
10. Herr, *Dispatches*, 163.

Bibliography

Books

Adler, B. M. *Letters Home: World War II Letters*. New York: St. Martin Press, 2002.

Alexander, B. *Korea: The First War We Lost*. New York: Hippocrene Books, 2003.

Appleman, R. E. *East of Chosin: Entrapment and Breakout in Korea, 1950*. College Station: Texas A&M University Press, 1987.

_______. *Escaping the Trap*. College Station: Texas A&M University Press, 1990.

_______. *South to the Naktong, North to the Yalu*. Washington, DC: Center of Military History, United States Army, 1992.

Ashton, P. *And Somebody Gives a Damn*. Santa Barbara: Self published, 1990.

_______. *Bataan Diary*. Self published, 1984.

Atkinson, R. *The Day of Battle: The War in Sicily and Italy, 1943-1944*. New York: Henry Holt, 2007.

Bahr, W., H. W. Bahr, O. Eberhard, & J. H. Meyer. *Kriegsbriefe gefallener Studenten 1939-1945*. Tubingen: R Wunderlich, 1952.

Barron, L. C. *No Silent Night: The Chrismas Battle For Bastogne*. New York: Penguin, 2012.

Bartimus, T., D. Fawcett, and J. Kazickas. *War Torn: The Personal Experiences of Women Reporters in the Vietnam War*. New York: Random House, 2004.

Beevor, A. *Ardennes 1944: Hitler's Last Gamble*. New York: Viking Penguin, 2015.

Bergsma, H. L. *Chaplains with Marines in Vietnam, 1962-1971*. Washington, DC: History and Museums Division, Headquarters, U.S. Marine Corps, 1985.

Blair, C. *The Forgotten War: America in Korea 1950-1953*. New York: Random House, 1987.

Blumenson, M. *The Patton Papers 1940-1945*. Boston: Da Capo Press, 1996.

Blythe, L. *38th EVAC: The Story of the Men and Women who Served in World War Two with the 38th Evacuation Hospital in North Africa and Italy*. Charlotte, NC: self published, 1966.

Brown, R. J. *Whirlybirds: U.S. Marine Helicopters in Korea*. Washington, DC: U.S. Marine Corps Historical Center, 2003.

Bumgarner, J. R. *Parade of the Dead*. Jefferson, NC: McFarland, 1995.

Buttinger, J. *Vietnam: A Dragon Embattled*. Vol. 1. New York: Praeger, 1967.

Buzo, A. *The Making of Modern Korea*. London: Routledge, 2002.

Caddick-Adams, P. *Snow and Steel: The Battle of the Bulge 1944-1945*. Oxford: Oxford University Press, 2015.

Carles, W. R. *Life in Corea*. London: Macmillan, 1888.

Cave, D. *Beyond Courage: One Regiment Against Japan, 1941-1945*. Las Cruces, NM: Yucca Tree Press, 1992.

Celli, A. *The History of Malaria in the Roman Campagna from Ancient Times*. London: John Bale, Sons, and Danielsson, 1933.

Churchill, E. D. *Surgeon to Soldiers*. Philadelphia: J. B. Lippincott, 1972.

Churchill, W. S. *Closing the Ring*. Boston: Houghton Mifflin, 1951.

Clark, M. W. *Calculated Risk*. New York: HarpersCollins, 1950.

_______. *Fifth Army History. Part IV: Cassino and Anzio*. Washington, DC: War Department, 1945.

Clarke, B. B. *Expendable Warriors: The Battle of Khe Sanh and the Vietnam War*. Mechanicsburg, PA: Stackpole Books, 2007.

Coates, J. B. *Surgery in World War II: Activities of the Surgical Consultants*. Washington, DC: U.S. Government Printing Office, 1962.

Cole, H. M. *The Ardennes: Battle of the Bulge*. Washington, DC: U.S. Government Printing Office, 1965.

Collins, M. *The Tigers of Bastogne: Voices of the 10th Armored Division in the Battle of the Bulge*. Havertown: Casemate, 2013.

Cooper, W. E. *Medical Department Activities in the Philippines from 1941 to 6 May 1942*. Washington, DC: Office of the Surgeon General, 1946.

Corsi, J. *No Greater Valor: The Siege of Bastogne and the Miracle that Sealed Allied Victory*. Nashville: Nelson Books, 2014.

Cosmas, G. A. *Medical Service in the European Theater of Operations*. Washington, DC: Center of Military History, United States Army, 1992.

Cowdry, A. E. *The Medics' War*. Honolulu: University Press of the Pacific, 2005.

D'Este, C. *Eisenhower: A Soldier's Life*. New York: Henry Holt, 2002.

_______. *Fatal Decision: Anzio and the Battle for Rome*. New York: HarperCollins, 1991.

Doll, J. G. *The Battling Bastards of Bataan*. Bennington, VT: Merriam Press, 1988.

Donovan, W. N. *P.O.W. in the Pacific: Memoirs of an American Doctor in World War II*. Wilmington, DE: SR Books, 1998.

Dorland, P. N. *Dust Off: Army Aeromedical Evacuation in Vietnam*. Darby, PA: Diane Publishing, 1982.

Drury, B. C. *The Last Stand of Fox Company: A True Story of U.S. Marines in Combat*. New York: Atlantic Monthly Press, 2009.

Dworak, D. D. *Victory's Foundation: US Logistical Support of the Allied Mediterranean Campaign, 1942-1945*. Syracuse: Syracuse University Press, 2011.

Edelman, B. *Dear America: Letters Home from Vietnam*. New York: W. W. Norton, 1985.

Eisenhower, D. D. *Crusade in Europe*. Baltimore: Johns Hopkins University Press, 1948.

Eisenhower, J. S. *The Bitter Woods: The Battle of the Bulge*. New York: G. P. Putnam's Sons, 1969.

Ent, U. W. *Fighting on the Brink: Defense of the Pusan Perimeter*. Paducah, KY: Turner Publishing, 1998.

Fall, B. B. *Hell in a Very Small Place: The Siege of Dien Bien Phu*. New York: Da Capo Press, 1966.

Fallaci, O. *Nothing And So Be It*. Garden City, NY: Doubleday, 1972.

Finnegan, J. O. *In the Company of Marines: A Surgeon Remembers Vietnam*. Philadelphia: self published, 2009.

Fitzgerald, D. *A History of the Irish Guards in the Second World War*. London: Gale and Polden, 1949.

Fussell, P. *The Boys' Crusade*. New York: Random House, 2003.

Futrell, R. F. *The United States Air Force in Southeast Asia: The Advisory Years to 1965*. Washington, DC: Office of Air Force History, 1981.

Gardner, I. *No Victory in Valhalla*. Oxford: Osprey Press, 2014.

Gellhorn, M. *The Face of War*. New York: Atlantic Monthly Press, 1988.

Giap, V. N. *People's War, People's Army*. Hanoi: Foreign Languages Publishing House, 1961.

Glusman, J. A. *Conduct Under Fire: Four American Doctors and Their Fight for Life as Prisoners of the Japanese 1941-1945*. London: Penguin Books, 2005.

Goodman, J. M. *M.D. P.O.W.: A Firsthand Account of 42 Months of Imprisonment in Japanese Hands*. New York: Exposition Press, 1972.

Graves, C. L.. *Front Line Surgeons: A History of the Third Auxiliary Group*. San Diego, CA: Frye and Smith, 1950.

Griffis, W. E. *Corea: The Hermit Nation*. New York: Charles Scribner's Sons, 1894.

Grossman, D. *On Killing*. Boston: Little, Brown, 1995.

Gugeler, R. A. *Combat Actions in Korea*. Army Historical Series. Washington, DC: Center of Military History, United States Army, 1987.

Halberstam, D. *The Coldest Winter: America and the Korean War*. New York: Hyperion, 2007.

Hammel, E. *Chosin: Heroic Ordeal of the Korean War*. Novato, CA: Presidio Press, 1981.

_______. *Khe Sanh: Siege in the Clouds. An Oral History*. Novato, CA: Presidio Press, 1989.

Harrison, M. *Medicine and Victory: British Military Medicine in the Second World War*. Oxford: Oxford University Press, 2004.

Herman, J. K. *Frozen in Memory: U.S. Navy Medicine in the Korean War*. Bangor, ME: Booklocker, 2006.

_______. *Navy Medicine in Vietnam: Oral Histories from Dien Bien Phu to the Fall of Saigon*. Jefferson, NC: McFarland, 2009.

Herr, M. *Dispatches*. New York: Vintage International, 1991.

Hess, G. R. *Presidential Decisions for War: Korea, Vietnam, the Persian Gulf, and Iraq*. Baltimore: Johns Hopkins University Press, 2009.

Hibbs, R. E. *Tell MacArthur to Wait*. Quezon City, P.I.: Giraffe Books, 1996.

Higgins, M. *War in Korea: The Report of a Woman Combat Correspondent*. New York: Doubleday, 1951.

Holloway, C. K. *Escape from Hell: A Navy Surgeon Remembers Pusan, Inchon, and Chosin Korea, 1950*. La Jolla, CA: self published, 1997.

Horwitz, D. G. *We Will Not Be Strangers: Korean War Letters Between A M.A.S.H. Surgeon And His Wife*. Champaign: University of Illinois Press, 1997.

Huebner, K. H. *Long Walk Through War*. College Station: Texas A&M University Press, 1987.

Jackson, C. G. *Diary of Col. Calvin G. Jackson, M.D.* Ada: Ohio Northern University Press, 1992.

Jacobs, E. C. *Blood Brothers: A Medic's Sketch Book*. New York: Carlton Press, 1985.

James, D. C. *The Years of MacArthur, Volume I, 1880-1941*. Boston: Houghton Mifflin, 1970.

Jolly, D. W. *Field Surgery in Total War*. London: Hamish Hamilton, 1940.

Junger, S. *Tribe: On Homecoming and Belonging*. New York: Hachette Book Group, 2016.

Karnow, S. *Vietnam: A History*. New York: Viking Press, 1983.

Kelly, F. J. *Vietnam Studies: U.S. Army Special Forces, 1961-1971*. Washington, DC: Department of the Army, 2004.

Kennedy, P. A. *Battlefied Surgeon: Life and Death on the Front Lines of World War II*. Lexington: University Press of Kentucky, 2016.

Keys, A. B. *The Biology of Human Starvation*. Vols. I and II. Minneapolis: University of Minnesota Press, 1950.

Knox, D. *The Korean War: An Oral History, Pusan to Chosin*. New York: Harcourt, Brace, Jovanovich Publishers, 1985.

Korson, G. *At His Side: The Story of the American Red Cross Overseas in World War II*. New York: Coward-McCann, 1945.

Koskimaki, G. *The Battered Bastards of Bastogne*. Philadelphia: Casemate, 2011.

Lea, H. *The Valor of Ignorance*. New York: Harper and Brothers, 1909.

Lech, R. B. *Broken Soldiers*. Champaign: University of Illinois Press, 2000.

Lee, H. G. *Nothing But Praise*. Hollywood: Murray & Gee, 1948.

Letterman, J. *Medical Recollections of the Army of the Potomac*. New York: D. Appleton, 1866

Littleton, M. R. *Doc: Heroic Stories of Medics, Corpsmen, and Surgeons in Combat*. Saint Paul, MN: Zenith Press, 2005.

MacArthur, D. *Reminiscences*. New York: McGraw-Hill, 1964.

MacDonald, C. B. *A Time for Trumpets: The Untold Story of the Battle of the Bulge*. New York: Quill, 1985.

Marshall, S. L. A. *Bastogne: The First Eight Days*. Washington, DC: Center of Military History, United States Army, 1946.

Massman, E. A. *Hospital Ships of World War II*. Jefferson, NC: McFarland, 1999.

May, A. *Witness to War: A Biography of Marguerite Higgins*. New York: Penguin Books, 1983.

McManus, J. C. *Alamo in the Ardennes*. Hoboken, NJ: John Wiley and Sons, 2007.

McWilliams, T. *The Chaplain's Conflict: Good and Evil in a War Hospital 1943-1945*. College Station: Texas A&M University Press, 2012.

Mead, E. V. *The Operations and Movements of the 31st Infantry Regiment (Philippine Division) 7 December 1941 to 9 April 1942*. Fort Benning, GA: Infantry School, 1947.

Miller, E. B. *Bataan Uncensored*. Long Prairie, MN: Hart Publications, 1949.

Monahan, N. and Neidel-Greenlee, R. *All This Hell: U.S. Nurses Imprisoned by the Japanese*. Lexington: University Press of Kentucky, 2000.

_______, and ______. *And If I Perish: Frontline U.S. Army Nurses in World War II*. New York: Anchor Books, 2003.

Montross, L. A. *U.S. Marine Operations in Korea 1950-1953*. Vol. III *The Chosin Reservoir Campaign*. Washington, DC: Historical Branch, G-3, Headquarters U.S. Marine Corps, 1957.

Morison, S. E. *History of United States Naval Operations in World War II*. Vol. 3, *The Rising Sun in the Pacific, 1931–April 1942*. New York: Little, Brown, 1948.

Morison, S. E. *History of United States Naval Operations in World War II*. Vol. 9, *Sicily, Salerno, Anzio, January 1943–June 1944*. New York: Little, Brown, 1954.

Morton, L. *The Fall of the Philippines*. Washington, DC: Center of Miliary History, United States Army, 1993.

Nalty, B. C. *Air Power and the Fight for Khe Sanh*. Washington, DC: Office of Air Force History, 1986.

Nealson, W. R. *The Operations of a Provisional Battalion, 41st Division (PA), at Abucay Hacienda (Bataan), 15–25 January 1942*. Fort Benning, GA: Advanced Infantry Officer Course, 1947.

Neel, S. *Vietnam Studies: Medical Support of the U.S. Army in Vietnam, 1965-1970*. Washington, DC: Department of the Army, 1991.

Nichols, D. J. *Ernie's War: The Best of Ernie Pyle's World War II Dispatches*. New York: Random House, 1986.

Norman, E. M. *We Band of Angels*. New York: Pocket Books, 1999.

Oberdorfer, D. *Tet!: The Turning Point in the Vietnam War*. Baltimore: Johns Hopkins University Press, 1971.

Peyton, F. W. *A Surgeon's Diary: 15th Evacuation Hospital; Experiences in World War II, North Africa–Sicily–Italy*. Crawfordsville, IN: self published, 1987.

Phibbs, B. *The Other Side of Time: A Combat Surgeon in World War II*. Boston: Little, Brown, 1987.

Pisor, R. *The End of the Line: The Siege of Khe Sanh*. New York: W. W. Norton, 1982.

Pitlyk, P. J. *Blood on China Beach: My Story as a Brain Surgeon in Vietnam*. Bloomington, IN: Universe, 2012.

Prados, J. S. *Valley of Decision: The Siege of Khe Sanh*. Annapolis: Naval Institute Press, 1991.

Pratt, J. C. *Vietnam Voices: Perspectives on the War Years, 1941-1975*. Athens: University of Georgia Press, 1984.

Pyle, E. *Brave Men*. Lincoln: University of Nebraska Press, reprint, 2001.

_______. *Here is Your War*. New York: Henry Holt, 1943.

Quezon, M. L. *The Good Fight*. New York: D. Appleton-Century, 1946.

Rapport, L. N. *Rendezvous with Destiny: History of the 101st Airborne Division*. Saybrook: Konecky and Konecky, 1948.

Reister, F. A. *Battle Casualties and Medical Statistics, U.S. Army Experience in the Korean War*. Washington, DC: Office of the Surgeon General, U.S. Army, 1973.

Rodman, J. S. *History of the American Board of Surgery*, 1937-1952. Philadelphia: J.B. Lippincott, 1956.

Russ, M. *Breakout: The Chosin Reservoir Campaign, Korea 1950*. New York: Penguin Books, 1999.

Sarnecky, M. T. *A History of the U.S. Army Nurse Corps*. Philadelphia: University of Pennsylvania Press, 1999.

Schorer, A. D. *A Half Acre of Hell: A Combat Nurse in WW II*. Lakeville, MN: Galde Press, 2000.

Schrijvers, P. *Those Who Hold Bastogne: The True Story of the Soldiers and Civilians Who Fought in the Biggest Battle of the Bulge*. New Haven: Yale University Press, 2014.

Shama, R. H. *Pulse and Repulse: Troop Carrier and Airborne Teams in Europe During World War II*. Austin: Eakin Press, 1995.

Shoemaker, R. C. *A Surgeon Remembers: Korea 1950-1951 and the Marines*. Victoria: Trafford Publishing, 2005.

Shore, M. S. *The Battle for Khe Sanh*. Washington, DC: History and Museums Division, Headquarters, U.S. Marine Corps, 1969.

Shrader, C. R. *A War of Logistics: Parachutes and Porters in Indochina, 1945-1954*. Lexington: University Press of Kentucky, 2015.

Shulimson, J. *U.S. Marines in Vietnam: The Defining Year, 1968*. Washington, DC: History and Museums Division, Headquarters, U.S. Marine Corps, 1997.

_______. *U.S. Marines in Vietnam: The Landing And The Buildup*. Washington, DC: History and Museums Division, Headquarters, U.S. Marine Corps, 1978.

Smith, C. R. *U.S. Marines in the Korean War*. Washington, DC: History Division, United States Marine Corps, 2007.

Stabler, H. D. *No One Ever Asked Me: The World War II Memoirs of an Omaha Indian Soldier*. Lincoln: University of Nebraska Press, 2005.

Stubbe, R. W. *Battalion of Kings*. Wauwatosa: Khe Sanh Veterans, 2008.

_______. *Pebbles in My Boots*, Volumes 1-4. Wauwatosa: self published, 2014.

Taithe, B. *Defeated Flesh: Medicine, Welfare, and Warfare in the Making of Modern France*. Lanham, MD: Rowman & Littlefield, 1999.

Taylor, T. H. *Rangers Lead the Way*. Nashville: Turner Publishing, 1997.

Telfer, G. L. *U.S. Marines in Vietnam: Fighting the North Vietnamese, 1967*. Washington, DC: History and Museums Division, Headquarters, U.S. Marine Corps, 1984.

Tobin, J. *Ernie Pyle's War: America's Eyewitness to World War II*. New York: Free Press, 2006.

Toland, J. *Battle: The Story of the Bulge*. Lincoln: University of Nebraska Press, 1959.

Tomblin, B. *G.I. Nightingales: The Army Nurse Corps in World War II*. Lexington: University Press of Kentucky, 1996.

Topmiller, R. J. *Binding Their Wounds: America's Assault on Its Veterans*. Abingdon-on-Thames: Routledge, 2015.

Tregaskis, R. *Invasion Diary*. New York: Random House, 1944.

Trueblood, H. W. *A Surgeon's War: My Year in Vietnam*. San Francisco: Astor & Lenox, 2015.

Verney, P. *Anzio 1944: An Unexpected Fury*. London: David and Charles, 1980.

Wandrey, J. *Bedpan Commando: The Story of a Combat Nurse During World War II*. Elmore: Elmore Publishing, 1989.

Articles

Bauchspies, R. L. "The Courageous Medics of Anzio." Part III. *Military Medicine* (1958), 122:119-128.

_______. "The Courageous Medics of Anzio." Part V. *Military Medicine* (1958), 122:338-359.

_______. "The Courageous Medics of Anzio." Part VI. *Military Medicine* (1958), 122:429-448.

Beecher, H. K. "Pain in Men Wounded in Battle." *Annals of Surgery* (1946), 123:96-105.

_______. "Preparation of the Battle Casualties for Surgery." *Annals of Surgery* (1945), 121:769-792.

Bowers, W. F. "The Present Story on Battle Casualties from Korea." *Surgery, Gynecology, and Obstetrics* (1951), 93:529-542.

Bricknell, M. C. "The Evolution of Casualty Evacuation in the British Army in the 20th Century (Part 2)—1918 to 1945." *Journal of the Royal Army Medical Corps* (2002), 148:314-322.

Brown, R. A. "Dateline: Vietnam." *Penn Medicine* (1968), 71:45-53.

Bruce-Chwatt, L. J. "Transmission of Malaria: 75th Anniversary of Ronald Ross's Great Discovery." *British Medical Journal* (1972), 3:464-466.

Burnett, M. W. "American Pediatricians at War: a Legacy of Service." *Pediatrics* (2012), 129 (Suppl): S33-S49.

Cahill, G. F. "Starvation in Man." *New England Journal of Medicine* (1970), 282:668-675.

Cannon, J. W. "Edward D. Churchill as a Combat Consultant." *Annals of Surgery* (2010), 251:566-572.

Churchill, E. D. "The Surgical Management of the Wounded in the Mediterranean Theater at the Time of the Fall of Rome." *Annals of Surgery* (1944), 120:268-283.

DeBakey, M. E. "Military Surgery in World War II." *New England Journal of Medicine* (1947), 236:341-350.

_______. "History, the Torch that Illuminates: Lessons from Military Medicine." *Military Medicine* (1996), 161:711-716.

Eiseman, B. "Combat Casualty Management in Vietnam." *Journal of Trauma* (1967), 7:53-63.

Finnegan, J. O. "Triage at Khe Sanh." *Surgery, Gynecology, and Obstetrics* (1972), 135:108-110.

Fisler, J. S. "Cardiac Effects of Starvation and Semistarvation Diets: Safety and Mechanisms of Action." *American Journal of Clinical Nutrition* (1992), 56:230S-240S.

Forsee, J. H. "Forward Surgery of the Severely Wounded." *American Surgery* (1951), 17:508-526.

George, C. R. "Blackwater Fever: the Rise and Fall of an Exotic Disease." *Journal of Nephrology* (2009), Suppl 14:120-128.

Gorter, R. R.-S. "Diagnosis and Management of Acute Appendicitis." *Surgical Endoscopy* (2016), 30:4668-4690.

Hanson, F. R. "Statistical Studies (Appendix I)." *Bulletin of the US Army Medical Department* (1949), 9(suppl):191-204.

Helling, T. S. "In Flanders Fields: the Great War, Antoine Depage, and the Resurgence of Debridement." *Annals of Surgery* (1998), 173-181.

Holloway, C. K. "The Military Surgical Aspects of the Chosin Reservoir Withdrawal." *Western Journal of Surgery, Obstetrics, and Gynecology* (1955), 63:308-311.

Holt, R. L. " Malaria and Anopheles Reconnaissance in the Philippines." *Philippine Journal of Science* (1932), 49:305-371.

Jones, D. F. "The Role of the Evacuation Hospital in the Care of the Wounded." *Annals of Surgery* (1918), 68:127-132.

Kalm, L. M. "They Starved So that Others be Better Fed: Remembering Ancel Keys and the Minnesota Experiment." *Journal of Nutrition* (2005), 135:1347-1352.

Lalich, J. J. "Resuscitation of Severely Wounded Casualties." *Surgery* (1945), 18:741-753.

Lally, J. "The Hill Battles of Khe Sanh: a Marine Corps Doctor Remembers." *Delaware Medical Journal* (2014), 86:377-379.

Leigh, O. C. "A Report on Trench Foot and Cold Injuries in the European Theater of Operations 1944-1945." *Annals of Surgery* (1946), 124:301-313.

Lewis, D. L. "The Organization and Operation of an Evacuation Hospital." *Annals of Surgery* (1919), 70:489-496.

Litvin, H. "Frozen in Memory: Recalling Chosin Reservoir." *Navy Medicine* (2000), 91:16-21.

Marble, S. "Forward Surgery and Combat Hospitals: the Origins of the MASH." *Journal of the History of Medicine* (2014), 69:68-100.

Masson, G. S. "Reaction Generale d'Adaption: Ses Indications Pratiques." *Canadian Journal of Comparative Medicine* (1938), 2:282-285.

McMurdo, H. B. "Malaria, 1940 Maneuvers, Luzon, Philippine Islands." *Military Surgery* (1940), 87:252-255.

Neel, S. H. "Medical Considerations in Helicopter Evacuation." *U.S. Armed Forces Medical Journal* (1954), 5:220-227.

Phalen, C. S. "Medical Service at Bastogne." *Military Surgeon* (1947), 100:37-42.

Ranson, S. W. "The Normal Battle Reaction: Its Relation to the Pathologic Battle Reaction." *Bulletin of the US Army Medical Department* (1949), 9(Suppl):3-11.

Ross, J. A. "Memoirs of an Army Surgeon." *Journal of the Royal Army Medical Corps* (1979), 125:32-38.

Russell, P. F. "Malaria and Anopheles Reconnaissance in the Philippines, II." *Philippine Journal of Science* (1934), 54:43-59.

_______. "Malaria and its Influence on World Health." *Bulletin of the New York Academy of Medicine* (1943), 19:599-630.

_______. "Malaria in the Philippine Islands." *American Journal of Tropical Medicine* (1933), 13:167-178.

Sallares, R. B. "The Spread of Malaria to Southern Europe in Antiquity: New Approaches to Old Problems." *Medical History* (2004), 48:311-328.

Snowden, F. "Latina Province, 1944-1950." *Journal of Contemporary History* (2008), 43:509-526.

Sobel, R. "Anxiety-depressive Reactions after Prolonged Combat Experience—the 'Old Sergeant Syndrome.'" *Bulletin of the US Army Medical Department* (1949), 9(suppl):137-149.

Swank R. L. "Combat Neuroses: Development of Combat Exhaustion." *Archives of Neurology and Psychiatry* (1946), 55:236-247.

Thornton, W. H. "The 24th Division Medical Battalion in Korea." *Military Surgeon* (1951), 109:110-120.

Tigertt, W. D. "Osler on Malaria." *Canadian Medical Association Journal* (1984), 131:1282-1284.

Van Buskirk, K. E. "Lessons Learned in a Mobile Surgical Hospital and Their Application in the Care of Mass Casualty Disaster." *Pennsylvania Medical Journal* (1956), 59:211-213.

Acknowledgments

THE PREPARATION OF A WORK SUCH AS THIS DEPENDS ON THE SUPPORT and assistance of a number of colleagues and associates to whom I am deeply grateful. First, I would like to thank my publisher, Bruce H. Franklin, and Westholme Publishing for recognizing the value of this project in illuminating the heroic deeds of many health care workers during the darkest of times. I would also like to extend my appreciation to Ron Silverman, whose thorough and meticulous review of the final manuscript allowed for focused editing and clarifications. Of course, navigating the National Archives and Records Administration in College Park, Maryland, can be a daunting task, and I would like to thank all the support staff there for assisting me. I would include in that group Don Budrejko for his assistance in investigating and procuring vital unit histories and his tireless efforts to track down hospital records from the Ardennes offensive and Korea. Suzette Robinson and her staff at the Rowlands Medical Library at the University of Mississippi Medical Center provided invaluable assistance in searching for and obtaining obscure medical literature on these events.

I would like to thank Carol Leadenham for generously sharing excerpts of Colonel Jarrett Huddleston's memoirs from the Norman Lee Baldwin collection of Stanford University. I am extremely grateful to Beverly Carver from the University of Texas, Arlington, for allowing me to use Henry Winans's collection of World War II essays, particularly his experiences with the 56th Evacuation Hospital in Italy. I am appreciative of Skip Gurnee's communications regarding his father, Quinby Gurnee, and his willingness to share anecdotes about Anzio.

I would extend my gratitude to the University of North Carolina Charlotte, Atkins Library, for their information concerning the 38th Evacuation Hospital and to Jessica Murphy, reference archivist at the Center for the History of Medicine of the Francis A. Countway Library of Medicine, Harvard Medical School. I would extend my appreciation to Sanders Marble, senior historian, Army Medical Department Center of History and Heritage for his expert counsel and advice regarding the Auxiliary Surgical Groups that played such a key role in the Mediterranean and European campaigns.

I am indebted to Howard "Chip" Serrell, Jr. for the information and diaries furnished about his Dad, Dr. Howard Serrell and the many friendly and informative exchanges we had concerning his illustrious father. My thanks to Martin King and his dogged pursuit of the amazing stories of Renée Lemaire and Augusta Chiwy, two nurses who lent an aura of the supernatural to the distinctly human tragedies of Bastogne. I would like to extend my appreciation to Reverend Ray Stubbe, former chaplain for the 26th Marines at Khe Sanh who provided many informative and tender anecdotes concerning his Marines during those trying times and who generously reviewed my chapter on Khe Sanh furnishing helpful comments and suggestions. He truly remains bound to the soil and the spirit of Khe Sanh. I was pleased to be able to portray the courageous wartime exploits of fellow surgeon and friend Dr. Jim Thomas, former chairman of surgery at the University of Kansas. I would like to thank Andre Sobocinski, historian for the Navy's Bureau of Medicine and Surgery in Falls Church, Virginia, for his help in procuring photographs and archival records. Thank you to Jan Thompson and the American Defenders of Bataan and Corregidor for help in procuring photographs of Bataan's hospitals.

To my lovely wife, thank you for the gracious and patient proofreading of my chapters and revisions.

I would remember in all this, my mentor, colleague, and friend Doctor Walton Ingham, combat surgeon for the 3rd Infantry Division, who survived Anzio and kept so many memories buried deep in his consciousness, rarely but proudly sharing bits and pieces over the years of our association. I would extend special thanks to Doctor Ed Feldman, one of the core physicians for "Charlie Med" who also reviewed my chapter on Khe Sanh. He passed away in October 2017. His loving wife, Patti, informed me of that sad event, and I sensed her deep grief but also an abiding adoration for her beloved hero.

Index